Bridging the Gap and Saving Lives - A Comprehensive Guide to Organ Donation

Edited by Samuel Jacob

Published in London, United Kingdom

Bridging the Gap and Saving Lives - A Comprehensive Guide to Organ Donation
http://dx.doi.org/10.5772/intechopen.1003458
Edited by Samuel Jacob

Contributors
Abdelrahman Balal, Aditya Kasina, Akash Shah, Ali Own, Anja Meyer, Antonio Paul, Arpit Amin, Chan Woo Cho, Chawannuch Ruaengsri, Chinedu Okoli, Ehtuish F.A. Ehtuish, Gyu-Seong Choi, Hetal Lad, Ivana Acan, Katarina Tomulić Brusich, Manuel Quiroz-Flores, Marc Leon, Mogahed Ismail Hassan Hussein, Mohammad Alomari, Mohsen Nafar, Nafiye Busra Celik, Noble Gracious, Obieze Nwanna-Nzewunwa, Pankaj Garg, Priya Walabh, Rajamony Chellammal Arun Dileep, Samuel Jacob, Saša Živković, Shiva Samavat, Siddhartha Banerjee, Si Pham, Sohel Mohamed Gamal Ahmed, Sujith Madambikattil Prabhakaran, Suresh Keshavamurthy, Tiffany Hsiung, Vivienne Pham, Wael Khalaf, Zia Mahmood Awan

First published in London, United Kingdom, 2025 by IntechOpen
IntechOpen is the global imprint of INTECHOPEN LIMITED, registered in England and Wales, registration number: 11086078, 167-169 Great Portland Street, London, W1W 5PF, United Kingdom

For EU product safety concerns: IN TECH d.o.o., Prolaz Marije Krucifikse Kozulić 3, 51000 Rijeka, Croatia, info@intechopen.com or visit our website at intechopen.com.

British Library Cataloguing-in-Publication Data
A catalogue record for this book is available from the British Library

Bridging the Gap and Saving Lives - A Comprehensive Guide to Organ Donation
Edited by Samuel Jacob
p. cm.
Print ISBN 978-1-83769-443-3
Online ISBN 978-1-83769-442-6
eBook (PDF) ISBN 978-1-83769-444-0

Meet the editor

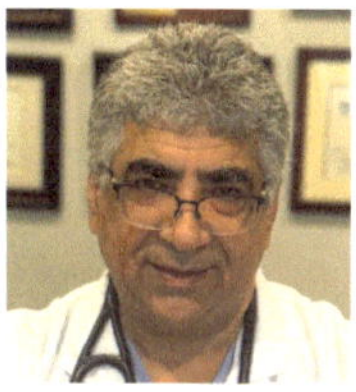

Dr. Samuel Jacob is a former Associate Professor of Surgery at Mayo Clinic, Florida, and a former Clinical Research Director for the Heart and Lung Transplant Program. Initially, he was trained in Great Britain with Sir Magdy Yacoub and became a member of the Royal College of Surgeons of Edinburgh. He was presented with the Eastman Golden Medal by Lady Limerick in the UK. He moved to the US and trained in General Surgery at the University of Illinois at Chicago, Masonic Medical Center. He started his cardiothoracic surgery training at Yale New Haven as a clinical researcher in heart transplant, then moved to Harvard in Boston, where he completed his cardiothoracic training. He was the first fellow in thoracic transplantation at Harvard and received the Golden Scissors. After that, he extended his training in heart transplant and mechanical support at Baylor University Medical Center in Dallas. Dr. Jacob was the winner of the T-Danny research fund, and his Lab is investigating the role of donor mitochondrial DNA and rejection. In addition, he has three innovation disclosures with the Mayo Clinic: a lung transplant retractor, an organ preservation and transportation device (Mayo Organs Preservation and Transport System), and a re-do sternotomy zipper. Furthermore, he performed the first DCD heart transplant on OCS at Mayo Clinic campuses. He served as the principal and director of multiple basic and clinical research projects. Dr. Jacob is active in academia; he has been published in high-impact surgical journals, authored multiple book chapters, and presented at several national and international conferences. He serves as a peer reviewer for multiple scientific journals, including BMJ, Chest, European Journal of Cardiothoracic Surgery, Interactive Journal of Cardiovascular and Thoracic Surgery, and Oxford publications. He is a fellow of the American College of Surgeons and the Royal College of Surgeons. In addition, he is a member of professional organizations and societies, including the International Society for Heart and Lung Transplantation, the American Thoracic Society, the American Medical Association, the American Society of Transplantation, Imperial College in London, and the Scottish Society of Experimental Medicine.

Contents

Preface

In human life, there exists a profound interdependence that moves beyond the boundaries of biology into the realm of profound kindness. Nowhere is this more evident than in the act of organ donation, a selfless gesture that transforms lives, bringing hope to the waiting and renewal to the weary. Yet, amidst this transformative potential, a pressing challenge persists: the lingering shortage of available organs. The scarcity is not merely a statistical concern; it touches lives, casting uncertainty over countless individuals and families. Resolving this crisis demands innovation and empathy in equal measure. Bridging the chasm between supply and demand involves not just awareness and willingness to donate, but also embracing advances in medical technology. Emerging techniques, such as normothermic machine perfusion, offer promising avenues to rejuvenate and preserve organs, extending their viability and availability. Such technologies, alongside concerted efforts to refine logistical frameworks, amplify outreach, and foster a robust donor community, are pivotal in expanding the organ donor pool. As we journey through this narrative, we uncover how science, compassion, and global cooperation converge to forge a hopeful path forward, one where each generous gift helps weave a future filled with possibilities.

Organ donation sits at the intersection of science, ethics, and humanity. It embodies the gift of life and second chances, yet complex decisions and profound emotions often accompany it. In this book, we seek to unravel the intricacies of organ donation, from medical procedures and public policy to the personal stories that breathe life into statistics and data.

This book is designed for everyone, from healthcare professionals seeking deeper insights to individuals contemplating the incredible act of donation, and for recipients who wish to understand the journey their new organs have undertaken. Together, we will explore advances in transplantation technology, the ethical considerations that shape donor systems worldwide, and effective strategies to increase donation rates.

However, more than that, this book is a testament to human resilience and the extraordinary bonds formed through the act of giving and receiving. It highlights the triumphs of successful transplants and the poignant tales of those waiting in hope. We aim to inspire informed conversations, encourage awareness, and advocate for compassionate action to ensure that no life poised for a second chance is left waiting in vain.

This book not only bridges knowledge gaps but also fosters a deeper appreciation for the lives being saved every day through organ donation. Together, we can transform understanding into action, hopes into reality, and contributions into life-saving outcomes.

Samuel Jacob, MD, FRCS, FACS
Chief of Surgical Operations,
Heart and Lung Transplant National Recovery Program,
Jacksonville, USA

Chapter 1

Perspective Chapter: Self-Sufficiency and Equitable Access in Organ, Tissue, and Cell Transplantation

Ehtuish F.A. Ehtuish

Abstract

This chapter, "Self-sufficiency and Equitable Access in Organ, Tissue, and Cell Transplantation," examines the critical issues of achieving self-sufficiency and ensuring equitable access within the transplantation field. The global demand for transplantable organs far exceeds the available supply, leading to severe shortages and disparities influenced by socio-economic factors, geographic locations, and healthcare infrastructure differences. Methodology used is a comprehensive literature review and policy analysis for analyzing case studies, stakeholder opinions, and an ethical review. These approaches were employed to understand the successful strategies and barriers in achieving self-sufficiency and equitable access, autonomy, and transparency. Results indicate significant disparities in transplantation access due to economic inequalities, geographic barriers, and variations in healthcare systems. The chapter concludes with actionable recommendations for policymakers, healthcare providers, and stakeholders. It aims to guide the development of more effective and equitable global transplantation systems. The chapter underscores the necessity of ethical frameworks, community engagement, and technological advancements in addressing the challenges of self-sufficiency and equitable access in organ, tissue, and cell transplantation. By implementing the recommended strategies, policymakers and healthcare providers can work towards reducing disparities, improving donor systems, and enhancing public awareness. These efforts are crucial for creating a more balanced and fair transplantation system worldwide, ensuring that all individuals have access to the life-saving treatments they need.

Keywords: organ donation, transplantation, self-sufficiency, ethical polices, equitable access, organ allocation

1. Introduction

The chapter "Self-sufficiency and Equitable Access in Organ, Tissue, and Cell Transplantation" addresses two pivotal issues in transplantation medicine:

IntechOpen

achieving self-sufficiency and ensuring equitable access. The global demand for transplantable organs, tissues, and cells far exceeds the available supply, leading to critical shortages and significant disparities. These disparities are often influenced by socioeconomic factors, geographic location, and differences in healthcare infrastructure [1–3].

Self-sufficiency in transplantation refers to a country or region's ability to meet its transplant needs through effective donor registration, allocation systems, and national policies. Achieving self-sufficiency is crucial to reducing dependency on international donations and ensuring a reliable supply of transplantable materials. However, this goal is complicated by various challenges, including cultural attitudes toward donation, regulatory and logistical barriers, and the need for sustained public awareness and education campaigns [4–7].

One of the primary motivations behind pursuing self-sufficiency is reducing dependency on international donations. While global cooperation is invaluable, reliance on organs from other countries can create unsustainable dependencies and introduce complexities in logistics, ethics, and equity. Self-sufficiency allows countries to develop and refine transplantation programs within their unique legal and ethical contexts, tailoring approaches to their population's needs and values [8–10].

The pursuit of self-sufficiency is also linked to combating organ trafficking, a grim and unethical practice of exploiting vulnerable populations. Ensuring a sufficient supply of legally donated organs within a country can significantly reduce the demand that fuels the black market, addressing critical ethical concerns and safeguarding the dignity and rights of all individuals, especially those most vulnerable to exploitation [11, 12].

Equitable access involves ensuring that all individuals have fair opportunities to receive transplants, regardless of socioeconomic status or geographic location. Achieving equitable access requires addressing systemic inequalities and implementing policies promoting fairness and inclusivity within the transplantation system. Factors such as economic disparities, rural-urban divides, and varying levels of healthcare development can all hinder equitable access to transplantation services [13–15].

This chapter explores these interconnected challenges, examining the strategies and policies that have been successful in promoting self-sufficiency and equitable access. By reviewing best practices from different regions [16–18], it seeks to provide a comprehensive understanding of how to build more effective and just transplantation systems. The ultimate goal is to offer actionable recommendations for policymakers, healthcare providers, and stakeholders to enhance the sustainability and fairness of transplantation practices globally (**Figure 1**).

In summary, self-sufficiency and equitable access in transplantation are multifaceted goals that touch on logistics, ethics, and social justice. Achieving these goals requires a concerted effort from governments, healthcare providers, and the community at large. Through initiatives aimed at increasing donor registration, improving medical technologies for transplantation, and fostering a culture of altruism and informed consent, countries can move closer to this ideal. The benefits of such efforts extend beyond the immediate recipients of transplants to society as a whole, reinforcing ethical standards in medical practice, combating illegal organ trafficking, and promoting equality in healthcare access (**Figure 2**).

DOI: http://dx.doi.org/10.5772/intechopen.1007602

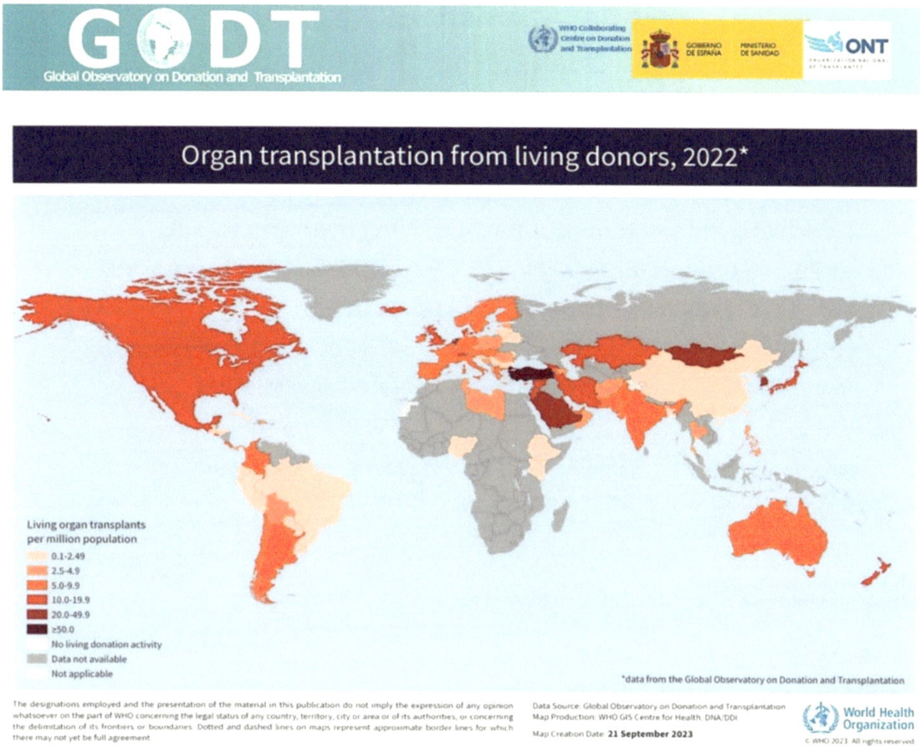

Figure 1.
Organ transplantation from living donors, 2022.

2. Strategies for achieving self-sufficiency

2.1 Improving donation rates

- Public awareness campaigns to educate on the importance of organ and tissue donation [1, 19].
- Implementing and promoting opt-out donation policies to increase potential donor pools [5–7, 20, 21].
- Enhancing the donor registration process to make it more accessible and straightforward.

2.2 Utilizing living donors

- Encouraging living donations for organs where possible (e.g., kidney, liver segments) through education and support programs for donors [1, 2, 9, 22, 23].
- Developing policies to protect and support living donors, including covering medical expenses and ensuring job security [9].

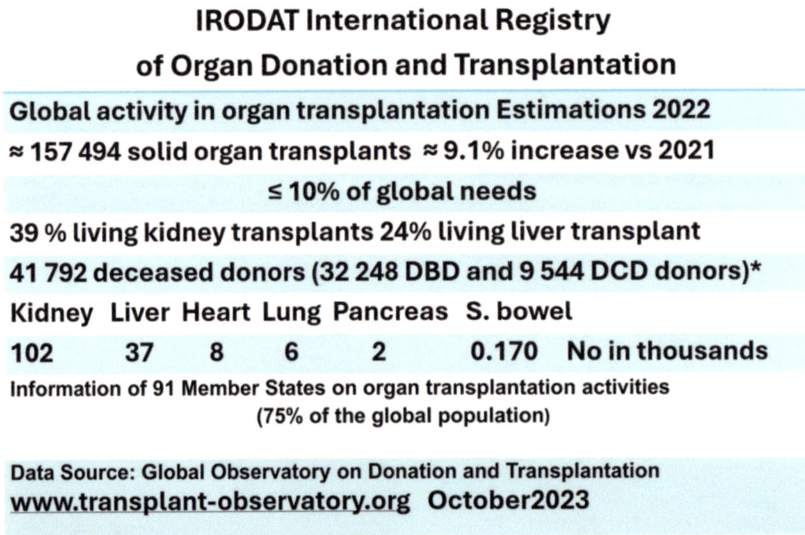

Figure 2.
Global activity in organ transplantation estimations 2022.

2.3 Developing regenerative medicine

- Investing in research on stem cells and tissue engineering to create lab-grown organs and tissues.

- Collaborating with biotech firms to accelerate the development of regenerative solutions.

2.4 Optimization of organ allocation systems

- Employing more efficient and equitable organ allocation systems to reduce wastage and improve transplant success rates.

- Utilizing technology and artificial intelligence to match donors with recipients more effectively [16, 18, 24–26].

3. Challenges to achieving self-sufficiency

3.1 Ethical challenges

- Balancing the need for more organs with the ethical treatment of donors, especially in the context of living donations and experimental treatments.

- Addressing disparities in access to transplantation services within the population.

DOI: http://dx.doi.org/10.5772/intechopen.1007602

3.2 Logistical challenges

- Ensuring the infrastructure is in place for a timely and efficient transplant process, from donor registration to organ transplantation.

- Overcoming geographical and regional disparities in organ availability and transplantation services.

3.3 Medical challenges

- Addressing the limitations of current medical technology in organ preservation and compatibility testing.

- Overcoming challenges in regenerative medicine, including ethical concerns and technical limitations in growing functional organs.

The push for self-sufficiency in organ donation is also fraught with ethical considerations. While the goal is to meet the transplant needs within a country or region to avoid exploiting international donors, questions about the means to achieve self-sufficiency arise. For instance, the ethics of implementing incentive programs for donors or the use of organs from executed prisoners are contentious issues that challenge ethical norms and principles.

4. Equitable access in transplantation

Equitable access in transplantation is a cornerstone of a just and effective health-care system, ensuring that organs, tissues, and cells are distributed fairly and without bias to all individuals in need. This principle rests on the ethical, social, and medical foundations that recognize the intrinsic value of every human life, irrespective of socioeconomic status, geography, or ethnicity. The pursuit of equitable access is not only a moral imperative but also a practical necessity to improve health outcomes across all segments of society [27–29].

Achieving equitable access in transplantation involves dismantling systemic barriers that impede fair access to transplant services. This requires policies that address not only medical suitability but also social determinants of health that may disadvantage certain groups. Efforts to create equitable access must grapple with the allocation policies that inadvertently favor certain populations over others, such as those with better access to healthcare or those more likely to be listed as candidates for transplant.

4.1 Foundational principles

The importance of equitable access is underpinned by ethical considerations of justice and fairness, ensuring that no individual is disadvantaged in their access to life-saving treatments. Socially, it addresses the broader determinants of health, acknowledging that disparities in healthcare access and outcomes often reflect underlying inequalities. Medically, equitable access is crucial for maximizing the utilization of available organs and tissues, ultimately saving more lives and reducing overall morbidity and mortality.

4.2 Goals of equitable access

The primary objectives include reducing health disparities across different population groups and ensuring that allocation systems are fair and transparent, and prioritize medical needs over other factors. Achieving these goals can lead to improved transplantation outcomes, a more trustful public perception of the transplantation system, and increased willingness among the public to donate organs.

4.3 Barriers to equitable access

Several barriers hinder the achievement of equitable access in transplantation.

4.3.1 Socioeconomic disparities

Individuals from lower-income backgrounds often face challenges in accessing transplantation services due to lack of insurance coverage, financial constraints, and limited access to information about transplantation [27–29].

4.3.2 Geographic disparities

People living in rural or remote areas may have limited access to specialized transplantation centers and face additional logistical challenges, such as the need for long-distance travel and accommodation near transplant centers [30].

4.3.3 Racial and ethnic disparities

Historical and systemic inequalities have led to lower transplantation rates among racial and ethnic minority groups. These disparities are compounded by biases in the healthcare system, cultural and linguistic barriers, and differences in organ donation rates.

4.4 Strategies to improve equitable access

Addressing these barriers requires a multifaceted approach.

4.4.1 Policy recommendations

Advocating for healthcare reforms to ensure comprehensive insurance coverage for transplantation and follow-up care. Policies should also aim to standardize transplantation practices across regions and healthcare providers to eliminate biases in the allocation process.

4.4.2 Awareness campaigns

Implementing targeted campaigns to raise awareness about organ donation and transplantation, especially in underserved communities. Efforts should focus on debunking myths, addressing fears, and highlighting the impact of transplantation on recipients' lives.

4.4.3 Changes in allocation systems

Revising organ allocation policies to prioritize medical urgency and compatibility over factors that may indirectly reflect socioeconomic status. The adoption of new technologies and data analytics can help create more sophisticated and fairer matching algorithms.

4.4.4 Strengthening community and healthcare provider education

Educating healthcare providers on the importance of equitable access and strategies to address their own biases. Additionally, empowering patients and families with comprehensive information about the transplantation process can help demystify it and encourage informed decision-making.

By addressing these barriers and implementing strategies for improvement, the healthcare community can make significant strides toward achieving equitable access in transplantation. This endeavor requires collaboration among policymakers, healthcare providers, patient advocacy groups, and the community at large. Ultimately, the goal is to create a transplantation system that serves all individuals fairly, respects their dignity and rights, and works tirelessly to save as many lives as possible [1, 2, 30].

5. Case studies and models of success

5.1 Case study 1: Spain's national transplant organization

5.1.1 Background

Spain is recognized globally for its success in organ donation and transplantation, consistently achieving one of the highest donation rates in the world. The foundation of its success lies in the national coordination system managed by the Organización Nacional de Trasplantes (ONT) [7, 10, 31–33].

5.1.2 Strategies

5.1.2.1 Opt-out donation policy

Spain operates an "opt-out" system, where all citizens are considered potential donors unless they have expressly registered their decision not to donate [33–35].

5.1.2.2 Decentralized coordination

The ONT works closely with regional coordinations and hospital transplant coordinators, ensuring a seamless process from donation to transplantation.

5.1.2.3 Public awareness

Continuous public education campaigns emphasize the importance of organ donation, fostering a culture of donation across the population.

5.1.3 Outcomes

Spain has sustained high rates of organ donation, significantly reducing waiting times for transplant surgeries. The model has demonstrated the effectiveness of combining legislative support with strong public education and a coordinated healthcare approach to improve organ donation rates.

5.1.4 Lessons learned

The importance of a well-organized, centrally coordinated transplant system that is integrated into the healthcare infrastructure. The role of societal attitudes and awareness in supporting organ donation [33, 35–37].

5.2 Case study 2: The US national kidney registry's paired exchange program

5.2.1 Background

The National Kidney Registry (NKR) in the United States has implemented an innovative paired kidney exchange program, aiming to increase the number of living donor kidney transplants and improve access for hard-to-match patients [38–40].

5.2.2 Strategies

5.2.2.1 Paired kidney exchanges

The program facilitates transplants by matching incompatible donor-recipient pairs with other pairs in similar situations.

5.2.2.2 Voucher program

The NKR introduced a "voucher" system, allowing donors to donate their kidney before their intended recipient needs the transplant. The recipient receives a "voucher" for priority in receiving a compatible kidney in the future.

5.2.2.3 Advanced matching algorithms

Utilizes sophisticated computer algorithms to identify potential matches across a wide network, optimizing the chances of finding compatible pairs.

5.2.3 Outcomes

Increase in the number of living donor transplants, particularly benefiting patients with rare blood types or antibodies that make finding a match challenging. The program has helped reduce waiting times and improve transplant outcomes by providing more timely access to compatible kidneys.

5.2.4 Lessons learned

Innovative approaches, such as paired exchanges and voucher programs, can significantly expand access to transplantation for patients facing barriers to finding a compatible donor. Leveraging technology for matching algorithms can optimize the pairing process, making transplantation more efficient and equitable [41].

6. Ongoing challenges in achieving equitable access

6.1 Resistance to policy changes

Efforts to reform organ donation and transplantation policies often encounter resistance from various quarters, including political entities, certain segments of the public, and even within the medical community. This resistance can stem from ethical concerns, cultural or religious beliefs about organ donation, and apprehensions about the implications of new policies, such as presumed consent or compensation for living donors. Overcoming this resistance requires sustained advocacy, transparent dialog, and education to build consensus and understanding.

6.2 Funding limitations

Transplantation programs require substantial financial investments in infrastructure, technology, and personnel. In many regions, funding limitations constrain the expansion of transplantation services, research into new technologies, and public education campaigns. These financial constraints are particularly acute in low- and middle-income countries, where the disparity in access to transplantation services is most pronounced. Addressing this challenge necessitates innovative funding models, international cooperation, and prioritization of healthcare resources to support transplantation services.

6.3 Need for ongoing education and advocacy

Public and professional education on organ donation and transplantation is critical for overcoming myths and misconceptions that hinder donation rates. Moreover, advocacy is needed to push for policy reforms, address disparities, and support research into new transplantation technologies. Continuous efforts are required to engage communities, empower patients and families, and educate healthcare providers about the latest advancements and ethical considerations in transplantation.

7. Future trends in transplantation medicine

7.1 Advancements in regenerative medicine

The burgeoning field of regenerative medicine, including stem cell therapy and tissue engineering, holds the promise of generating bioengineered organs for transplantation. These technologies could potentially alleviate the shortage of available organs, offering a renewable source of transplantable materials. However, their impact on equitable access will depend on the affordability and availability of such treatments, necessitating policies to ensure these innovations benefit all segments of society.

7.2 Precision medicine and immunomodulation

Future advancements in precision medicine and immunomodulation promise to enhance the success rates of transplants and reduce the need for lifelong immunosuppression, which carries significant side effects and costs. Personalized approaches to matching donors and recipients, based on genetic and immunological profiles, could improve outcomes and efficiency. Ensuring that these sophisticated technologies are accessible to diverse populations will be crucial for equitable access.

7.3 Global collaboration and ethical frameworks

As transplantation medicine advances, international collaboration will become increasingly important for sharing best practices, resources, and innovations. Ethical frameworks that guide the global exchange of organs, technologies, and knowledge will be essential to prevent exploitation and ensure that advancements in transplantation benefit humanity as a whole.

7.4 Challenges of new technologies

The integration of new technologies, such as artificial intelligence (AI) and machine learning, in the matching and allocation processes could improve efficiency and fairness. However, these technologies also raise ethical and privacy concerns that must be addressed. Ensuring that AI algorithms are transparent, unbiased, and designed with ethical considerations in mind will be paramount [42–44].

8. Ethical considerations

8.1 Ethical dilemmas in transplantation and allocation of scarce resources

The heart of the ethical dilemma in organ allocation lies in the principle of distributive justice—how to fairly distribute a very limited resource. The ethical challenge is not only in deciding who gets an organ but also in determining the criteria for that decision. Age, life expectancy, quality of life post-transplant, and the concept of "fair innings" often come into play. These considerations raise ethical questions about preferential treatments and the role of social worth assessments, such as prioritizing patients based on their perceived contribution to society or penalizing them based on lifestyle choices.

8.2 Consent for donation

The ethical terrain of consent in organ donation is nuanced by cultural, legal, and personal beliefs. Informed consent is a cornerstone, requiring transparency about the process, risks, and potential outcomes. The transition to presumed consent in some jurisdictions aims to increase organ availability but introduces ethical concerns about autonomy and the right to choose. The role of the family in the consent process adds another layer of complexity, especially in cases where the donor's wishes are unknown or conflicted with the family's sentiments [42, 44].

8.3 Living donations

Living donation poses unique ethical challenges, particularly concerning the potential coercion of donors and the risks they face. The ethical principle of non-maleficence must be carefully weighed against the potential benefits to the recipient. Ethical scrutiny is required to ensure that decisions are free from undue influence, especially in situations where there might be emotional, financial, or social pressure to donate. The advent of paired kidney exchanges and altruistic donations expands the ethical discourse around living donation, introducing questions about anonymity, reciprocity, and the role of incentives [9].

Living donations raise ethical concerns regarding potential harm to the donor, the voluntariness of the donation, and the risk of coercion. Ensuring the donor's informed consent and safeguarding their well-being is paramount, alongside evaluating the ethical implications of donations directed to specific recipients versus non-directed, altruistic donations. Ethical Frameworks and Principles Guiding Ethical Decision-Making Four principal ethical frameworks guide decision-making in transplantation.

8.4 Autonomy

Respecting the decision-making capacities of individuals, requiring that donors and recipients are informed and consent freely [30, 42].

8.5 Beneficence

Acting in the best interest of the patient, which includes both saving lives and ensuring the well-being of donors.

8.6 Non-maleficence

"Do no harm" principle, emphasizing the need to minimize risks and harm, especially to living donors.

8.7 Justice

Ensuring fair and equitable access to transplantation resources, including fair allocation systems.

8.8 Ethical frameworks and principles

The ethical landscape of transplantation is navigated using key frameworks and principles, providing a structured approach to ethical decision-making.

9. Navigating ethical dilemmas "case studies"

In-depth case studies can provide insights into how these ethical principles are applied in real-world scenarios. For example, the debate around pediatric vs. adult liver transplant candidates offers a window into how ethical principles clash and coalesce in practice. Similarly, the use of organs from high-risk donors, such as those with a history of drug use, presents ethical dilemmas in balancing the risk of disease transmission with the urgent need for organs.

Certainly, providing in-depth case studies within the ethical landscape of organ, tissue, and cell transplantation can illuminate the practical applications of ethical principles and the real-world challenges encountered. Here are two hypothetical case studies that explore these dynamics.

9.1 Case study 1: The allocation of a pediatric liver transplant

9.1.1 Background

In a large metropolitan hospital, two candidates are awaiting a pediatric liver transplant: an 8-year-old child with rare genetic liver disease and a 17-year-old teenager who developed liver failure due to a history of substance abuse. Both are in urgent need of a transplant, but there is currently only one liver available from a pediatric donor [43, 44].

9.1.2 Ethical dilemmas

9.1.2.1 Justice and fairness

How to equitably allocate the available liver when both candidates have pressing needs but different circumstances leading to their conditions. Allocation policies are crucial for ensuring that organs are distributed equitably among patients in need. Criteria such as medical urgency, waiting time, and compatibility are commonly used to prioritize recipients. However, disparities can arise from socioeconomic factors, geographic location, and systemic biases. Policies that prioritize local or regional recipients can hinder equitable access and self-sufficiency at a national level [30, 33, 45].

9.1.2.2 Social worth and medical history

Considering the teenager's substance abuse in the decision-making process raises questions about responsibility, social worth, and the potential for recurrence of liver failure post-transplant.

9.1.2.3 Beneficence and non-maleficence

Balancing the benefits of the transplant to each candidate against the potential risks, including the risk of transplant rejection and the ethical imperative to do no harm.

9.1.3 Resolution

The hospital's transplant ethics committee, comprising healthcare professionals, ethicists, and patient advocates, convenes to review the cases. They decide to prioritize based on medical urgency and the likelihood of transplant success, as determined by objective clinical criteria. The committee emphasizes the importance of nondiscrimination and the principle that past behavior should not penalize candidates in the allocation process. After careful consideration, the liver is allocated to the teenager due to a slightly higher urgency level and compatibility match, coupled with a comprehensive post-transplant support plan to address substance abuse issues.

9.1.4 Lessons learned

This case study highlights the complexities of organ allocation decisions and the importance of applying ethical principles such as justice, non-maleficence, and beneficence. It also underscores the need for support systems that address underlying issues facing transplant recipients [40, 41].

9.2 Case study 2: Consent in living donor kidney transplantation

9.2.1 Background

A 30-year-old woman with end-stage renal disease is informed that her best chance for a quality life is to receive a kidney transplant. Her 55-year-old mother, in excellent health, immediately offers to donate one of her kidneys. The transplantation center's protocol requires thorough medical and psychological evaluation of potential living donors to ensure informed consent and minimize risks.

9.2.2 Ethical dilemmas

9.2.2.1 Autonomy and informed consent

Ensuring that the mother's decision to donate is free from coercion and that she fully understands the risks involved in the donation [44, 45].

9.2.2.2 Beneficence and non-maleficence toward the donor

Balancing the potential benefits to the recipient against the risks to the donor, who will have to live with one kidney after the surgery [30].

9.2.2.3 Family dynamics

Navigating the emotional and psychological complexities inherent in family donations, where familial pressure or a sense of obligation might influence the decision to donate.

9.2.3 Resolution

The transplantation center conducts comprehensive evaluations, including medical, psychological, and social assessments, to ensure the mother is a suitable donor and is making an informed decision. Ethical consultations are offered to discuss the potential risks and benefits, and family counseling is provided to address any underlying pressures or concerns. Following a thorough review process, the mother is cleared to donate her kidney, and the transplant proceeds successfully with both parties fully informed and consenting.

9.2.4 Lessons learned

This case underscores the critical importance of autonomy and informed consent in living donor transplants, highlighting the need for rigorous evaluation processes to protect the well-being and rights of donors. It also demonstrates the value of psychological and social support services in navigating the emotional complexities of living donations.

9.3 Case study 3: Utilizing organs from high-risk donors

9.3.1 Background

A regional hospital faces a significant shortage of organs for transplantation. A potential donor, who recently passed away, was identified, but the individual had a history of intravenous drug use, raising concerns about the risk of transmitting infections such as HIV or Hepatitis C to the recipient. Advances in medical treatments have made it possible to treat these infections more effectively than in the past, yet the use of organs from high-risk donors remains a contentious issue.

9.3.2 Ethical dilemmas

9.3.2.1 Beneficence vs. non-maleficence

Weighing the potential benefit of saving a life with the transplant against the risk of transmitting a serious infection to the recipient.

9.3.2.2 Autonomy and informed consent

Ensuring that recipients are fully informed about the risks associated with accepting an organ from a high-risk donor and are able to make a voluntary, informed decision [30, 44, 45].

9.3.2.3 Justice and equity

Addressing potential biases and stigmas that may influence the decision-making process, such as unfairly devaluing the lives of individuals with histories of substance abuse [42, 43].

9.3.3 Resolution

The transplant ethics committee, along with infectious disease specialists, reviews the case, considering recent medical advancements in treating and managing HIV and Hepatitis C. They develop guidelines for the use of organs from high-risk donors, emphasizing informed consent and the autonomy of recipients to accept or decline such organs based on a clear understanding of the risks and benefits. The committee decides to offer the organ to a recipient who has been waiting for a transplant for an extended period and for whom the risk of waiting longer for another organ outweighs the potential risk of infection. The recipient is provided with detailed information about the donor's history, the risks involved, and the availability of treatments for infections. After thorough counseling and consideration, the recipient consents to the transplant.

9.3.4 Lessons learned

This case highlights the importance of balancing ethical principles when considering the use of organs from high-risk donors. It underscores the necessity of informed consent, where recipients are empowered to make decisions based on comprehensive information. Furthermore, it illustrates the potential to expand the donor pool and save more lives by carefully assessing and managing the risks associated with high-risk donors, coupled with advancements in medical treatments for infections. The case also stresses the importance of nondiscrimination and ensuring equitable access to transplantation opportunities, regardless of a donor's past behaviors or health history.

These case studies illustrate the multifaceted nature of ethical dilemmas in transplantation, offering insights into the application of ethical principles and the importance of a holistic, patient-centered approach in resolving these challenges.

10. Legal and policy frameworks

10.1 Legal and policy frameworks in transplantation: A comparative analysis

The legal and policy frameworks governing organ transplantation vary significantly across the globe, deeply influencing the success of national programs in achieving self-sufficiency and equitable access. These frameworks encompass consent laws, allocation policies, and regulations on living donations, each tailored to address the ethical, cultural, and logistical challenges inherent in transplantation. By examining the approaches of different countries, we can gain insights into the effectiveness of various legal and policy strategies [30, 45].

10.2 Consent laws and their impact opt-in vs. opt-out systems

Countries typically follow either an opt-in system, where individuals must actively register their consent to donate organs, or an opt-out system, where consent is presumed unless an individual has registered their refusal. Spain and Austria, for example, employ opt-out systems and boast high donation rates, suggesting that such frameworks can significantly enhance organ supply. Conversely, countries like the United States and Canada, which use opt-in systems, face challenges in meeting the demand for organs, despite extensive public awareness campaigns [30, 44, 46].

10.3 Legal implications

The choice between opt-in and opt-out systems has profound legal and ethical implications, influencing public perceptions of autonomy and state authority over individuals' bodies. The effectiveness of either system in achieving self-sufficiency in organ donations is also influenced by cultural attitudes, healthcare infrastructure, and the implementation of supportive policies. The United States operates the United Network for Organ Sharing (UNOS), which manages a complex, data-driven allocation system designed to maximize the fairness and efficiency of organ distribution. In contrast, countries like India have implemented a tiered system that allocates organs first to local, then regional, and finally national recipients, aiming to balance local needs with broader access.

11. Regulations on living donations

11.1 Safeguarding donors

Living donations, particularly of kidney and liver segments, play a crucial role in transplantation. Legal frameworks that protect living donors are essential for ensuring that donations are voluntary and free from coercion or financial inducement. Many countries have established rigorous screening and consent processes for living donors, as well as policies to provide donors with healthcare support and financial protection against the costs associated with donation [9, 36].

11.2 International policies

Iran's regulated system for compensated kidney donations from living donors is unique, allowing for direct financial compensation to donors within a legal and regulated framework. This approach has virtually eliminated the waiting list for kidney transplants in Iran but remains controversial internationally due to ethical concerns about commodification and exploitation [30, 31, 44, 45].

12. International cooperation and standards

12.1 Sharing best practices

International cooperation is pivotal for advancing global transplantation medicine. Organizations such as the World Health Organization (WHO) and the Transplantation Society work to promote ethical standards and share best practices among countries. The Declaration of Istanbul on Organ Trafficking and Transplant Tourism represents a significant international effort to combat illegal practices and promote ethical donation and transplantation policies.

12.2 Cross-border organ sharing

Some regions have established cross-border organ-sharing agreements to enhance access to transplantation. The European Union, for example, has mechanisms in place for sharing organs across member states, facilitating better matches and improving patient outcomes (**Figure 3**) [16–18].

13. Future directions

Legal and policy frameworks in transplantation are continually evolving to address new ethical dilemmas, technological advancements, and changes in societal attitudes. The future of transplantation law and policy will likely focus on enhancing global cooperation, refining consent and allocation systems to increase organ supply, and ensuring that innovations in transplantation medicine are accessible to all, regardless of geographical or socioeconomic barriers.

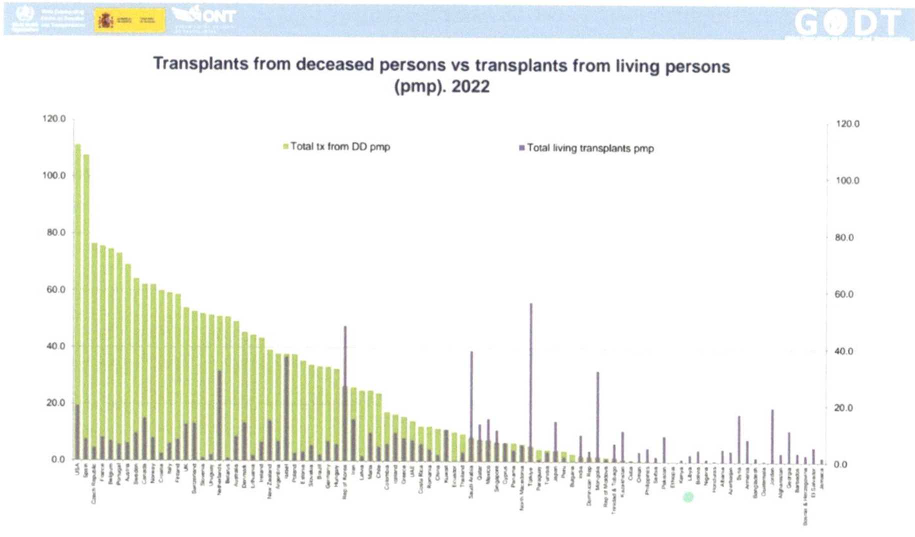

Figure 3.
Transplants from deceased donors vs. transplants from living donors.

14. Recommendations

14.1 For policymakers

14.1.1 Implement opt-out consent laws

Countries should consider adopting opt-out consent frameworks and customizing them with their religion and culture to increase organ donation rates, supported by public education campaigns to ensure community understanding and acceptance.

14.1.1.1 Detail

Opt-out consent laws, also known as presumed consent, automatically register all citizens as potential organ donors unless they choose to opt out. This approach has been successful in countries like Spain and Belgium, significantly increasing organ donation rates.

14.1.1.2 Challenges

Resistance may come from cultural, religious, or personal beliefs about organ donation. There is also the need to ensure that the public is fully informed and that the system respects individual autonomy in religion, culture, and choice.

14.1.1.3 Solutions

Public education campaigns are critical in addressing concerns and misinformation. These campaigns can highlight the personal stories of donors and recipients, showcasing the life-saving impact of organ donation. Additionally, making the opt-out process straightforward and accessible ensures that those who wish to opt out can easily do so.

14.1.2 Enhance legal and financial protections for living donors

Establish comprehensive policies that safeguard living donors from financial burden and health risks, encouraging more individuals to consider living donation.

14.1.2.1 Detail

Providing comprehensive health coverage and financial compensation for expenses incurred due to donation can encourage living donations. Iran's system offers an example, where living donors receive compensation and health coverage, contributing to a high rate of living donations.

14.1.2.2 Challenges

There's a fine line between compensating donors for their expenses and unethical payments that could coerce individuals into donating. Additionally, such programs require substantial funding and oversight to ensure fairness and transparency.

14.1.2.3 Solutions

Establishing clear guidelines and caps on compensation can help avoid ethical pitfalls. Implementing robust oversight mechanisms and ensuring transparent communication about the compensation process can build trust in the system. Fundraising efforts and government subsidies could support the financial aspects of these protections.

14.1.3 Promote international collaboration

Foster partnerships between countries to share best practices, innovations, and resources, and work toward harmonizing legal and ethical standards in transplantation.

14.1.3.1 Detail

International collaboration can take the form of shared databases for organ matching across borders, joint research projects on transplantation technologies, and harmonized standards for donor care. The Euro-transplant and Scandia-transplant networks provide successful models of regional collaboration, enhancing organ allocation efficiency and outcomes.

14.1.3.2 Challenges

Differences in legal, ethical, and medical standards can complicate international cooperation. There's also the risk of unequal benefits, where wealthier countries might disproportionately benefit from shared resources.

14.1.3.3 Solutions

Establishing international agreements that outline shared principles and goals can provide a foundation for collaboration. Mechanisms for equitable sharing of resources, along with joint funding models for research and development, can ensure that all participants benefit. Regular meetings and conferences can facilitate ongoing dialog and adjustment of collaborative efforts.

14.1.4 Invest in healthcare infrastructure

Ensure that all regions within a country have access to transplantation services, reducing geographic disparities in access. Investing in healthcare infrastructure to ensure equitable access to transplantation services across all regions addresses one of the critical challenges in the field of organ transplantation is geographic disparities in access. This recommendation focuses on the development and distribution of resources and facilities that can support transplantation services, from donor identification and organ procurement to post-transplant care.

14.1.4.1 Details

Investment in healthcare infrastructure encompasses building or enhancing transplant centers, laboratories for immunological testing, organ preservation facilities, and transportation systems for organs. It also involves training medical personnel specialized in transplant medicine, including surgeons, immunologists, coordinators, and support staff. An integrated approach ensures that patients, regardless of their geographic location, have timely access to transplantation services.

14.1.4.2 Challenges

1. *High costs*: The establishment and maintenance of transplantation infrastructure require significant financial investment. In resource-limited settings, prioritizing such investment can be challenging.

2. *Distribution and maintenance*: Ensuring even distribution of facilities and services across urban and rural areas is complex. Additionally, maintaining state-of-the-art facilities and technologies outside major urban centers can be challenging due to lower patient volumes and revenue.

3. *Workforce training and retention*: Training healthcare professionals in transplant medicine is resource-intensive, and retaining these highly specialized professionals in less urbanized regions poses an additional challenge.

14.1.4.3 Solutions

1. *Public-private partnerships (PPPs)*: Leveraging PPPs can mobilize additional funding sources for infrastructure development and operational costs. Collaborations with non-governmental organizations (NGOs) and international health organizations can also support infrastructure development, especially in underserved areas.

2. *Telemedicine and mobile units*: Implementing telemedicine programs can extend the reach of transplant services, allowing for remote consultations, patient monitoring, and even remote participation in transplant evaluations. Mobile units equipped with necessary medical technologies can travel to remote areas for screening, evaluation, and follow-up care, reducing the need for patients to travel.

3. *Decentralized training programs*: Developing decentralized training programs for transplant specialists can help address workforce challenges. Utilizing online education and remote mentorship programs can facilitate the training of medical personnel in less urbanized areas. Offering incentives, such as loan forgiveness, scholarships, or guaranteed positions, can attract and retain talent in these regions.

4. *National and regional coordination*: Establishing a national coordination body can help oversee the equitable distribution of resources and services. This body can work alongside regional coordinations to identify needs, allocate resources effectively, and ensure that all regions have access to transplantation services. Implementing a centralized organ allocation system that operates transparently across the entire country can also help minimize geographic disparities in access.

5. *Community engagement*: Engaging local communities in the planning and development of healthcare infrastructure can ensure that the services meet the specific needs of the area. Community involvement can also promote organ donation awareness and support for transplantation programs.

By addressing these challenges with targeted solutions, countries can work toward reducing geographic disparities in access to transplantation services. Investing in healthcare infrastructure is not only a commitment to improving health outcomes for patients in need of transplants but also a step toward achieving greater equity within the healthcare system.

14.2 For healthcare providers

14.2.1 Strengthen education on ethical allocation

14.2.1.1 Details

Strengthening education on ethical allocation involves creating comprehensive training programs for healthcare providers, focusing on the ethical principles that should guide the allocation of organs. This includes understanding the principles of equity, justice, and nondiscrimination, as well as the application of these principles in the complex decision-making process of organ allocation. Training should cover the ethical frameworks used to prioritize patients, the importance of transparency in the allocation process, and the role of healthcare providers in advocating for fair practices.

14.2.1.2 Challenges

a. *Complexity of ethical decision-making*: The multifaceted nature of ethical decision-making in organ allocation poses a challenge. Healthcare providers must balance medical urgency, patient compatibility, and broader ethical considerations, sometimes under pressing time constraints [30, 44].

b. *Varied interpretations of equity*: Different stakeholders may have varied interpretations of what constitutes equitable access, leading to disagreements and ethical dilemmas in the allocation process.

c. *Resistance to change*: Established practices and ingrained biases may lead to resistance among healthcare professionals to adopt new ethical guidelines or allocation principles.

d. *Lack of standardized training*: The absence of standardized, universally accepted training programs on ethical allocation can result in inconsistent practices and understandings among healthcare providers across different institutions and regions.

14.2.1.3 Solutions

a. *Development of standardized curriculum*: Collaborate with ethical bodies, transplantation societies, and educational institutions to develop a standardized curriculum for training healthcare providers. This curriculum should cover ethical theories, principles of equitable allocation, and practical case studies to illustrate ethical dilemmas and resolutions.

b. *Continuing education programs*: Implement mandatory continuing education programs for all healthcare professionals involved in the transplantation process. These programs can be delivered through workshops, online courses, and annual conferences to ensure ongoing learning and adaptation to new ethical guidelines.

c. *Interdisciplinary collaboration*: Foster interdisciplinary collaboration among ethicists, transplant coordinators, surgeons, and other healthcare providers to facilitate a holistic understanding of ethical allocation. Such collaboration can promote a shared commitment to equity and justice in organ allocation.

d. *Simulation-based training*: Utilize simulation-based training tools to allow healthcare providers to practice decision-making in hypothetical scenarios. This method can help participants understand the consequences of different allocation decisions and the importance of adhering to ethical principles.

e. *Promote ethical leadership*: Encourage the development of ethical leadership within transplant teams, where senior members model ethical decision-making and mentor junior staff. Ethical leaders can also serve as advocates for fair allocation policies within their institutions and the broader medical community.

f. *Evaluate and refine practices*: Regularly evaluate the effectiveness of training programs and the impact on allocation practices. Use feedback from healthcare providers and outcomes data to refine training programs and address emerging ethical challenges in organ allocation.

By addressing these challenges with comprehensive solutions, the transplantation community can enhance the understanding and implementation of ethical allocation principles. Strengthening education on ethical allocation is essential for building a fair and transparent transplantation system that upholds the dignity and rights of all patients.

14.2.2 Implement culturally sensitive outreach programs

14.2.2.1 Details

Implementing culturally sensitive outreach programs entails designing and delivering education initiatives that are specifically tailored to the cultural, linguistic, and social contexts of diverse communities. These programs aim to address and dismantle cultural barriers, myths, and misconceptions about organ donation and transplantation, thereby increasing awareness and willingness to donate. Effective outreach involves collaboration with community leaders, use of culturally relevant materials, and respectful communication strategies that honor the values and beliefs of each community.

14.2.2.2 Challenges

1. *Cultural diversity and sensitivity*: Communities are culturally diverse, with varying beliefs, practices, and attitudes toward organ donation and transplantation. Designing programs that respect this diversity while effectively conveying the importance of organ donation is challenging.

2. *Language barriers*: Providing information in multiple languages and ensuring that the messaging is not only translated but also culturally nuanced can be resource-intensive.

3. *Myths and misconceptions*: Deeply ingrained myths and misconceptions about organ donation can be difficult to overcome, particularly when they are tied to religious or cultural beliefs.

4. *Trust in healthcare systems*: Historical or ongoing healthcare disparities and injustices can lead to mistrust in healthcare messages and initiatives, making community engagement challenging.

14.2.2.3 Solutions

a. *Community engagement and partnerships*: Partner with community leaders, religious organizations, and cultural institutions to co-create outreach programs. Their endorsement can lend credibility and facilitate deeper engagement with community members.

b. *Culturally tailored materials*: Develop educational materials that are culturally relevant and sensitive, including testimonials and stories from community members who have been donors or recipients. Ensure materials are available in the predominant languages of the community and are accessible in various formats (print, digital, and video). Training for cultural competency: Train healthcare providers and outreach staff in cultural competency to ensure they can effectively communicate with and engage diverse communities. Understanding cultural nuances can help tailor conversations about organ donation in a respectful and impactful manner.

c. *Leveraging social media and technology*: Use social media platforms popular within specific communities to spread awareness and counter myths about organ donation. Technology can also facilitate virtual discussions and Q&A sessions with healthcare providers, donors, and recipients.

d. *Addressing mistrust*: Acknowledge and address historical mistrust in healthcare systems by being transparent about the organ donation and allocation process. Collaborate with trusted community healthcare providers to deliver messages about organ donation.

e. *Monitoring and evaluation*: Continuously monitor and evaluate the effectiveness of outreach programs in different communities. Use feedback to refine strategies and ensure that the programs are meeting the needs and addressing the concerns of each community.

By overcoming these challenges with thoughtful and inclusive solutions, healthcare systems can significantly improve organ donation awareness and consent rates among diverse communities. Culturally sensitive outreach programs not only promote equity in organ donation but also strengthen community relations with the healthcare sector, fostering a more inclusive and understanding environment for all.

14.2.3 Adopt precision medicine approaches in transplantation

Utilize advances in genetic and immunological testing to improve matching processes and outcomes in transplantation, making the best use of available organs.

14.2.3.1 Detail

Precision medicine involves tailoring medical treatment to the individual characteristics of each patient, which in transplantation could mean detailed genetic and immunological matching between donors and recipients. This approach can increase transplant success rates and reduce rejection incidents.

14.2.3.2 Challenges

Implementing precision medicine in transplantation requires advanced technology and significant investment in research. There is also the need for specialized training for healthcare providers in genetics and immunology.

14.2.3.3 Solutions

Governments and healthcare institutions can invest in the necessary technologies and training programs. Collaborations with academic institutions and private sector partners can accelerate research and development. Public-private partnerships might offer a viable model for funding precision medicine initiatives in transplantation.

14.3 For communities

14.3.1 Engage in public awareness campaigns

Communities should actively participate in campaigns that promote organ donation awareness, highlighting the impact of transplantation on individuals' lives and the societal benefits of increased donation rates.

14.3.1.1 Detail

Effective public awareness campaigns can demystify organ donation and address misconceptions, using various media platforms to reach broad audiences. The "Don't take your organs to heaven, heaven knows we need them here" campaign in the United States serves as a poignant example of leveraging emotional appeal and humor to promote organ donation.

14.3.1.2 Challenges

Crafting messages that resonate across diverse cultural and demographic groups can be challenging. There is also the potential for campaign fatigue if messages become too repetitive or are not effectively targeted.

14.3.1.3 Solutions

Tailoring campaigns to specific communities using cultural insights can enhance relevance and impact. Employing a mix of traditional and social media platforms ensures broader reach. Engaging influencers, religious and community leaders as campaign ambassadors can lend credibility and foster grassroots support.

14.3.2 Support transplant recipients and donors

Establish community-based support networks for individuals and families navigating the transplantation process, offering emotional, logistical, and informational support.

14.3.3 Advocate for equitable access

Community leaders and patient advocacy groups should lobby for changes in policies and practices that currently hinder equitable access to transplantation services.

15. Conclusions

This chapter explored the multifaceted challenges and opportunities in achieving self-sufficiency and equitable access in organ, tissue, and cell transplantation. From the foundational understanding of transplantation's significance in modern medicine to the intricate legal and policy frameworks governing it globally, several key themes have emerged.

15.1 The vital role of transplantation

Transplantation stands as a critical life-saving intervention, offering hope to those with organ failure or tissue damage. Despite advancements, a gap remains between the demand for and the supply of transplantable organs and tissues.

15.2 Barriers to equitable access

Socioeconomic status, geographic location, and racial or ethnic disparities significantly impact access to transplantation. These barriers underscore the need for systemic changes to ensure fairness in transplantation services, along with recapitulation of the imperative for equitable access in transplantation and the multifaceted approach required to overcome existing barriers.

15.3 Self-sufficiency

Achieving self-sufficiency in organ donation within countries or regions is essential to reduce reliance on international donations, address organ trafficking, and improve equitable access to transplantation services (**Figure 4**) [16–18].

15.4 Legal and policy frameworks

Diverse approaches to consent laws, allocation policies, and regulations on living donations illustrate the complexity of creating effective systems that balance ethical considerations with the goal of increasing organ availability, that needs a call to action for policymakers, healthcare providers, and the community at large to commit to the principles of equity and justice in the provision of life-saving transplantation services.

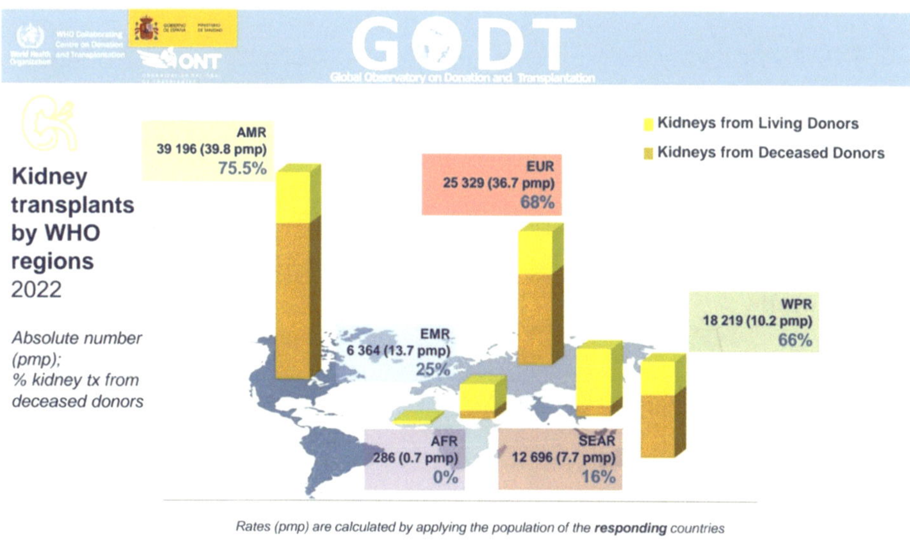

Figure 4.
Kidney transplants by WHO regions 2022.

15.5 Innovations and challenges ahead

Emerging technologies and treatments promise to revolutionize transplantation. However, ethical, logistical, and financial challenges must be navigated to realize their full potential.

The ethical considerations in transplantation are deeply complex, touching on profound questions about life, death, and what it means to act justly within a constrained system. As transplantation medicine continues to advance, the ethical frameworks that guide it must be continually revisited and refined. Through ongoing dialog among ethicists, medical professionals, patients, and the public, the field can strive to uphold the principles of justice, autonomy, beneficence, and non-maleficence at the heart of ethical medical practice.

Author details

Ehtuish F.A. Ehtuish
Surgery Department, Libyan Transplant Authority, Central Hospital Tripoli, Libya

*Address all correspondence to: ehtuish@gmail.com

IntechOpen

References

[1] Ehtuish EF. In: Ortiz J, editor. Ethical Controversies in Organ Transplantation, Understanding the Complexities of Kidney Transplantation. London, UK: InTech; 2011. ISBN: 978-953-307-819-9. Available from: http://www.intechopen.com/books/show/title/understanding-the-complexities-of-kidney-transplantation

[2] Ehtuish EF, Abouna GM, Shebani AH, Abdulmola TS, Shawesh TZ. Kidney transplantation in Libya: A North African and middle eastern perspective. Experimental and Clinical Transplantation. 2006;**4**(1):425-428

[3] Alashek W, Ehtuish E, Elhabashi A, Emberish W, Mishra A. Reasons for unwillingness of Libyans to donate organs after death. Libyan Journal of Medicine LJM. 2009;**4**:110-113. DOI: 10.3402/ljm.V4/3.4827

[4] Rosenblum AM, Horvat LD, Siminoff LA, Prakash V, Beitel J, Garg AX. The authority of next-of-kin in explicit and presumed consent systems for deceased organ donation: an analysis of 54 nations. Nephrol Dial Transplant. Jun 2012;**27**(6):2533-2546. DOI: 10.1093/ndt/gfr619. Epub 2011 Nov 25

[5] Wendler D, Dickert N. The consent process for cadaveric organ procurement: how does it work? How can it be improved? JAMA. Jan 2001 17;**285**(3):329-333. DOI: 10.1001/jama.285.3.329

[6] Sharif A. Competing wishes of next-of-kin versus the deceased when it comes to organ donation consent. Evidence-Based Nursing. Apr 2023;**26**(2):72. DOI: 10.1136/ebnurs-2022-103684. Epub 2023 Feb 6

[7] Molina-Pérez A, Delgado J, Frunza M, Morgan M, Randhawa G, de Wijdeven JR, et al. Should the family have a role in deceased organ donation decision-making? A systematic review of public knowledge and attitudes towards organ procurement policies in Europe. Transplantation Reviews. (Orlando). Jan 2022;**36**(1):100673. DOI: 10.1016/j.trre.2021.100673. Epub 2021 Nov 26

[8] Delgado J. The role of the family in deceased organ procurement: A guide for clinicians and policymakers. Transplantation. 2019

[9] Chon WJ, Josephson MA, Gordon EJ, Becker YT, Witkowski P, Arwindekar DJ, et al. When the living and the deceased cannot agree on organ donation: a survey of US organ procurement organizations (OPOs). American Journal of Transplantation. Jan 2014;**14**(1):172-177. DOI: 10.1111/ajt.12519

[10] Sandal S. Advancing a paradigm shift to approaching health systems in the field of living-donor kidney transplantation: An opinion piece. Canadian Journal of Kidney Health and Disease. 2022

[11] Rithalia A, McDaid C, Suekarran S, Norman G, Myers L, Sowden A. A systematic review of presumed consent systems for deceased organ donation. Health Technology Assessment. May 2009;**13**(26):iii, ix-xi, 1-95. DOI: 10.3310/hta13260

[12] Ramalingam ND, Gordon EJ, Ross L. Attitudes and practices in postmortem organ procurement. JAMA. Apr 2001 18;**285**(15):1958; author reply 1959-60

[13] Capron AM. Re-examining organ transplantation. JAMA. 17 Jan 2001;**285**(3):334-366. DOI: 10.1001/jama.285.3.334

[14] Horvat LD, Cuerden MS, Kim SJ, Koval JJ, Young A, Garg AX. Informing the debate: Rates of kidney transplantation in nations with presumed consent. Annals of Internal Medicine. 16 Nov 2010;**153**(10):641-649. DOI: 10.7326/0003-4819-153-10-201011160-00006

[15] Wilkinson TM. Individual and family consent to organ and tissue donation: is the current position coherent? Journal of Medical Ethics. Oct 2005;**31**(10):587-590. DOI: 10.1136/jme.2004.009654

[16] WHO publications. 2022

[17] ONT. The National Organisation of Transplantation in Spain, 2022 publications

[18] IRODAT. International Registry of Organ Donation and Transplantation. 2022

[19] Cowie S, et al. Healthcare System Impact on Deceased Organ Donation and Transplantation: A Comparison Between the Top 10 Organ Donor Countries With 4 Countries in Southeast Asia. Transplant International. 2023

[20] Van Oosterhout SPC. How clinicians discuss patients' donor registrations of consent and presumed consent in donor conversations in an opt-out system: A qualitative embedded multiple-case study. Critical Care. 2023

[21] Toews M. Legislation and policy recommendations on organ and tissue donation and transplantation from an international consensus forum. Transplantation direct. 2023

[22] Molina-Pérez A. Differential impact of opt-in, opt-out policies on deceased organ donation rates: A mixed conceptual and empirical study. BMJ Open. 2022

[23] Aubrey P, Arber S, Tyler M. The organ donor crisis: The missed organ donor potential from the accident and emergency departments. Transplantation Proceedings. 2008;**40**:1008-1011

[24] Kirste G. Organ exchange in Europe–barriers and perspectives for the future. Annals of Transplantation. 2006;**11**:52-55

[25] Santiago-Delpin EA. The organ shortage: A public health crisis. What are Latin American governments doing about it? Transplantation Proceedings. 1997;**29**:3203-3204

[26] Langone AJ, Helderman JH. Disparity between solid-organ supply and demand. The New England Journal of Medicine. 2003;**349**:704-706

[27] Bendorf A, Pussell BA, Kelly PJ. Socioeconomic, demographic and policy comparisons of living and deceased kidney transplantation rates across 53 countries. Nephrology. 2013;**18**:633-640. DOI: 10.1111/nep.12101

[28] e-Statistics Report on Transplant, Waiting List and Donor Statistics. Canadian Institute for Health Information; 2010. Canadian Institute for Health Information

[29] Urquhart R. Nurse knowledge and attitudes towards organ donation and deemed consent: The human organ and tissue donation act in Nova Scotia. Canadian Journal of Anaesthesia. 2023

[30] Beraldo S, Karpus J. Nudging to donate organs: Do what you like or like what we do? Medicine, Health Care, and Philosophy. 2021;**24**:329-340. DOI: 10.1007/s11019-021-10007-6

[31] Tennankore KK. Perspectives on opt-out versus opt-In legislation for deceased organ donation: An opinion

piece. Canadian Journal of Kidney Health and Disease. 2021

[32] Shepherd L. When do next-of-kin opt-in? Anticipated regret, affective attitudes and donating deceased family member's organs. Journal of Health Psychology. 2014

[33] Ahmad MU, Hanna A, Mohamed A-Z. A systematic review of opt-out versus opt-in consent on deceased organ donation and transplantation (2006-2016). World Journal of Surgery. 2019;**43**:3161-3171. DOI: 10.1007/s00268-019-05118-4

[34] Walton P, Pérez-Blanco A, Beed S, Glazier A, Ferreira Salomao Pontes D, Kingdon J, et al. Organ and tissue donation consent model and intent to donate registries: Recommendations from an international consensus forum. Transplantation direct. May 2023;**9**(5):p e1416. DOI: 10.1097/TXD.0000000000001416

[35] Martinez-Lopez MV, Coll E, Cruz-Quintana F, Dominguez-Gil B, Hannikainen IR, Lara Rosales R, et al. Family bereavement and organ donation in Spain: a mixed method, prospective cohort study protocol. BMJ Open. 6 Jan 2023;**13**(1):e066286. DOI: 10.1136/bmjopen-2022-066286

[36] Martínez-López MV, McLaughlin L, Molina-Pérez A, et al. Mapping trust relationships in organ donation and transplantation: a conceptual model. BMC Med Ethics. 2023;**24**:93. DOI: 10.1186/s12910-023-00965-2

[37] Shaw D, Georgieva D, Haase B, Gardiner D, Lewis P, Jansen N, et al. ELPAT Working Group on Deceased Donation. Family Over Rules? An Ethical Analysis of Allowing Families to Overrule Donation Intentions. Transplantation. Mar 2017;**101**(3):482-487. DOI: 10.1097/TP.0000000000001536

[38] Gunderson S. Donation Starts With a Decision: The Role of the Individual and Family in Organ Donation. Transplantation. May 2019;**103**(5):864-865. DOI: 10.1097/TP.0000000000002623

[39] NHS. Transplant Activity Report. NHS Organ Donation. 2019. Available from: http://helping-you-to-decide/about-organ-donation/statistics-about-organ-donation/transplant-activity-report/ [Accessed: 6 August 2020]

[40] Nolin T, Mårdh C, Karlström G. Identifying opportunities to increase organ donation after brain death. An observational study in Sweden 2009-2014. Acta Anaesthesiologica Scandinavica. 2017;**61**(1):73-82. DOI: 10.1111/aas.12831

[41] Thybo KH, Eskesen V. The most important reason for lack of organ donation is family refusal. Danish Medical Journal. 2013;**60**(1):A4585

[42] Qurashi GM. Opt-out paradigms for deceased organ donation are ethically incoherent. Journal of Medical Ethics. 2021. DOI: 10.1136/medethics-2021-107630. [Epub ahead of print: 11 Sep 2021]

[43] Morla-González M, Moya-Guillem C, Delgado J, et al. European and comparative law study regarding family's role in deceased organ procurement. Revista General de Derecho Público Comparado. 2021:29. Available from: https://www.iustel.com//v2/revistas/detalle_revista.asp?id_noticia=423928&popup=

[44] Bagheri A. Organ transplantation laws in Asian countries: A comparative study. Transplantation Proceedings. 2005;**37**:4159-4162. DOI: 10.1016/j.transproceed.2005.11.016

[45] Coppen R, Friele RD, Gevers SKM. The impact of donor policies in Europe: A steady increase, but not everywhere. BMC Health Services Research. 2008;**8**:235. DOI: 10.1186/1472-6963-8-235

[46] Molina-Pérez A, Delgado J, Rodríguez-Arias D. Defining consent: Autonomy and the role of the family. In: Hansen SL, Schicktanz S, editors. Ethical Challenges of Organ Transplantation: Current Debates and International Perspectives. Transcript Verlag; 2021. pp. 43-64

Chapter 2

Desensitization Strategies in Kidney Transplantation

Mohsen Nafar and Shiva Samavat

Abstract

Desensitization protocols offer a promising approach to increase the pool of kidney transplant recipients by enabling transplantation with HLA-incompatible kidneys. This chapter explores the rationale for desensitization, considering the growing number of highly sensitized patients and the limitations of compatible donor availability. We discuss various desensitization strategies, including plasmapheresis, intravenous immunoglobulin, B-cell targeting agents, proteasome inhibitors, costimulatory blockers, and CAR T-cell therapy. Each strategy has its own mechanisms of action, efficacy rates, and potential complications. The chapter also highlights the challenges associated with desensitization, including limited efficacy, antibody rebound, increased risk of infections and malignancies, and significant treatment costs. Cost-effectiveness analyses of desensitization remain a subject of debate. The decision to pursue desensitization requires careful consideration of various factors, including patient characteristics, transplant center expertise, and the availability of safe and effective protocols. While advancements in virtual crossmatch techniques and allocation systems represent the most cost-effective approaches to transplantation, desensitization offers a valuable tool for expanding access to transplantation for patients with limited options.

Keywords: kidney transplantation, desensitization, highly sensitized, apheresis, memory B-cell, costimulatory blocker, anti-CD38, interleukin-6, treatment strategies, complications

1. Introduction

Sensitization, defined by the presence of antibodies against Human Leukocyte Antigens (HLA), is a major barrier to kidney transplantation. Individuals waiting for a kidney transplant are considered sensitized if their calculated panel-reactive antibody (cPRA) is greater than 1%. According to the OPTN/SRTS 2022 annual data report, 38.6% of adults on the kidney transplant waiting list are sensitized, and 11% have a cPRA above 80% [1]. Eurotransplant (ET) data from 2019 indicates that 5.6% of adults waiting for a transplant had a cPRA ≥85% [2]. Patients with a cPRA ≥80% are classified as highly sensitized, and those with a cPRA ≥98% are considered very highly sensitized, placing them in the category of un-transplantable patients [2–4].

Factors contributing to sensitization include previous transplantation, prior pregnancies and abortions, transfusion, and rarely, bacterial or viral infections like COVID-19. Recently, SARS-CoV-2 vaccination has also been linked to sensitization [5]. Different sensitizing events have various effects on anti-HLA antibody formation and the outcome of transplantation. The strongest sensitizing event is prior transplantation; even transplant nephrectomy shortly after graft loss due to vascular thrombosis may result in detectable class I and class II anti-HLA antibodies in 60% of patients [6]. Additionally, when comparing miscarriage and pregnancy as sensitizing events, prior miscarriage results in lower alloimmunization than a successful pregnancy [7]. Previous transplantation results in a vigorous antibody response compared to pregnancy, which in turn causes a stronger response than transfusion. It also leads to antibody formation against both class I and class II, while pregnancy and transfusion predominantly result in anti-class I antibodies [8]. In a recent study using machine learning consensus clustering, highly sensitized kidney transplant recipients who were younger, male, and had a history of previous transplantation had lower graft survival and higher rejection rates than those who were older with no history of transplantation [4]. These studies point out the fact that the type of sensitizing event has an impact on the degree of sensitization, type of antibody, and even the prognosis of the patient and graft after transplantation.

2. Immunologic basis of sensitization

When the body is exposed to HLA antigens, a series of cells and mediators work together to produce antibodies and cause sensitization, regardless of how the exposure occurs. Upon recognition of HLA antigens by antigen-presenting cells (APCs) such as B cells in the indirect pathway and dendritic cells in direct and semidirect pathways, the alloantigen is presented to $CD4^+$ T cells. The indirect pathway leads to the activation of follicular helper $CD4^+$ T cells (Tfh), which in turn activate antibody-producing B cells and $CD8^+$ cytotoxic T cells. Interestingly, while direct pathway-activated $CD4^+$ T cells can activate cytotoxic T cells, they are not capable of helping B cells to produce alloantibodies. T-cell activation requires both T-cell receptor and costimulatory signaling. This costimulation occurs via CD80/86 and CD28 interaction. Indirect pathway-activated Tfh migrate to follicular regions in secondary lymphoid organs, where they interact with pre-germinal center (pre-GC) B cells and promote the proliferation of antigen-specific B cells in the germinal center (GC). The effect of Tfh on B cells is mediated by IL-6 and IL-21. The activated GC B cells can then differentiate into either low-affinity antibody-producing plasmablasts or memory B cells and long-lived plasma cells (LLPCs). B-cell maturation, development, and hemostasis are regulated by the interaction of BAFF (B-cell activating factor) and APRIL (a proliferation-inducing ligand) with BCMA (B-cell maturation antigen) on B cells (**Figure 1**).

Memory B cells remain in circulation for years, independent of the antigen's presence, and can respond to future exposures even years later [9]. Long-lived plasma cells (LLPCs) residing in bone marrow niches continue antibody production for decades [10]. Additionally, the type of sensitizing event influences the persistence of memory B cells. There would be no or little detectable memory B cells after transfusion when compared to transplantation or pregnancy [11]. All these players in the process of sensitization could be potential targets for desensitization, and we may need to hit multiple targets to overcome the immunologic barriers in transplantation.

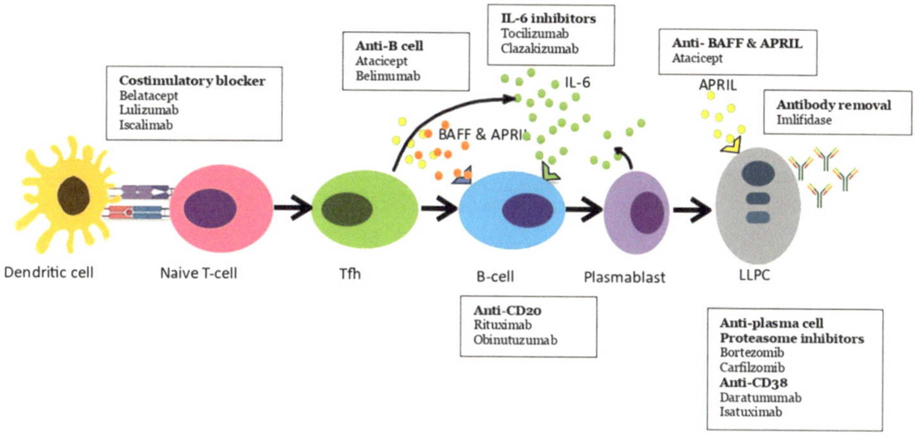

Figure 1.
Immunologic basis of sensitization and potential treatments.

3. Choosing the best candidate for desensitization

To achieve successful transplantation outcomes, careful selection of both the patient and the antibody is crucial. Two categories of transplant candidates may benefit from desensitization: (1) patients on the waiting list with cPRA >85% and a low likelihood of finding an HLA-compatible donor. Desensitization might increase the chance of transplantation for these patients. (2) Patients with only one positive crossmatch HLA-incompatible living donor who cannot be changed [12, 13].

Once we have identified a patient who might benefit from antibody removal strategies, we need to determine which antibody characteristics can predict the response to treatment. One of the predictors is antibody strength measured by single antigen bead (SAB) assay or mean fluorescence intensity (MFI). However, the SAB assay has limitations that can lead to overestimation of the amount of antibodies. These limitations include decreased antigen density on the beads, which can underestimate antibody titer, interfering factors such as high-titer antibodies or the prozone effect, nonspecific binding to the beads, and shared epitopes that can result in a lower estimated MFI of an antibody. Dilution of the sample is one way to overcome the prozone effect, potentially providing a better estimation of antibody level than the absolute MFI [14]. Furthermore, diluted titers might be a predictor of response to antibody removal processes. In a study by Pinelli et al., antibodies with an initial titer greater than 1:512 did not respond to repeated cycles of treatment [15]. Therefore, dilution can be used to predict response, especially when the undiluted antibody titer is more than 12,000 [16].

One of the flaws of antibody titer is the lack of a standardized solid-phase assay, which results in inconsistency in test results. To address this, Cedars-Sinai Medical Center developed a scoring system based on the MFI of DSAs, called DSA-RIS (Relative Intensity Scale). The scale assigns zero points for no DSA, 2 points for each DSA with MFI < 5000, 5 points for each DSA between 5000 and 10,000, and 10 points for each DSA with MFI above 10,000. This scale helps predict treatment response and define a threshold for successful desensitization. A DSA-RIS score ≤ 17 is considered a positive determinant for response, as scores above 17 have been shown to have a 91% positive predictive value for antibody-mediated rejection (AMR) after transplantation [17, 18].

Another factor influencing treatment response is the HLA loci targeted by the antibodies. Several reports suggest that HLA antibodies against DQ and DP antigens are more resistant to desensitization strategies than DR and class I anti-HLA antibodies [19]. However, further investigation is warranted, as the Pinelli study showed similar response rates for HLA-B, DR, and DQ antibodies, though HLA-A antibodies had a lower response rate [15]. Additionally, C1q-positive antibodies have been shown to have a weaker response to desensitization strategies [15].

Based on current data, low titer, C1q-negative, and class I anti-HLA antibodies appear to be more favorable candidates for desensitization.

4. Treatment strategies

The current standard of care desensitization protocol typically includes apheresis and rituximab, with or without intravenous immune globulin (IVIG). Based on what was discussed earlier, treatment strategies can be categorized into four sections: (I) antibody removal, (II) targeting B cells and maturation factors like BAFF and APRIL, (III) targeting plasma cells and $CD38^+$ cells, and (IV) inhibition of cytokines such as IL-6.

One of the main challenges we face during the process of desensitization is the "transient" effect of desensitization, which is particularly problematic for patients on deceased donor waiting lists. The other limitation in this process is variability in response and lack of specific tests to precisely predict the response rate. High cost and complications of overimmunosuppression are other major drawbacks of desensitization [20]. Thus, a treatment strategy with a durable and sustained response and a low rate of complication is the aim of most studies.

The following section will discuss ongoing clinical trials aimed at achieving these goals and introduce some novel desensitization strategies currently in the early stages of investigation.

4.1 Antibody removal techniques

Apheresis and imlifidase are two available options for antibody removal.

4.1.1 Apheresis

Three apheresis techniques are available for antibody removal: therapeutic plasma exchange (TPE), double-filtration plasmapheresis (DFPP), and semi-specific immunoadsorption (IA). The choice of apheresis technique and subsequent response depends on factors like the MFI, class, and HLA locus of the targeted HLA antibodies. HLA antibodies with MFI > 20,000 are generally considered resistant to all removal techniques. Removing class II antibodies, particularly HLA-DQ antibodies, appears more challenging with apheresis techniques [21]. However, this may be due to their higher MFI, requiring longer removal sessions for significant reduction [22].

The TPE technique (either centrifugal or membrane) is readily available, inexpensive, and removes ABO, HLA, and non-HLA antibodies like vascular endothelial cell antibodies. However, its nonspecific nature leads to the loss of essential components like coagulation factors, antimicrobial antibodies, and hormones. DFPP, while depleting coagulation factors and immunoglobulins, requires less replacement fluid compared to TPE, resulting in a lower risk of allergic reactions and infections. The IA technique utilizes specific columns designed to adsorb HLA antibodies, avoiding coagulopathy and infection risks associated with other methods [23]. Each technique is typically implemented daily or every other day for five sessions, with MFI reassessment after the fifth session. Malvezzi et al. proposed an algorithm based on initial MFI to guide apheresis technique selection. IA, DFPP, and TPE are recommended for antibodies with MFI > 12,000, 9000 < MFI < 12,000, and MFI ≤ 9000, respectively (**Figure 2**) [24].

Apheresis alone is insufficient because it removes the inhibitory effects of antibodies on B cells, lifting the negative feedback and leading to a rapid rise in antibody production (rebound). However, recent data suggest this increase in antibody levels after apheresis is due to a decreased catabolism rate rather than increased production [15]. Regardless of the mechanism, additional strategies are necessary to reduce antibody levels alongside apheresis.

The advantage of apheresis in addition to decreasing antibody level is its immunomodulatory effects. It increases regulatory T cells (Tregs) and sensitizes B cells and plasma cells to immunosuppressants [25]. The consequences of apheresis on cytokines are unclear, though some studies revealed increased plasma levels of IL-10 and IL-6 and decreased levels of IL-8 and TNF-α [20].

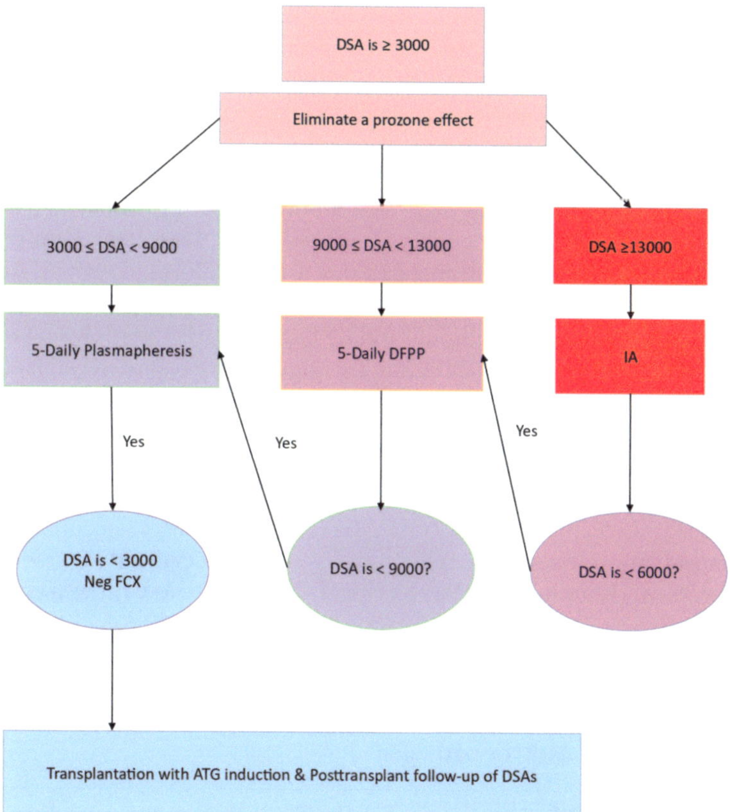

Figure 2.
Choosing the appropriate apheresis technique. ATG: anti-thymocyte globulin; DFPP: double filter plasmapheresis; DSA: donor specific antibody; FCX: flowcytometric crossmatch; IA: immunoadsorption.

4.1.2 Imlifidase

Imlifidase is a cysteine protease that specifically cleaves the heavy chain of all IgG subclasses but not IgM, IgA, or IgE. This rapid removal of IgG anti-HLA antibodies inhibits antibody-dependent cellular cytotoxicity (ADCC) of natural killer (NK) cells and complement-dependent cytotoxicity (CDC). Imlifidase has a half-life of 8–12 hours, and its activity persists for up to 4 days. During this period, it cleaves all IgG antibodies in the circulation, including IVIG, rituximab, and anti-thymocyte globulin (ATG), except for horse ATG [10]. Therefore, administration of these medications should be delayed for at least 4–5 days after imlifidase to avoid potential interference. The drug's primary purpose is to induce an antibody-free window. However, antibody rebound typically occurs within 3–7 days after drug elimination, especially in patients who have not received pre-transplant IVIG and rituximab [12, 26]. Imlifidase can also be immunogenic, making re-administration challenging and typically restricted to the first 24 hours after the initial dose [13].

In addition to IgG destruction, imlifidase cleaves B-cell antigen receptors on memory B cells, limiting their antigen recognition capacity and differentiation into plasma cells [27]. A study by Kjellman et al. reported promising 3-year post-transplant outcomes in positive crossmatch recipients desensitized with imlifidase before transplantation. Among 39 patients, 15 experienced AMR, with most episodes occurring within the first post-transplant month. Overall patient and graft survival at 3 years were 90 and 84%, respectively. Even patients with AMR had a favorable outcome, with 93% death-censored graft survival and 85% patient survival [28]. These promising results suggest that imlifidase can be a potent and rapid-acting option for desensitization, particularly for highly sensitized patients on deceased donor waiting lists.

To overcome the post-imlifidase DSA rebound, Kanbay et al. proposed an immunosuppressive protocol combining high-dose steroids (500 mg on day 0, 250 mg on days 1–3, 125 mg on day 4, 20 mg on day 5), rabbit ATG 1.5 mg/kg/day for five daily doses starting on the fourth post-transplant day, 2 g/kg IVIG on days 4–5, Rituximab 375 mg/m^2 on the seventh post-transplant day, and a standard triple maintenance regimen with prednisolone, tacrolimus, and mycophenolate mofetil [27]. While this approach appears promising, clinical trials are ongoing to explore the efficacy, cost-effectiveness, and safety of imlifidase in both desensitization protocols and treatment of AMR after transplantation.

4.2 B-cell targeting strategies

The humoral immune response relies heavily on the specialized functions of B cells. These versatile lymphocytes play a critical role in three key processes:

- **Antigen presentation:** B cells can act as antigen-presenting cells (APCs), capturing and displaying foreign invaders (antigens) on their surface to T cells. This crucial step initiates the adaptive immune response by allowing T cells to recognize and eliminate the pathogen.

- **Antibody production:** Upon activation by T cells and antigen binding, B cells differentiate into antibody-secreting plasma cells. These plasma cells churn out vast quantities of highly specific antibodies that can directly neutralize pathogens or flag them for destruction by other immune cells.

- **Memory B-cell survival:** A subset of activated B cells develop into memory B cells. These immunological "reservoirs" persist long after the initial infection. Upon encountering the same antigen again, memory B cells can rapidly mount a stronger and more targeted antibody response, providing long-term immunity.

Consequently, due to their central role in both the primary and secondary immune response, B cells have become a major target for therapeutic strategies, including desensitization protocols.

4.2.1 Rituximab

For decades, rituximab has been a cornerstone of desensitization protocols. A 2014 systematic review, although based on limited-quality evidence, suggested that rituximab was comparable to splenectomy in reducing panel-reactive antibodies (PRA) and offered benefits in terms of graft survival and rejection prevention [29].

4.2.2 Obinutuzumab

Obinutuzumab, a third-generation anti-CD20 monoclonal antibody, induces B-cell destruction primarily through antibody-dependent cellular cytotoxicity. A phase 1b study showed that obinutuzumab resulted in more effective depletion of B cells in the peripheral blood and lymph nodes compared to rituximab. Obinutuzumab combined with IVIG also appeared to reduce the population of memory B cells and plasmablasts [30]. NasrAllah et al. demonstrated that obinutuzumab had a B-cell depleting effect and, unlike rituximab, did not lead to a false-positive B-cell CDC crossmatch [31]. While obinutuzumab offers a more durable and complete impact on B cells compared to rituximab, its effect on cPRA and anti-HLA antibodies remains limited, similar to rituximab [17, 30].

4.2.3 Belimumab and atacicept

B-lymphocyte stimulator (BLyS)/BAFF and APRIL are factors that influence B-cell activation, development, and homeostasis. These factors bind with the BAFF receptor (BAFF-R), B-cell maturation antigen (BCMA), and transmembrane activator and CAML interactor (TACI) on B cells. Premature B cells require BLyS binding to TACI for their development. Memory B cells express TACI independent of BLyS or APRIL, and long-lived plasma cells (LLPCs) express BCMA and depend on APRIL for survival [32]. Because memory B cells and LLPCs can hinder the elimination of anti-HLA antibodies by anti-CD20 therapies, targeting BLyS or specific B-cell receptors, particularly APRIL and TACI, might be a promising approach. Belimumab, a monoclonal antibody that blocks BLyS, and Atacicept, a fusion protein that blocks both BAFF and APRIL, are being explored for this purpose. Belimumab is already approved for the treatment of systemic lupus erythematosus (SLE), and Atacicept is a fusion protein that blocks not only BAFF but also APRIL [33].

The research on belimumab for desensitization shows mixed results. In a study by Banham et al. belimumab used as an add-on therapy to standard immunosuppression in low immunological risk kidney transplant recipients resulted in a decline in both naive and memory B cells, plasmablasts, and preformed IgG levels [34]. However, a pilot trial by Agrawal et al. using belimumab to desensitize patients failed to show a reduction in cPRA [35]. The authors suggest that the lack of effect might be due to the presence of APRIL or IL-21, which can work with BAFF to maintain humoral immunity and support the survival of LLPCs. Targeting both APRIL and IL-21 might be necessary for a more significant reduction in alloantibodies. This hypothesis is supported by a rat model experiment where dual knockout of APRIL and BLyS resulted in a significant decrease in DSA generation [36]. Similarly, Atacicept showed a drop in the B-cell population and lower DSA levels in a murine model [37]. These findings suggest promise, but further studies and clinical trials are needed to confirm the efficacy of Belimumab, Atacicept, or a combination approach in desensitization strategies.

4.3 Plasma cell targeting strategies

Long-lived plasma cells (LLPCs) residing in bone marrow niches are a major challenge in desensitization because they can continue antibody production even without antigen exposure. These anti-HLA-specific memory B cells and LLPCs are considered the Achilles' heel of desensitization therapies. Cytokines like IL-6, IL-21, and factors such as BAFF and APRIL play a role in the development, maturation, and bone marrow homing of LLPCs [20].

Anti-plasma cell therapies, including proteasome inhibitors (bortezomib and carfilzomib) and anti-CD38 antibodies (daratumumab, felzartamab, and isatuximab), are being explored to overcome this transplant barrier.

4.3.1 Proteasome inhibitors

4.3.1.1 Bortezomib

Bortezomib is the most studied agent among proteasome inhibitors for desensitization. Its inhibitory effect on proteasomes is reversible, leading to more neurotoxicity compared to carfilzomib, an irreversible proteasome inhibitor [12]. Woodle et al. reported a promising outcome in 2015 using desensitization with rituximab, plasmapheresis, and 6–8 doses of bortezomib. This approach resulted in a durable and consistent reduction in anti-HLA antibodies [38]. Similar to treatment for multiple myeloma, intravenous methylprednisolone is administered before bortezomib to sensitize plasma cells [20]. However, using higher or more frequent doses of bortezomib is associated with increased toxicity without a significant additional decrease in cPRA [39]. The response to bortezomib therapy can also depend on the underlying cause of sensitization. For instance, chronic sensitization due to previous transplantation or pregnancy is more resistant to treatment because of a larger number of bone marrow LLPCs [20].

4.3.1.2 Carfilzomib

Carfilzomib, a new-generation proteasome inhibitor with potentially less neurotoxicity, is being studied for desensitization due to its irreversible potency and potential to reduce antibody relapse. This is because it offers irreversible inhibition of proteasomes compared to bortezomib's reversible effect.

Tremblay et al. conducted the only study on kidney transplant recipients using carfilzomib. While they observed a significant reduction in incompatible antibodies, there was a rapid rebound within 81 to 141 days [40]. Other studies using carfilzomib are ongoing in heart transplant candidates [41, 42]. The limited sample sizes and conflicting results from these studies highlight the need for further investigations on carfilzomib for desensitization.

However, preclinical studies on non-human primates (NHP) using carfilzomib in combination with lulizumab (a costimulatory blocker) showed promising results. This combination led to a decrease in DSA, Tfh cells, and B cells, while preserving regulatory T cells (Tregs) [43]. A clinical trial named Carfilzomib and Belatacept for Desensitization (ADAPT) (NCT05017545) is currently underway to evaluate this approach in highly sensitized prospective kidney transplant recipients.

4.3.2 Anti-CD38 antibodies

Anti-CD38 antibodies represent another strategy for targeting plasma cells. Studies on daratumumab, an anti-CD38 antibody, have shown a significant decrease in bone marrow plasma cells and natural killer (NK) cells. However, this treatment also depletes Tregs and regulatory B cells (Bregs) [10, 44]. The depletion of Tregs and Bregs raises concerns about an increased risk of T-cell-mediated rejection following transplantation [12].

4.3.2.1 Daratumumab

Data on the use of daratumumab in desensitization is scarce, primarily limited to case reports involving highly sensitized heart and lung transplant candidates [45]. A case report described a successful kidney transplant in a third-time recipient with cPRA >99% who received daratumumab, plasmapheresis, and IVIG to achieve a significant reduction in anti-HLA antibodies [46]. The most recent case report details a successful desensitization approach in an ABO-incompatible (ABOi) and HLA-incompatible (HLAi) second transplant candidate. This approach involved imlifidase followed by daratumumab, a single dose of rituximab, IVIG, and a second dose of daratumumab administered after transplantation [47]. Overall, daratumumab appears to be more effective than bortezomib in depleting DSA-producing cells [10]. Two ongoing clinical trials are investigating the role of daratumumab in highly sensitized kidney transplant recipients: Desensitization in Kidney Allograft Using Daratumumab (DARDAR) (ClinicalTrials.gov ID NCT04204980) and the Safety/Efficacy of Daratumumab with Belatacept in Highly HLA-Sensitized Patients Awaiting Kidney Transplantation (COMBAT) (ClinicalTrials.gov ID NCT05145296). The results of these trials will be crucial in determining the efficacy of daratumumab for desensitization.

4.3.2.2 Isatuximab

Isatuximab is another anti-CD38 monoclonal antibody with the potential for a sustained depleting effect on LLPCs. An open-label, single-arm phase 1/2 study investigated isatuximab in two cohorts of highly sensitized kidney transplant candidates with cPRA ≥99.9% and 80- < 99.9%. The drug demonstrated an acceptable safety profile with no reports of treatment-related infections. The study results showed a significant decrease in plasmablasts, plasma cells, NK cells, and memory B cells [48]. While proteasome inhibitors can lead to a compensatory increase in memory B cells after treatment, potentially hindering sustained reductions in antibody levels [30], the effect of isatuximab on memory B cells appears to lead to a more sustained (at least 26 weeks after stopping treatment) decline in the mean fluorescence intensity

(MFI) of anti-HLA antibodies, even if the change in cPRA is minimal. The risk of T-cell-mediated rejection with isatuximab therapy requires further investigation because the drug efficiently depletes $CD38^+$ Tregs and Bregs, potentially increasing this risk [10, 48]. Given that isatuximab monotherapy results in partial desensitization, combining it with other strategies like anti-IL-6 therapy might be a promising approach. Felzartamab, another anti-CD38 antibody, has not yet been studied in desensitization protocols.

4.4 Cytokine targeting strategies

IL-6 and IL-21 are two key cytokines involved in sensitization and memory B-cell development. IL-6 plays a critical role in sensitization and memory B-cell development. In the presence of IL-6, naive $CD4^+$ T cells differentiate into Tfh cells. Tfh cells then release IL-21, which promotes B-cell maturation and the development of memory B cells, plasmablasts, and plasma cells. Additionally, IL-6, in cooperation with TGF-β, promotes Th17 cell formation. On the other hand, IL-6 prevents naive T cells from differentiating into regulatory T cells (Tregs). The combined effects of IL-6 lead to antibody formation, impaired tolerance, and allograft rejection. Because of this central role, IL-6 has become a target of interest in desensitization strategies and rejection treatment [49].

Tocilizumab (anti-IL-6 receptor antibody) and clazakizumab (anti-IL-6 antibody) are being studied in desensitization protocols.

4.4.1 Tocilizumab (TCZ)

A single-center uncontrolled trial by Vo et al. evaluated the efficacy and safety of TCZ in desensitization. The study involved 10 highly sensitized kidney transplant candidates who did not respond to standard treatments. They received 8 mg/kg monthly doses of TCZ. Five patients received a transplant within an average of 8.1 months after starting TCZ treatment. One patient experienced colonic diverticulitis, a possible side effect of TCZ. Encouragingly, no DSA or antibody-mediated rejection (AMR) was reported 6 months post-transplantation in these patients [50].

Following these promising initial results, TCZ was studied as a monotherapy in patients who had not undergone prior desensitization attempts. However, the clinical results were disappointing, with only one patient receiving a kidney transplant. Additionally, TCZ showed only a marginal effect on the mean fluorescence intensity (MFI) of anti-HLA antibodies [51].

Jouve et al. later investigated the immune response to TCZ. They concluded that while TCZ treatment hindered B-cell maturation in germinal centers (GCs), it did not significantly affect Tfh cells or IL-21 levels. Interestingly, the study also observed an increase in soluble IL-6 receptor (s-IL6R) and IL-6 levels [52]. These findings suggest that TCZ monotherapy may not be sufficient for desensitization. Recently, researchers have explored combining TCZ with agents that target other aspects of the immune response. A study on highly sensitized non-human primates (NHPs) showed that dual treatment with carfilzomib (a proteasome inhibitor) and TCZ resulted in a decline in DSA compared to carfilzomib alone. This combination therapy also prevented B-cell expansion. However, it was not effective in preventing antibody rebound after transplantation [53].

4.4.2 Clazakizumab

Tocilizumab (TCZ) blocks the IL-6 receptor, which can lead to a paradoxical increase in IL-6 levels, potentially dampening the intended effects of TCZ. Clazakizumab, an anti-IL-6 antibody, directly targets IL-6 and might offer improved efficacy over TCZ [53].

A single-arm trial investigated the effectiveness of clazakizumab in desensitization. The study included patients with cPRA ≥50% who received the drug alongside five sessions of plasmapheresis and high-dose intravenous immune globulin (IVIG). The clazakizumab treatment involved 25 mg subcutaneous injection every 4 weeks for up to 270 days before transplantation, followed by continuation for at least 6 months post-transplantation. The treatment was well-tolerated, and both classes of anti-HLA antibodies significantly decreased. Additionally, no DSA was detected up to 6 months post-transplantation. Interestingly, the study also observed a significant increase in both Tregs and Bregs after transplantation, which could contribute to improved graft tolerance [54].

These promising initial findings from a single-arm trial warrant further evaluation in larger, randomized controlled trials to confirm the efficacy and safety of clazakizumab for desensitization.

4.5 Novel strategies

The limitations of current desensitization strategies include limited efficacy, lack of complete target specificity, and the involvement of multiple factors in the immune response to HLA antigens. These limitations highlight the need for novel therapeutic approaches, including the development of new therapies and combination regimens.

4.5.1 Complement inhibitors

Complement activation can lead to tissue damage, making complement inhibitors a potential therapeutic target in highly sensitized patients. However, results so far have been mixed. Eculizumab, a terminal complement pathway inhibitor, reduced the incidence of AMR episodes during the first post-transplantation year but failed to prevent chronic AMR in crossmatch-positive kidney transplant recipients. Additionally, the five-year death-censored graft survival rates were not significantly different from historical controls [55]. C1-esterase inhibitor, on the other hand, showed promise in a preventive study. This placebo-controlled trial investigated the use of C1-esterase inhibitor in 20 highly sensitized transplant recipients who had undergone desensitization with plasmapheresis, IVIG, and rituximab due to positive crossmatches. The study reported no AMR episodes, and there was a decrease in C1q + HLA antibodies [56].

4.5.2 Costimulatory blockade

4.5.2.1 Belatacept

Since activation of naive B cells by Tfh cells in germinal centers (GCs) requires a costimulatory signal (signal 2), costimulatory blockers are a potential target in desensitization protocols. Following treatment with plasma cell-depleting agents like proteasome inhibitors or anti-CD38 antibodies, the removal of negative feedback can lead to germinal center activation. Therefore, a dual blockade targeting both plasma cells and the costimulatory signal has gained attention [44]. Studies on non-human primates (NHPs) have explored the effects of combining belatacept (a costimulatory blocker) with carfilzomib or bortezomib (proteasome inhibitors) [10, 57, 58]. Early results from the ATTAIN trial (ITN090st) are promising. This trial investigated the safety and efficacy of daratumumab (anti-CD38 antibody) and belatacept in kidney transplant candidates with cPRA = 100%. The treatment resulted in a significant and sustained decline in anti-HLA antibodies, with no observed rebound [59].

4.5.2.2 Lulizumab and iscalimab

Lulizumab, another costimulatory inhibitor, has been studied in combination with either carfilzomib or tocilizumab (IL-6 receptor antibody) for desensitization [43, 60]. However, the lulizumab plus TCZ study in highly sensitized patients failed to show efficacy, likely due to a low Treg count. This is because anti-CD28 agents like lulizumab can suppress Tregs, which play a crucial role in inducing tolerance to the graft [60].

Iscalimab, an anti-CD40 monoclonal antibody, offers a different approach. CD40-CD154 interaction is a key part of the costimulatory pathway, and its inhibition in GCs can prevent memory B-cell differentiation. Additionally, CD40 signaling also induces cytokine secretion that contributes to dendritic cell maturation. A significant advantage of iscalimab is the non-B lymphocytes depleting effect. It does not activate platelets, thereby reducing the risk of thromboembolic events [61]. A combination therapy involving iscalimab, belatacept, and bortezomib in NHP desensitization demonstrated improved graft survival, a lower risk of rejection-related graft loss, but also a higher incidence of cytomegalovirus (CMV) infection [62].

Further human clinical trials are needed to evaluate the efficacy and safety of costimulatory inhibitors for desensitization in kidney transplantation.

4.5.3 CAR T-cell therapy

Chimeric antigen receptor (CAR) T-cell therapy represents a cutting-edge technology in immunomodulation. CAR T cells are engineered T cells equipped with synthetic receptors that allow them to recognize and attack specific target cells. These engineered T cells possess unique immunological properties, enabling them to react against target cells, proliferate, and potentially provide long-term protection. Compared to monoclonal antibodies, CAR T cells offer a potential advantage of a longer half-life, potentially leading to a more durable and sustained effect. CAR T-cell therapy has been successfully implemented for the treatment of certain malignancies [63].

Preclinical studies have explored the use of CAR T cells targeting CD19 and BCMA in patients with multiple myeloma. However, the results were not conclusive. CAR T-cell therapy targeting CD19 did not significantly reduce anti-HLA antibodies in sensitized patients. The study on BCMA-targeted CAR T cells involved non-sensitized patients, so the effects on anti-HLA antibodies could not be evaluated [60].

A recent study by Jarmi et al. investigated the potential of MC10029 CAR T cells, which recognize the B-cell activating factor receptor (BAFF-R), to target B cells in highly sensitized kidney transplant candidates. The study's preliminary results demonstrated the cytotoxicity of these CAR T cells against autologous B cells. The investigators have received FDA approval for MC10029 CAR T-cell therapy and are planning to launch a clinical trial to assess its efficacy and safety in transplant patients [64]. While these initial findings are promising, CAR T-cell therapy for desensitization in transplantation is still in its early stages of development.

5. Cons, complications, and costs

Despite the advancements in desensitization strategies and medications, there are still limitations and challenges associated with this approach.

5.1 Lack of efficacy and antibody rebound

One of the major drawbacks of desensitization is its limited efficacy and, more importantly, the potential for antibody rebound after transplantation. This rebound can lead to acute and chronic rejection episodes, ultimately decreasing graft survival. However, the use of newer agents with potentially more durable effects, such as isatuximab and CAR T-cell therapy, might offer solutions to overcome this issue.

Meticulous monitoring of DSA levels and regular protocol biopsies are crucial tools for identifying rejection episodes early during the post-transplant period. Early detection and effective treatment interventions can improve response rates and graft survival [18].

5.2 Complications

Desensitization protocols can also lead to several concerning complications, including post-transplant infections, malignancies, and drug-specific adverse effects.

5.2.1 Infections

The reported incidence, causative agents, and severity of infections following desensitization vary significantly. These variations are often linked to differences in the intensity of desensitization protocols and the specific immunosuppressive agents used. Generally, more intense desensitization regimens are associated with a higher risk of infections. This includes an increased incidence of urinary tract infections, other bacterial infections like pneumonia and surgical site infections, and even opportunistic infections. Patients who receive more than ten sessions of plasmapheresis, with or without additional agents, appear to be at a higher risk of developing infections. Importantly, recurrent infections, particularly during the first post-transplantation year, are associated with a significant increase in death-censored graft loss [65].

To mitigate the risk of infections, several key strategies are crucial:

- Thorough screening for latent infections before desensitization.
- Complete vaccination of the recipient prior to desensitization.
- Implementation of appropriate prophylactic measures.
- Careful monitoring for infections following treatment [66].

5.2.2 Cancer

The use of intensive immunosuppressive therapy before and after transplantation with HLA-incompatible (HLAi) kidneys is a theoretical concern, as it could increase the risk of malignancies by impairing the body's immunosurveillance mechanisms. However, existing research provides mixed results. A study on ABO-incompatible (ABOi) transplant recipients did not observe an increased incidence of cancer [67].

A more recent study by Motter et al. compared the risk of cancer in HLAi-desensitized patients to HLA-compatible living donor kidney recipients. The study followed patients for a median of 6.7 years and found no significant differences in the overall risk, type, or stage of cancers. However, the study did report a higher incidence of colorectal cancer in the HLAi recipient group. This finding suggests that more intensive screening for colorectal cancer might be warranted for HLAi transplant recipients while acknowledging the importance of routine cancer screening for all transplant patients [68]. It is important to note that this data was collected before the widespread use of some newer desensitization agents. Therefore, further research is needed to assess the long-term cancer risk associated with these newer therapies.

5.2.3 Drug-related adverse events

Beyond infusion-related side effects, desensitization protocols can lead to drug-specific adverse events that are often dose-dependent. Examples of reported complications include:

- Lung disease after repeated rituximab doses
- Gastrointestinal symptoms and peripheral neuropathy associated with bortezomib use
- Diverticulitis and spondylolisthesis linked to TCZ treatment
- Bleeding complications can occur soon after plasmapheresis [66]

5.2.4 Cost

The cost-effectiveness of desensitization strategies remains a subject of debate. A key factor influencing success is the likelihood of achieving durable desensitization and ultimately, transplantation. As discussed earlier, the rate of successful desensitization depends on various patient-specific characteristics, the type of antibodies present, the desensitizing agents used, and the overall treatment strategy employed.

Studies investigating the survival benefit of incompatible kidney transplantation have yielded conflicting results. A study in the United States reported a significant survival advantage for recipients of HLA-incompatible transplants compared to those who remained on the waiting list. However, a study in the United Kingdom did not observe a similar survival benefit. These discrepancies likely stem from differences in study design [69].

The financial burden of desensitization treatment is another critical consideration when deciding between desensitization and remaining on dialysis. A recent study in Japan evaluated the two-year medical costs associated with maintenance hemodialysis and transplantation in highly sensitized patients. The desensitization protocol included plasmapheresis, intravenous immune globulin (IVIG), and rituximab. The findings demonstrated favorable outcomes in terms of both patient and graft survival. However, due to the higher risk of antibody-mediated rejection (AMR) and the associated costs of DSA monitoring and AMR treatment, the initial post-transplantation year resulted in higher transplantation costs than hemodialysis. Interestingly, the study showed that by year three, the cost of maintenance hemodialysis became equivalent to the cost of HLA-incompatible transplantation, suggesting that the financial burden of desensitization might be acceptable in the long term [70].

6. Conclusion

The increasing number of highly sensitized patients and retransplant candidates, coupled with the limited pool of HLA-compatible donors, creates a significant challenge in kidney transplantation. Several options exist to expand access to transplantation, including kidney-paired exchange programs, transplants from HLA-matched siblings, acceptable mismatch program, revisions in allocation systems, and virtual crossmatch techniques.

The decision to pursue desensitization requires careful consideration of several factors, including cost-effectiveness, the limited donor pool, potential long-term outcomes, and the safety of the desensitization protocol itself. The expertise of the transplant center, patient preferences, the capacity to monitor and manage potential complications, and the availability of safe and effective desensitization protocols all play a crucial role in this decision-making process.

While virtual crossmatch techniques, improved allocation systems, and acceptable mismatch programs represent the most cost-effective approaches to transplantation, considering the recent advancements in therapeutic options, desensitization offers a viable option for patients with little to no chance of receiving an HLA-compatible donor kidney.

Acknowledgements

The authors would like to thank Dr. Marieh Farokhi Moghaddam for her assistance.

Conflict of interest

The authors declare no conflict of interest.

Author details

Mohsen Nafar[1] and Shiva Samavat[2*]

1 Chronic Kidney Disease Research Center (CKDRC), Shahid Labbafinejad Medical Center, Shahid Beheshti University of Medical Sciences (SBMU), Tehran, Iran

2 Urology and Nephrology Research Center (UNRC), Shahid Labbafinejad Medical Center, Shahid Beheshti University of Medical Sciences (SBMU), Tehran, Iran

*Address all correspondence to: shsamavat@gmail.com; samavat@sbmu.ac.ir

References

[1] Lentine KL, Smith JM, Lyden GR, Miller JM, Dolan TG, Bradbrook K, et al. OPTN/SRTR 2022 annual data report: Kidney. American Journal of Transplantation. 2024;**24**(2S1):S19-S118. DOI: 10.1016/j.ajt.2024.01.012

[2] Heidt S, Haasnoot GW, van der Linden-van Oevelen MJH, Claas FHJ. Highly sensitized patients are well served by receiving a compatible organ offer based on acceptable mismatches. Frontiers in Immunology. 2021;**12**:687254. DOI: 10.3389/fimmu.2021.687254

[3] Bestard O, Thaunat O, Bellini MI, Böhmig GA, Budde K, Claas F, et al. Alloimmune risk stratification for kidney transplant rejection. Transplant International. 2022;**35**:10138. DOI: 10.3389/ti.2022.10138

[4] Thongprayoon C, Miao J, Jadlowiec CC, Mao SA, Mao MA, Vaitla P, et al. Differences between very highly sensitized kidney transplant recipients as identified by machine learning consensus clustering. Medicina (Kaunas, Lithuania). 2023;**59**(5):977. DOI: 10.3390/medicina59050977

[5] Roll GR, Bray RA, Cooper M, Eagar TN, Gebel HM, Vranic GM, et al. COVID-19 infection and vaccination rarely impact HLA antibody profile in waitlisted renal transplant candidates- a multicenter cohort. Human Immunology. 2023;**84**(4):278-285. DOI: 10.1016/j.humimm.2023.02.005

[6] Martínez Díaz M, Torío Ruíz A, Lorenzo González I, Martínez RR, Llamas Fuentes F, Gonzalvo Díaz C, et al. Anti-HLA antibodies after precocious Transplantectomy by vascular thrombosis. Transplantation Proceedings. 2018;**50**(2):546-549. DOI: 10.1016/j.transproceed.2018.01.002

[7] Triulzi DJ, Kleinman S, Kakaiya RM, Busch MP, Norris PJ, Steele WR, et al. The effect of previous pregnancy and transfusion on HLA alloimmunization in blood donors: Implications for a transfusion-related acute lung injury risk reduction strategy. Transfusion. 2009;**49**(9):1825-1835. DOI: 10.1111/j.1537-2995.2009.02206.x

[8] Pandey P, Pande A, Mandal S, Devra AK, Sinha VK, Bhatt AP, et al. Effects of different sensitization events on HLA alloimmunization in renal transplant cases; a retrospective observation in 1066 cases. Transplant Immunology. 2022;**75**:101680. DOI: 10.1016/j.trim.2022.101680

[9] Hickey MJ, Valenzuela NM, Reed EF. Alloantibody generation and effector function following sensitization to human leukocyte antigen. Frontiers in Immunology. 2016;**7**:30. DOI: 10.3389/fimmu.2016.00030

[10] Jordan SC, Ammerman N, Choi J, Huang E, Peng A, Sethi S, et al. The role of novel therapeutic approaches for prevention of allosensitization and antibody-mediated rejection. American Journal of Transplantation. 2020;**20**(Suppl. 4):42-56. DOI: 10.1111/ajt.15913

[11] Scornik JC, Meier-Kriesche HU. Blood transfusions in organ transplant patients: Mechanisms of sensitization and implications for prevention. American Journal of Transplantation. 2011;**11**(9):1785-1791. DOI: 10.1111/j.1600-6143.2011.03705.x

[12] Schinstock C, Tambur A, Stegall M. Current approaches to desensitization

in solid organ transplantation. Frontiers in Immunology. 2021;**12**:686271. DOI: 10.3389/fimmu.2021.686271

[13] Mamode N, Bestard O, Claas F, Furian L, Griffin S, Legendre C, et al. European guideline for the management of kidney transplant patients with HLA antibodies: By the European society for organ transplantation working group. Transplant International. 2022;**35**:10511. DOI: 10.3389/ti.2022.10511

[14] Konvalinka A, Tinckam K. Utility of HLA antibody testing in kidney transplantation. Journal of the American Society of Nephrology. 2015;**26**(7):1489-1502. DOI: 10.1681/ASN.2014080837

[15] Pinelli DF, Zachary AA, Friedewald JJ, Gjertson DW, Evans MA, Chatroop EN, et al. Prognostic tools to assess candidacy for and efficacy of antibody-removal therapy. American Journal of Transplantation. 2019;**19**(2):381-390. DOI: 10.1111/ajt.15007

[16] Tambur AR, Bestard O, Campbell P, Chong AS, Barrio MC, Ford ML, et al. Sensitization in transplantation: Assessment of risk 2022 working group meeting report. American Journal of Transplantation. 2023;**23**(1):133-149. DOI: 10.1016/j.ajt.2022.11.009

[17] Sethi S, Choi J, Toyoda M, Vo A, Peng A, Jordan SC. Desensitization: Overcoming the immunologic barriers to transplantation. Journal of Immunology Research. 2017;**2017**:6804678. DOI: 10.1155/2017/6804678

[18] Vo AA, Aubert O, Haas M, Huang E, Zhang X, Choi J, et al. Clinical relevance of posttransplant DSAs in patients receiving desensitization for HLA-incompatible kidney transplantation. Transplantation. 2019;**103**(12):2666-2674. DOI: 10.1097/TP.0000000000002691

[19] Khuu T, Cadeiras M, Wisniewski N, Reed EF, Deng MC. Reduced HLA class II antibody response to proteasome inhibition in heart transplantation. The Journal of Heart and Lung Transplantation. 2015;**34**(6):863-865. DOI: 10.1016/j.healun.2015.01.982

[20] May FNJ, Rees MT, Griffin S, Fildes JE. Understanding immunological response to desensitisation strategies in highly sensitised potential kidney transplant patients. Transplantation Reviews (Orlando, Fla.). 2021;**35**(2):100596. DOI: 10.1016/j.trre.2021.100596

[21] Jambon F, Merville P, Guidicelli G, Taton B, De Précigout V, Couzi L, et al. Efficacy of plasmapheresis and semi-selective immunoadsorption for removal of anti-HLA antibodies. Journal of Clinical Apheresis. 2021;**36**(3):291-298. DOI: 10.1002/jca.21858

[22] Chen X, Wang Y, Dong P, Wang J, Yu X, Yu B. Efficacy of combined desensitization therapy based on protein a immunoadsorption on anti-human leukocyte antigen antibodies in sensitized kidney transplant recipients: A retrospective study. Cureus. 2022;**14**(9):e28661. DOI: 10.7759/cureus.28661

[23] Melexopoulou C, Filiopoulos V, Marinaki S. Therapeutic apheresis in renal transplantation: An update. Transfusion and Apheresis Science. 2024;**63**(1):103844. DOI: 10.1016/j.transci.2023.103844

[24] Malvezzi P, Jouve T, Noble J, Rostaing L. Desensitization in the setting of HLA-incompatible kidney transplant. Experimental and Clinical Transplantation. 2018;**16**(4):367-375. DOI: 10.6002/ect.2017.0355

[25] Jacob S, Mazibrada G, Irani SR, Jacob A, Yudina A. The role of

plasma exchange in the treatment of refractory autoimmune neurological diseases: A narrative review. Journal of Neuroimmune Pharmacology. 2021;**16**(4):806-817. DOI: 10.1007/s11481-021-10004-9

[26] de Weerd AE, Roelen DL, van de Wetering J, Betjes MGH, Heidt S, Reinders MEJ. Imlifidase desensitization in HLA-incompatible kidney transplantation: Finding the sweet spot. Transplantation. 2024;**108**(2):335-345. DOI: 10.1097/TP.0000000000004689

[27] Kanbay M, Copur S, Guldan M, Topcu AU, Ozbek L, Hasbal B, et al. Imlifidase in kidney transplantation. Clinical Kidney Journal. 2024;**17**(3):sfae033. DOI: 10.1093/ckj/sfae033

[28] Kjellman C, Maldonado AQ, Sjöholm K, Lonze BE, Montgomery RA, Runström A, et al. Outcomes at 3 years posttransplant in imlifidase-desensitized kidney transplant patients. American Journal of Transplantation. 2021;**21**(12):3907 3918. DOI: 10.1111/ajt.16754

[29] Macklin PS, Morris PJ, Knight SR. A systematic review of the use of rituximab for desensitization in renal transplantation. Transplantation. 2014;**98**(8):794-805. DOI: 10.1097/TP.0000000000000362

[30] Redfield RR, Jordan SC, Busque S, Vincenti F, Woodle ES, Desai N, et al. Safety, pharmacokinetics, and pharmacodynamic activity of obinutuzumab, a type 2 anti-CD20 monoclonal antibody for the desensitization of candidates for renal transplant. American Journal of Transplantation. 2019;**19**(11):3035-3045. DOI: 10.1111/ajt.15514

[31] Nasr Allah MM, Elalfy M, El Ansary M, Elmeseery Y, Amer I, Malvezzi P, et al. Obinutuzumab in kidney transplantation: Effect on B-cell counts and crossmatch tests. Transplantation. 2022;**106**(2):369-372. DOI: 10.1097/TP.0000000000003686

[32] Treml JF, Hao Y, Stadanlick JE, Cancro MP. The BLyS family: Toward a molecular understanding of B cell homeostasis. Cell Biochemistry and Biophysics. 2009;**53**(1):1-16. DOI: 10.1007/s12013-008-9036-1

[33] Cogollo E, Silva MA, Isenberg D. Profile of atacicept and its potential in the treatment of systemic lupus erythematosus. Drug Design, Development and Therapy. 2015;**9**:1331-1339. DOI: 10.2147/DDDT.S71276

[34] Banham GD, Flint SM, Torpey N, Lyons PA, Shanahan DN, Gibson A, et al. Belimumab in kidney transplantation: An experimental medicine, randomised, placebo-controlled phase 2 trial. Lancet. 2018;**391**(10140):2619-2630. DOI: 10.1016/S0140-6736(18)30984-X

[35] Agarwal D, Luning Prak ET, Bharani T, Everly M, Migone TS, Cancro M, et al. BLyS neutralization results in selective anti-HLA alloantibody depletion without successful desensitization. Transplant Immunology. 2021;**69**:101465. DOI: 10.1016/j.trim.2021.101465

[36] Bath NM, Verhoven BM, Wilson NA, Zeng W, Zhong W, Coons L, et al. APRIL/BLyS deficient rats prevent donor specific antibody (DSA) production and cell proliferation in rodent kidney transplant model. PLoS One. 2022;**17**(10):e0275564. DOI: 10.1371/journal.pone.0275564

[37] Wilson NA, Bath NM, Verhoven BM, Ding X, Boldt BA, Sukhwal A, et al. APRIL/BLyS blockade reduces donor-specific antibodies in allosensitized mice.

Transplantation. 2019;**103**(7):1372-1384. DOI: 10.1097/TP.0000000000002686

[38] Woodle ES, Shields AR, Ejaz NS, Sadaka B, Girnita A, Walsh RC, et al. Prospective iterative trial of proteasome inhibitor-based desensitization. American Journal of Transplantation. 2015;**15**(1):101-118. DOI: 10.1111/ajt.13050

[39] Moreno Gonzales MA, Gandhi MJ, Schinstock CA, Moore NA, Smith BH, Braaten NY, et al. 32 doses of bortezomib for desensitization is not well tolerated and is associated with only modest reductions in anti-HLA antibody. Transplantation. 2017;**101**(6):1222-1227. DOI: 10.1097/TP.0000000000001330

[40] Tremblay S, Driscoll JJ, Rike-Shields A, Hildeman DA, Alloway RR, Girnita AL, et al. A prospective, iterative, adaptive trial of carfilzomib-based desensitization. American Journal of Transplantation. 2020;**20**(2):411-421. DOI: 10.1111/ajt.15613

[41] Sriwattanakomen R, Xu Q, Demehin M, Shullo MA, Mangiola M, Hickey GW, et al. Impact of carfilzomib-based desensitization on heart transplantation of sensitized candidates. The Journal of Heart and Lung Transplantation. 2021;**40**(7):595-603. DOI: 10.1016/j.healun.2021.03.001

[42] Sobhanian M, Saltarrelli J, Weeks P, Nathan S, Radovacevic R, Kar B, et al. Comparative efficacy of bortezomib and carfilzomib desensitization protocols in highly sensitized cardiac transplant candidates. The Journal of Heart and Lung Transplantation. 2019;**38**(4):S35-S36

[43] Schroder PM, Schmitz R, Fitch ZW, Ezekian B, Yoon J, Choi AY, et al. Preoperative carfilzomib and lulizumab based desensitization prolongs graft survival in a sensitized non-human primate model. Kidney International. 2021;**99**(1):161-172. DOI: 10.1016/j.kint.2020.08.020

[44] Joher N, Matignon M, Grimbert P. HLA desensitization in solid organ transplantation: Anti-CD38 to across the immunological barriers. Frontiers in Immunology. 2021;**12**:688301. DOI: 10.3389/fimmu.2021.688301

[45] Lemal R, Blandin L, Uro-Coste C, Philipponnet C, Geoffroy E, Heng AE, et al. Daratumumab treatment in six highly sensitised solid organ transplant recipients: A case series and literature review. HLA. 2024;**103**(4):e15458. DOI: 10.1111/tan.15458

[46] Zhao D, Guo Z, Zhao G, Sa R, Zhu L, Chen G. A novel daratumumab-based regimen for desensitization in highly HLA-presensitized patients awaiting kidney transplantation. Transplant International. 2023;**36**:11771. DOI: 10.3389/ti.2023.11771

[47] Schrezenmeier E, Choi M, Globke B, Dorner T, Leimbach A, Osmanodja B, et al. Successful desensitization with imlifidase and daratumumab in a highly immunized, crossmatch positive, blood group-incompatible living-donor re-transplant recipient with systemic lupus erythematosus and antiphospholipid syndrome. Transfusion Medicine and Hemotherapy. 2024;**51**:1-6. DOI: 10.1159/000538513

[48] Vincenti F, Bestard O, Brar A, Cruzado JM, Seron D, Gaber AO, et al. Isatuximab monotherapy for desensitization in highly sensitized patients awaiting kidney transplant. Journal of the American Society of Nephrology. 2024;**35**(3):347-360. DOI: 10.1681/ASN.0000000000000287

[49] Weinhard J, Noble J, Jouve T, Malvezzi P, Rostaing L. Tocilizumab and desensitization in kidney transplant candidates: Personal experience and literature review. Journal of Clinical Medicine. 2021;**10**(19):4359. DOI: 10.3390/jcm10194359

[50] Vo AA, Choi J, Kim I, Louie S, Cisneros K, Kahwaji J, et al. A phase I/II trial of the interleukin-6 receptor-specific humanized monoclonal (tocilizumab) + intravenous immunoglobulin in difficult to desensitize patients. Transplantation. 2015;**99**(11):2356-2363. DOI: 10.1097/TP.0000000000000741

[51] Daligault M, Bardy B, Noble J, Bourdin A, Masson D, Naciri Bennani H, et al. Marginal impact of tocilizumab monotherapy on anti-HLA alloantibodies in highly sensitized kidney transplant candidates. Transplantation direct. 2021;**7**(5):e690. DOI: 10.1097/TXD.0000000000001139

[52] Jouve T, Laheurte C, Noble J, Weinhard J, Daligault M, Renaudin A, et al. Immune responses following tocilizumab therapy to desensitize HLA-sensitized kidney transplant candidates. American Journal of Transplantation. 2022;**22**(1):71-84. DOI: 10.1111/ajt.16709

[53] Anwar IJ, Ezekian B, DeLaura I, Manook M, Schroder P, Yoon J, et al. Addition of interleukin-6 receptor blockade to carfilzomib-based desensitization in a highly sensitized nonhuman primate model. American Journal of Transplantation. 2022;**22**(Suppl. 4):1-11. DOI: 10.1111/ajt.17208

[54] Vo AA, Huang E, Ammerman N, Toyoda M, Ge S, Haas M, et al. Clazakizumab for desensitization in highly sensitized patients awaiting transplantation. American Journal of Transplantation. 2022;**22**(4):1133-1144. DOI: 10.1111/ajt.16926

[55] Schinstock CA, Bentall AJ, Smith BH, Cornell LD, Everly M, Gandhi MJ, et al. Long-term outcomes of eculizumab-treated positive crossmatch recipients: Allograft survival, histologic findings, and natural history of the donor-specific antibodies. American Journal of Transplantation. 2019;**19**(6):1671-1683. DOI: 10.1111/ajt.15175

[56] Vo AA, Zeevi A, Choi J, Cisneros K, Toyoda M, Kahwaji J, et al. A phase I/II placebo-controlled trial of C1-inhibitor for prevention of antibody-mediated rejection in HLA sensitized patients. Transplantation. 2015;**99**(2):299-308. DOI: 10.1097/TP.0000000000000592

[57] Manook M, Olaso D, Anwar IJ, Yoon J, Delaura I, Bae Y, et al. Desensitization and belatacept-based maintenance therapy in pregnancy-sensitized monkeys receiving a kidney transplant. Science Advances. 2023;**9**(20):eadg1448. DOI: 10.1126/sciadv.adg1448

[58] Kitchens WH, Larsen CP, Badell IR. Costimulatory blockade and solid organ transplantation: The past, present, and future. Kidney International Reports. 2023;**8**(12):2529-2545. DOI: 10.1016/j.ekir.2023.08.037

[59] Vincenti F, Chandran S, Raja R, Mason K, Mall S, Maruthamuthu S, et al. Impact of daratumumab and belatacept on Hla antibodies in kidney transplant candidates with 100% cPRA: Early results of ATTAIN (ITN090ST). Nephrology, Dialysis, Transplantation. 2023;**38**(Suppl. 1):gfad063a_6402. DOI: 10.1093/ndt/gfad063a_6402

[60] Vo A, Ammerman N, Jordan SC. Advances in desensitization for human leukocyte antigen incompatible

kidney transplantation. Current Opinion in Organ Transplantation. 2024;**29**(2):104-120. DOI: 10.1097/MOT.0000000000001131

[61] van Vugt LK, Schagen MR, de Weerd A, Reinders ME, de Winter BC, Hesselink DA. Investigational drugs for the treatment of kidney transplant rejection. Expert Opinion on Investigational Drugs. 2022;**31**(10):1087-1100. DOI: 10.1080/13543784.2022.2130751

[62] Olaso D, Manook M, Moris D, Knechtle S, Kwun J. Optimal immunosuppression strategy in the sensitized kidney transplant recipient. Journal of Clinical Medicine. 2021;**10**(16):3656. DOI: 10.3390/jcm10163656

[63] Alnefaie A, Albogami S, Asiri Y, Ahmad T, Alotaibi SS, Al-Sanea MM, et al. Chimeric antigen receptor T-cells: An overview of concepts, applications, limitations, and proposed solutions. Frontiers in Bioengineering and Biotechnology. 2022;**10**:797440. DOI: 10.3389/fbioe.2022.797440

[64] Jarmi T, Luo Y, Attieh RM, Qie Y, Gadd ME, Hundal T, et al. CAR T-cell therapy-paving the way for sensitized kidney transplant patients. Kidney International. 2024;**105**(5):1124-1129. DOI: 10.1016/j.kint.2024.02.008

[65] Avery RK, Motter JD, Jackson KR, Montgomery RA, Massie AB, Kraus ES, et al. Quantifying infection risks in incompatible living donor kidney transplant recipients. American Journal of Transplantation. 2021;**21**(4):1564-1575. DOI: 10.1111/ajt.16316

[66] Han DJ. Complication from Desensitization. In: Han D, editors. Kidney Transplantation in Sensitized Patients. Singapore: Springer; 2020. DOI: 10.1007/978-981-10-7046-4_6

[67] Hall EC, Engels EA, Montgomery RA, Segev DL. Cancer risk after ABO-incompatible living-donor kidney transplantation. Transplantation. 2013;**96**(5):476-479. DOI: 10.1097/TP.0b013e318299dc0e

[68] Motter JD, Massie AB, Garonzik-Wang JM, Pfeiffer RM, Yu KJ, Segev DL, et al. Cancer risk following HLA-incompatible living donor kidney transplantation. Transplantation direct. 2023;**9**(8):e1505. DOI: 10.1097/TXD.0000000000001505

[69] Clayton PA, Coates PT. Are sensitized patients better off with a desensitization transplant or waiting on dialysis? Kidney International. 2017;**91**(6):1266-1268. DOI: 10.1016/j.kint.2017.04.004

[70] Maenosono R, Unagami K, Oki R, Fujiwara Y, Banno T, Okada D, et al. The medical cost and outcome of desensitization protocol in kidney transplantation recipients with high immunological risks. International Journal of Urology. 2024;**31**(4):422-429. DOI: 10.1111/iju.15383

Chapter 3

A Comprehensive Guide to Optimize Thoracic Organ Recovery

Chinedu Okoli, Obieze Nwanna-Nzewunwa and Suresh Keshavamurthy

Abstract

This section delves into the concept of Donation After Circulatory Determination of Death (DCDD) as a way to tackle the severe shortage of organs for transplantation. It explains the key differences between DCDD and traditional Donation after Brain-Death (DBD) and how they help address the organ shortage. The section also outlines the criteria for selecting suitable DCDD donors and discusses the two main types of DCDD, along with the ethical considerations and protocols for each type. The focus then shifts to thoracic organs, specifically lungs and increasingly hearts due to advancements in the field. It highlights the challenges of warm ischemia time in traditional DCD and delves into recent breakthroughs in organ preservation techniques. These include *Ex-situ* perfusion with EVLP (static), EVLP (mobile) such as TransMedics OCS, and NRP, as well as advancements in transportation using devices like Paragonix Lung guard. These advancements pave the way for the potential expansion of DCD transplantation.

Keywords: donation after circulatory death (DCD), organ transplant, organ preservation, organ perfusion, innovation transplant

1. Introduction

Organ transplantation is a lifesaving intervention and has become a successful worldwide practice with improved outcomes due to increasingly refined surgical techniques, the evolution of immunosuppressive therapy, and other medical advances. As transplantation outcomes improve, the number of transplant candidates listed for transplantation has increased dramatically. According to the United Network for Organ Sharing (UNOS), in 2023, more than 100,000 patients were added to the transplantation waitlist, while more than 46,000 organs were transplanted, and more than 6000 patients died while waiting for a suitable organ [1]. With this high mortality rate on the waiting list, searching for new sources of transplantable organs is a necessity. Thus, centers are accepting more expanded criteria donors to enhance organ transplantation of patients who need transplants.

Various approaches have been implemented to expand the organ donor pool as organ scarcity remains a challenge. One means of extending the donor pool is to use donations after circulatory death (DCD) organs for transplant. Presently, deceased donors comprise seventy percent of organ donors, and 35 percent of the deceased donors are DCDs; thus, DCD is a potential source of transplantable organs that has yet to be fully utilized [1].

2. Deceased donors

2.1 Donation after brain death (DBD)

Traditionally, death is characterized by the permanent cessation of the three vital functions: circulation, respiration, and brain function [2]. This definition of death changed after the development of cardiopulmonary resuscitation (CPR) and positive pressure ventilation (PPV), which could allow the maintenance of respiratory and circulatory functions in the presence of the irreversible cessation of brain function [3]. This led to the development of criteria for brain death because of the loss of the interdependence of the three vital functions. In the context of donation after brain death, brain death is declared once a physician has established the irreversible cessation of brain function, including the brainstem, in the absence of any factor that could affect the assessment, such as abnormal temperature or blood pressure, the influence of toxins or medications or electrolyte or acid-base imbalances [4]. Ancillary testings are performed if confounding factors cannot be eliminated or the examination cannot be safely or entirely performed. These tests include Transcranial Doppler (TCD), digital subtraction cerebral angiography and single photon emission computed tomography (SPECT), and electrophysiological tests such as electroencephalography (EEG) and evoked potentials (EPs) [5]. Ancillary testing can also be done to supplement the clinical examination in young children. Cerebral angiography best approximates a "gold standard" test but has some limitations. In addition to being invasive and risky, it may be inaccurate in cases of profound hypotension and breached cranial vault, as seen in trauma, open cranial sutures, post-surgery, and ventricular drain placement. Under these conditions, an electrophysiologic test may be superior to cerebral angiography [6]. The use of therapeutic hypothermia or extracorporeal membrane oxygenation complicates but does not preclude the determination of brain death. See **Table 1** for prerequisites and criteria for diagnosis of brain death.

2.2 Donation after circulatory determination of death (DCD)

DCD was formally known as non-heart-beating-donation and later donation after cardiac death. The current term, donation after circulatory death, refers to donation after 'permanent cessation of circulatory and respiratory function [7]. DCD donors were the source of organ transplantation in the early years before brain-death criteria were defined in the 1960s. The first human clinical lung and heart transplantations, in 1963 by James Hardy and in 1967 by Christian Barnard, respectively, used DCD donors [8, 9]. However, the definition of brain death criteria, together with the better outcomes from using organs retrieved from cadavers with a heartbeat, resulted in the initial cessation of most of the early DCD programs. With the increasing organ shortages, there has been a rekindled interest in DCD donors to help reduce the difference between the supply of organs and the demand for organs for transplantation. This is illustrated by the over 9000 DCD donors reported globally [10]. The persisting shortfall in the availability of organ transplants and the repeated demonstration of comparable outcomes from DCD donors have fueled the growing interest in DCD transplants [11, 12]. Not only are the numbers of DCD donations increasing [10], but

Prerequisites
1. Clinical or neuroimaging evidence of an acute central nervous system (CNS) condition(e.g., traumatic brain injury, subarachnoid hemorrhage)
2. Exclusion of medical conditions that may confound clinical assessment (severe electrolytes, acid–base, endocrine, etc.).
3. No drug intoxication or poisoning that can confound the clinical assessment.
4. Core temperature > 36°C
5. Systolic blood pressure >100 mmHg
Examination findings
1. Coma
2. Absence of brain-originating motor response, including response to pain stimulus above the neck or other brain-originating movements (e.g., seizures, decerebrate or decorticate posturing)
3. Absence of brain stem reflexes, including pupillary, corneal, oculocephalic, and oculovestibular, gag reflexes.
4. Apnea as demonstrated by apnea test
Adapted from: Ref. [6].

Table 1.
Clinical diagnosis of brain death: Prerequisites and criteria.

the transplantable organs from DCD donors have also extended beyond kidneys and livers to the pancreas [13], lungs [14], and, most recently, hearts [11]. In addition, DCD makes it possible for patients who did not meet the criteria for neurological death to meet their wish to donate their organs after death [15].

Potential DCD donors are patients who would die within 60 minutes after removal of life support in the presence of irreversible cerebral injuries, high spinal cord injuries, or end-stage musculoskeletal disorders [16]. The United Network for Organ Sharing (UNOS) oversees organ transplantation and donation in the United States. As a federal entity, UNOS ensures best practices for organ transplant programs and organ procurement organizations (OPOs). **Table 2** shows the potential DCD donor characteristics and contraindications. The latter includes some infective and malignant conditions.

An international workshop on non-heart-beating donors (NHBD) in Maastricht (Netherlands) in 1995 defined the original four-category classification of DCD (**Table 3**) [19]. This was subsequently revised to include the location of cardiac arrest and a fifth category (**Table 3**) [18]. The change was made because the location of cardiac arrest is linked to different additional health conditions and varying durations of warm ischemia time in potential donors.

2.2.1 Controlled DCD (cDCD)

cDCD refers to organ donation from persons following the decision to withdraw life-sustaining treatments (WLST), which are no longer considered to be in the best interests of the patients (Maastricht III, IV& V) [18]. These donors include patients with non-recoverable neurologic damage who are dependent on advanced life support therapies but do not fulfill all brain-death criteria [20] **Figures 1** and **2** show the clinical pathway of controlled DCD. The decision to withdraw life-supporting treatment may be based on a patient's advance directive or the decision of a surrogate decision-maker.

Following withdrawal of life-sustaining treatment (WLST), transplant teams wait for the donor to progress to circulatory arrest. This must occur within a specific time,

Potential DCD donor characteristics [17]
Any mechanically ventilated patient with any of the following: 1. Glasgow Coma Scale s,m,core <5 without sedation due to catastrophic brain injury or other illness such as end-stage musculoskeletal disease, pulmonary disease, or spinal cord injury 2. Patients in consideration for Brain death examinations, Withdrawal of life support, Do-not-resuscitate, or comfort care order. 3. The family brings up the topic of organ donation. 4. Brain death criteria are not met (except in rare circumstances), although a potential DCD donor may progress to become a DBD donor. 5. No expectation of meaningful survival, as determined by the patient's treating physician 6. Medically suitable for donation
The contraindications of deceased organ donation include
1. Age >90 years 2. Not on a ventilator 3. history of active metastatic cancer 4. active hematologic malignancy 5. active melanoma 6. Creutzfeldt-Jakob disease

Adapted from Ref. [16].

Table 2.
DCD donor characteristics and contraindications.

Categories	The original Maastricht Classification	Modified Maastricht
I	Dead on arrival at hospital	Found dead: • IA - Out of hospital • IB - In-hospital
II	Death with unsuccessful resuscitation	Witnessed cardiac arrest • IIA - Out of hospital • IIB - In-hospital
III	Awaiting cardiac death	WLST
IV	Cardiac arrest while brain-dead	Cardiac arrest in a brain-dead patient prior to organ recovery
V		Euthanasia

Categories I and II - Uncontrolled donation after circulatory death. Categories III, IV, and V - Controlled donation after circulatory death. Adapted from: Ref. [18].

Table 3.
Donation after circulatory death classification.

or the organ is declined. The maximum time teams are willing to wait to follow the WLST varies between countries, as does the designated stand-off period and definitions of functional warm ischemic time [21].

Thus, in the cDCD setting, circulatory death is defined as the permanent cessation of circulation (which will not return) rather than the irreversible (which cannot

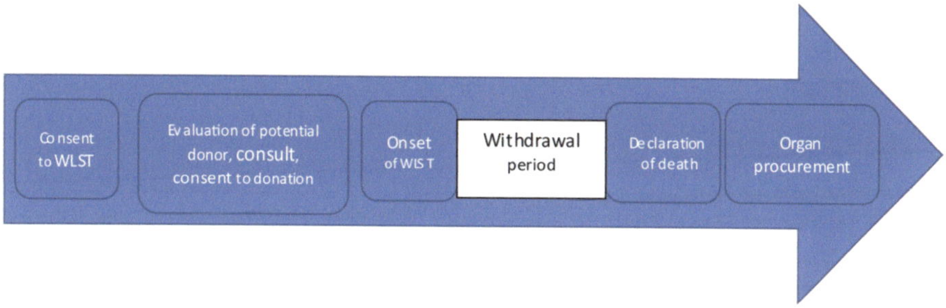

Figure 1.
The clinical pathway for controlled DCD.

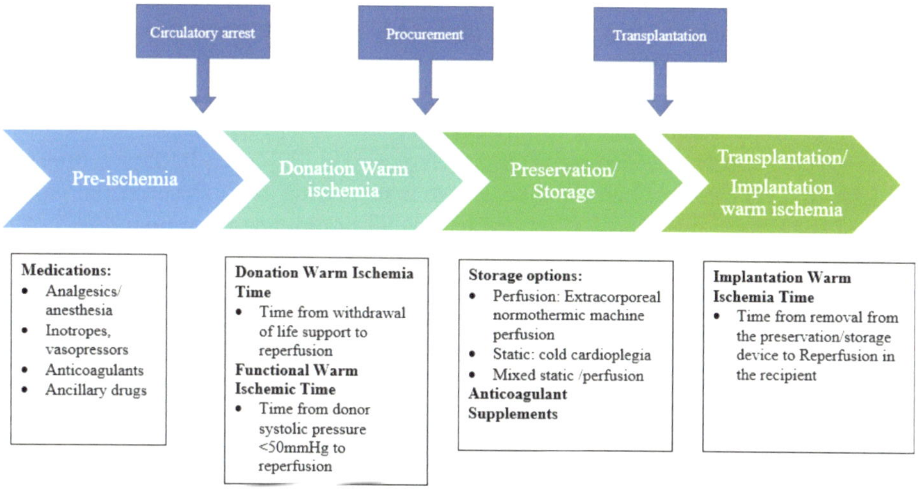

Figure 2.
Clinical protocol for DCD. Adapted from: Ref. [18].

return) cessation of circulation [22]. Following circulatory arrest, an ethically necessary "no-touch" period is required between the occurrence of circulatory arrest and declaration of death to ensure permanence. The no-touch period of at least 2 minutes and not more than 5 minutes is observed for autoresuscitation. The Society of Critical Care Medicine recommends at least 2 min, while the Institute of Medicine recommends 5 min [23]. Of interest, some countries have extended periods ranging from 10 minutes (Austria, Czech Republic, and Switzerland) to 20 minutes for transplant programs in Italy [24]. Although adequate time is needed to ensure the permanent cessation of circulatory function, this period must be balanced with the need to minimize the ischemic insult to the organs. After 5 minutes of circulatory arrest following the withdrawal of life-sustaining therapies, no autoresuscitation has been described [25].

After this period, death is declared after the clinician reassesses the patient for the permanence of circulatory arrest, apnea, and unresponsiveness [22]. This is followed by expeditious organ harvesting. Depending on the local protocol, if the patient does not expire after a particular timeframe from the withdrawal of ventilatory support, the patient is no longer considered a potential donor; they are returned to the intensive care unit, and comfort care is continued.

Depending on the hospital's facilities and policy, the transplant team must be available before extubation, which can occur in the operating room, perioperative area, or intensive care unit (ICU). Transplant surgical teams are not only prohibited from the patient's room but also not involved in the comfort care or death declaration of the patient [17].

2.2.2 Uncontrolled DCD (uDCD)

uDCD is defined as an organ donation from a person who was unsuccessfully resuscitated and died following an unexpected uncontrolled cardiac arrest (CA) [4, 18]. It is less common than controlled DCD and is more common in European countries, including France, Spain, and Russia, where it has been used to expand the donor pool [26]. In the United States, only a few studies have been reported [27]. Some programs initiated uDCD practices in the late 1990s and early 2000s but have discontinued them for different reasons. uDCD has a vast potential to help bridge the organ donor–recipient deficit, as the EuReCa study showed. This study identified almost 7000 cases of out-of-hospital cardiac arrest in 27 European countries treated by emergency medical services (EMS) over a month [28]. Successful CPR was recorded in only 28.6% of these patients, revealing a considerable missed potential for uDCD. Despite its potential, UDCD practices are on the decline after peaking in 2010 [29], even in the European countries that have established practice, which is surprising given the clear recommendation of the European Resuscitation Guidelines. The guideline recommends considering uDCD when advanced cardiopulmonary resuscitation (aCPR) is terminated [30].

For a patient to be considered a potential uDCD donor, they must have had unsuccessful advanced CPR and met strict inclusion criteria, as shown in **Table 2**. After a witnessed cardiac arrest outside the hospital, CPR is done according to national protocols that are aligned with international standards aiming for a return of spontaneous circulation (ROSC) [31]. If the CPR is unsuccessful, the emergency care services will contact the donor coordinator at the recipient hospital for a joint evaluation to determine the suitability of the donation [29]. The uDCD protocol is only activated after the donor suitability is determined and family consent is obtained. Countries have different practices for consent. For instance, Spain does not require family consent for uncontrolled donation [32], whereas in Canada, family consent is required even for registered donors [33]. After obtaining or waiving family consent, the potential donor is reintubated, allowing for mechanical ventilation and oxygenation (to minimize lung ischemia). Mechanical ventilation and cardiac compression are continued during transfer to the hospital and thus retain the option of organ donation until their wishes are known [34]. The uDCD protocol is only activated in some countries for cardiac arrest that occurs in-hospital settings following the transfer of the patient to the hospital for treatment [29]. In the Spanish program, mechanical ventilation and cardiac compressions are continued until legal permission for *in-situ* organ preservation is obtained [35]. Once consent has been obtained and legal permission granted, organ recovery is performed. Organs are validated similarly to donation after brain death (DBD) donor organs, based on function, macroscopic appearance, and histology, when appropriate [29]. See the process of uncontrolled DCD **Figure 3**.

2.3 Thoracic organs suitable for DCD donations

2.3.1 Heart transplants from DCD donors

The first adult heart transplantation in 1967 in South Africa was performed using a DCD donor as the procurement strategy; since then, brain-dead donors have been

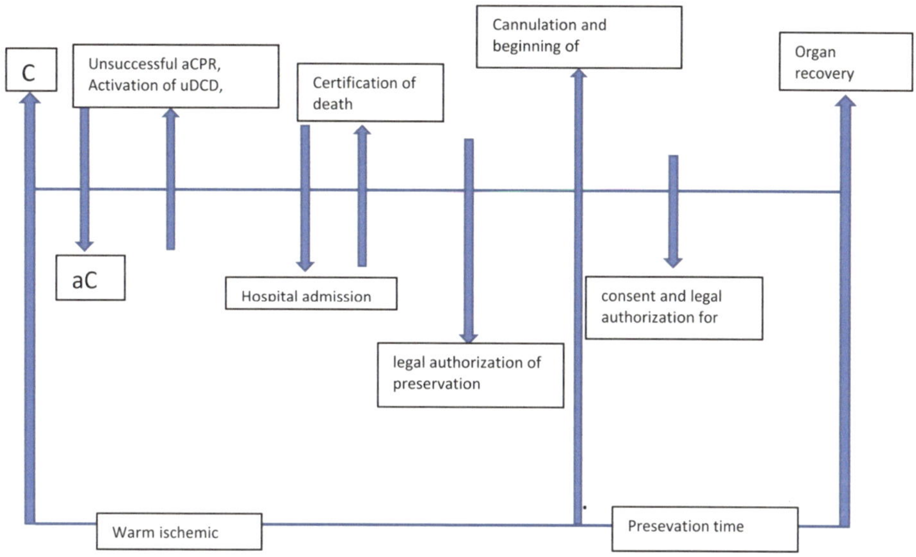

Figure 3.
The process of uncontrolled donation after circulatory death (uDCD). aCPR, advanced cardiopulmonary resuscitation; CA, cardiac arrest. Adapted from: Ref. [29].

the only donors for heart transplantation until recently. Brain death donors have two advantages over DCD donors. Firstly, it allows *in-situ* assessment of the graft viability and function of the heart. Secondly, the grafts are not subject to the detrimental effect of warm ischemic time. DCD donors are exposed to an unquantifiable warm ischemic injury between the withdrawal of life-sustaining therapy (WLST) and between circulatory arrest (CA) and heart procurement [36] Consequently, during procurement, the DCD heart is distended and non-beating. This raised concerns about the organ quality and function [37]. This was challenged in 2008; Boucek et al. [38] reported the successful transplantation of 3 DCD pediatric hearts using simple cold storage. Boucek et al. [39] reported that the 6-month survival, post-transplant inotropic support, rejection episodes, and ventricular function were similar to control infants who underwent DBD heart transplant during the same period. Following this finding, a group from Sydney, Australia, reported three successful DCD heart transplants in adults. This group utilized normothermic blood perfusion of the DCD hearts, instead of cold static storage, during transportation from donor to recipient hospitals [39]. They did not assess cardiac function before transplantation and lactate metabolism was used as a surrogate marker of heart quality. After transplantation, the group reported a 30% reliance on extracorporeal membrane oxygenation (ECMO) support for primary graft dysfunction (PGD).

The development of broad policies to tackle the ethical dilemma of DCD and advancements in machine perfusion technology allowed for the transplantation of hearts from more circulatory-death donors in adults. The growing clinical experience from different heart transplant programs has provided conclusive evidence that hearts from DCD donors are both possible and safe. This thought was confirmed by the Proceed II trial, which showed that normothermic machine perfusion with TransMedics organ care system (Andover MA, USA) was non-inferior to cold static storage in the setting of BDD-HT recipients [40]. At present, several protocols allow for the revival of organs and the evaluation of the viability of DCD hearts, either outside or inside the body. The protocol for retrieving hearts from DCD donors will vary depending on local regulations. However, the reported outcomes for DCD heart transplant recipients have been excellent so far.

2.3.2 Lung transplants from DCD donors

At present, lung transplantation from DCD is in its infancy but has been associated with good outcomes. The lung may be ideal for DCD because, unlike other solid organs, it is tolerant to warm ischemia at substantial time, provided they are inflated with oxygen because of its low metabolic requirement in the absence of circulation [41]. A detailed review of an international multicenter registry study of lung transplantation outcomes and a systematic review showed no difference in short- or long-term survival between DCD and DBD [14, 42]. A follow-up meta-analysis including 2570 patients who received a graft from DBD persons and 403 patients who received a graft from DCD donors showed no difference in 1-year survival, chronic lung allograft dysfunction, and grade 2–3 primary graft dysfunction [43]. Although the airway complications were higher with lower pooled 5-year survival in the DCD lungs, the validity of the airway result was limited by different institutional definitions of airway complications and small cohort size. Bobba et al. [44] reviewed the Scientific Registry of Transplant Recipients database and constructed three 5-year intervals of lung transplantation. They found no difference in overall survival when DCD was compared with DBD. Though Sabashnikov et al. [45] found a higher risk of bronchiolitis obliterans syndrome (BOS) and a higher incidence of primary graft dysfunction (grade 3) in the long-term follow-up post-DCD transplantation, the overall cumulative survival was not significantly different.

2.4 DCD organ evaluation, procurement, and management

The pathway for DCD can be divided into multiple phases, as shown below:

Identification & referral: Effective DCD protocol requires collaboration among different healthcare workers. Before withdrawing life support, the local organ procurement organization should be contacted for any patient who fulfills the following criteria stated in **Table 2**. The hospital record should initially be reviewed for eligibility. If eligible, further evaluation is done to ascertain if circulatory death is likely to occur within a specified period as predetermined by the caregiving team and OPO after WLS. If a patient or their surrogates elect for end-of-life care, trained requestors should undertake subsequent approaches for organ donation, as this improves authorization rates [46]. The donation coordination staff should only become involved after it has been decided that end-of-life care is appropriate for registered donors.

In case of uncontrolled DCD, donor coordinators must evaluate the patient's position toward organ donation through advanced directive registries and family interviews. Discussion about donation opportunities may happen at any point from when aCPR is terminated to after initiating organ preservation.

2.4.1 Preliminary evaluation

Once the care team supports the withdrawal of care and has communicated a grave prognosis to the family, the DCD procedure is reviewed with the local Organ Procurement Coordinator (OPC). The organ procurement and transplantation network (OPTN) has mandated specific tasks that the organ procurement organization

(OPO) must perform on every organ. As part of the initial evaluation, the OPO coordinator obtains a detailed medical and social history from the patient's family or next-of-kin. The history includes but is not limited to a history of smoking, alcohol consumption, and use of nonprescription drugs. The clinical history will consist of the history of malignancy, infections including viral hepatitis and HIV, laboratory testing, and procedures. The United States Public Health Service (USPHS) guidelines identify donors who have risk factors for transmissible viral infections, including HIV, HBV, and HCV infection [47].

Plasma and serum samples are usually drawn within 24 hours of organ procurement and preserved for 10 years. These samples are retrospectively used to detect donor-derived infections and diseases in the recipient after transplantation.

2.4.2 Family discussion and consent

With the care team agreeing to proceed with WLST, support services are offered to the family. The OPC will approach the family about donation options. The Legal next-of-kin (NOK) or the surrogate decision-maker is informed of donation options and recovery procedures. If in agreement, the Legal NOK grants consent for DCD following the withdrawal of support. The OPC will obtain witnessed consent from legal NOK for DCD. Informed consent includes consent for any pre-recovery procedures or drug administration specific to organ donation. The medical examiner/coroner will also be notified. The transplant process is terminated if the Family or the ME/Coroner denies consent. Also, if the patient is deemed an unsuitable candidate for DCD. If the patient progresses to brain death during evaluation, the brain-dead pathway is activated.

2.4.3 Comprehensive evaluation and donor management

Following family consent, the physician implements management guidelines in collaboration with OPO. The location of the withdrawal of support depends on the hospital policy. The usual locations for WLST are the intensive care unit (ICU) or the operating theater complex, such as the anesthetic bay, recovery, or operating theater. As part of explaining the process for donation and obtaining consent from families, it should be conveyed where WLST will occur and what this will mean if family members wish to be present with their relatives during this time. DCD organ procurements in which stopping WLST occurred in the ICU had more prolonged mean donor warm ischemia time (DWIT) than cases in which WLST occurred in the operating room (OR) [48]. This is due to the extra time needed to move the donor to the OR, position, prep, and drape after confirmation of circulatory death. In addition, WLST occurring outside of the OR will need additional personnel to ensure efficient donor transport and positioning. There should also be a plan for continued supportive care if the patient survives more than 1 hour or a predetermined time interval after withdrawal of support.

2.4.4 Withdrawal of life-sustaining treatment/pronouncement of death

The decision to withdraw care should be made in the absence of the transplant team. Depending on the institutional protocol, the withdrawal of life-sustaining treatment can occur in the OR or ICU, either in the presence or absence of the family. Several studies have evaluated the impact of the location of WLST on successful

DCD donation for specific organs. Cao et al. [48], in their meta-analysis, reported that WLST in the OR and premortem heparin administration improved outcomes of DCD liver transplants. The expert consensus statement by the International Liver Transplantation Society, which recommended WLST in the OR, supported their finding [49].

Before WLST, the arterial line should be placed. An arterial line allows for accurate time monitoring of blood pressure throughout the withdrawal process. It also enables the transplant teams to make appropriate organ viability decisions accurately based on specific hemodynamic thresholds. Pulseless electrical activity (PEA) is an acceptable criterion for death and cessation of cardiorespiratory function because it represents an undetectable pulse in the presence of measurable electrical discharge [50]. PEA can be noted on the arterial line. Furthermore, in cases involving DCD thoracic organ procurement using normothermic regional perfusion (NRP), a radial arterial line will help to ensure no upper extremity and brain perfusion.

The withdrawal of life support is carried out per the hospital practice guidelines in the absence of the transplant team. The vital signs are monitored and recorded every minute until death to ensure that f-DWIT can be accurately determined for all transplant centers involved. A mandatory wait time of no more than 5 minutes is recommended to avoid unnecessary warm ischemic injury. However, some European DCD programs extend this time to 20 minutes [23, 51]. The transplant team initiates surgical recovery at the prescribed time following the pronouncement of death and the mandatory wait period. If cardiac death is not established within 1 hour or after a predetermined time interval following withdrawal of support, the transplant process is stopped. The patient is transported to a predetermined area for continuation of supportive care.

2.4.5 Organ recovery

Four different DCD pathways exist for organ procurement and preservation. The first two pathways involve normothermic regional perfusion (NRP) before organ retrieval. Subsequently, cold storage or an *ex-vivo* perfusion machine is utilized during transport to the recipient institution. The other two pathways involve direct organ procurement immediately after the declaration of death and the mandatory wait period. The organ is then preserved with cold storage or an *ex-vivo* perfusion (EVP) system [52]. Using NRP or direct procurement with a subsequent EVP system allows organ evaluation to determine viability before transplantation. NRP involves cardiopulmonary bypass (CPB) or extracorporeal membrane oxygenation (ECMO) with cerebral perfusion exclusion in both cases. The use of direct procurement techniques and cold storage systems is less common.

2.5 Thoracic organs preservation and transport techniques

2.5.1 Static cold storage transport

For over 50 years, the traditional method of most organ preservation and transport, including kidneys and liver, has been static cold storage (SCS) in ice. This offers a simple and effective way to preserve and transport organs. It is also the most cost-efficient and easiest way to provide hypothermal environments. It consists of three plastic bags and an ice box. The first plastic bag includes the organ immersed in a preservation solution. SCS works by reducing the metabolic rate of organs, but because this happens in an oxygen-deprived environment, it leads to anaerobic metabolism. This gradually depletes the cellular energy in the form of adenosine triphosphate (ATP) and results in the accumulation of succinate. The latter drives the production of the reactive oxygen species that cause ischemia and reperfusion injury [53]. The theoretical optimal temperature for organ preservation is 4–8°C, with higher temperatures leading to hypoxic organ injury because of inefficient reduction in the metabolism, while temperatures lower than 4°C increase the risk of cold injury with protein denaturation [54]. Different preserving solutions have been developed to preserve organ function using static cold storage. These solutions differ in their electrolyte content, additives, and antioxidant concentrations. The University of Wisconsin (UW), Histidine-Tryptophan-Ketoglutarate (HTK), and the Celsior solutions are the most common heart-preserving solutions used in current practice. The post-transplant outcome studies to evaluate these three solutions have not shown the superiority of any solutions [55]. This contrasts with whole lung preservation, which is mainly preserved with Perfadex® (XVIVO Perfusion, Goteborg, Sweden), which is a low-potassium dextran solution [56]. Also, cold static preservation only allows short-term storage in whole lung preservation. However, the optimal duration of storage varies. While some authors report that lungs transplanted after undergoing cold static preservation for longer than 5 hours resulted in poorer recipient outcomes [57, 58], others report no difference in recipient outcomes for up to 9 hours of cold storage [59]. Regardless, lungs are only used if preservation time using cold static storage is less than 8 hours [60].

Static cold storage is adequate for short-term preservation when DBD and living donor organs are used. However, with the growing use of marginal organs from extended-criterion donors, the static cold storage method is no longer adequate. Some studies report inferior rates of primary non-function and delayed graft function when DCD donor grafts are compared with DBD donor grafts [61, 62].

2.5.2 Temperature-controlled donor organ transport system

The disadvantage of the Static cold storage preservation and transport method is that the organ may get too cold. To circumvent this limitation of SCS, particularly when the donor and the recipient do not reside in the same hospital, a series of medical devices were developed by Paragonix Technologies, Inc. These devices intended for use for transporting donor hearts, lungs, and kidneys to recipients for an implant include the Sherpa Pak™ Cardiac Transport System (CTS), Paragonix Lung guard system, the Sherpa Pak™ Cardiac Transport System, and the Sherpa Pak™ Kidney Transport System (KTS). The Sherpa Pak™ System was designed to provide a safe, consistent method for cold ischemic storage and transport of donor organs. Existing data suggest encouraging outcomes with these new transport devices. The GUARDIAN-Lung study evaluated two methods of hypothermic storage: patients with donor lungs transported with the LUNGguard and patients with donor lungs transported by conventional preservation methods in 797 patients (389 ice storage patients, 408 LUNGguard patients). It showed statistically significant improvements in the controlled hypothermic preservation group, including a 38% reduction of primary graft dysfunction at 24 hours, a 39% reduction of extracorporeal membrane oxygenation post-transplant, and a 51% reduction in the need for dialysis at discharge [59]. A multivariable logistic regression analysis showed that using the Paragonix SherpaPak® CTS was associated with a significantly reduced risk of primary graft dysfunction (44% reduction, $P = 0.045$) and the severity of primary graft dysfunction (69% reduction, $P = 0.009$).

The preservation management in the Sherpa Pak™ System for the kidneys and hearts are similar, except that the heart is connected to a connector in the inner rigid shell assembly, and the kidney is not [54]. The Sherpa Pak™ Cardiac Transport System maintains organ temperature from 4 to 8 degrees Celsius with temperature sensors and special ice packs. Some studies have shown that organs transported within this temperature-controlled system have reduced freezing injury and reduced protein denaturation, decreased metabolic rate, and reduced rates of tissue reperfusion injury [55, 63]. It also provides continuous real-time temperature monitoring and transmits temperature and geographic data via Bluetooth connected to a cell phone. A case series by Radakovic et al. [64] analyzed the donor heart temperature during transportation, donor heart function, and systemic infection rate among recipients after transplantation regarding the transportation method used; they found that the SherpaPak™ Cardiac Transport System maintained a constant temperature during transportation with permanent monitoring, never dropping below 4°C as well as normal perioperative function [64].

2.6 *Ex-vivo* organ perfusion

Although a relatively new concept in the field of organ transplant, the foundation of machine perfusion can be traced to Alexis Carrel and Charles Lindbergh, whose collaboration resulted in the Carrel–Lindbergh Perfusion device in the twentieth century. *Ex-vivo* heart perfusion was developed based on the Langendorff perfusion model, which demonstrated that coronary artery perfusion could resuscitate a dead heart. This concept resulted in the first commercial normothermic *ex-vivo* heart perfusion system (Transmedics Organ Care System, OCS). With the OCS, the heart can be successfully resuscitated, preserved, assessed, and possibly reconditioned before transplantation [65]. It allows continuous monitoring of the graft's aortic pressure, lactate level, and coronary blood flow [66]. Using the OCS, the heart viability can be evaluated by examining the lactate trends in arterial and venous blood samples taken from the OCS circuit. The effectiveness of the OCS was evaluated in the EXPAND trial. In this study, of the 93 marginal hearts, 75 hearts were transplanted (81% utilization rate) with average cross-clamp time and OCS perfusion time of 381 minutes and 279 minutes, respectively. The incidence of severe primary graft dysfunction within 24 hours of transplant was 11%, with a 30-day survival of 95%. The overall graft survival at 24 months was 82 and 95%, respectively [67]. Nevertheless, the absence of a comparative group somewhat limits these findings' robustness and applicability in clinical practice. Another ex- vivo machine preservation technique is currently being evaluated in a multi-centered randomized clinical trial in Europe to explore the safety and potential advantages of the NVivo® (XVivo Perfusion AB, Göteborg, Sweden) (HMP) (NCT03991923) [68]. Unlike the OCS, NVivo® perfuses the heart at a colder temperature with a specialized preservation solution. The clinical significance of these devices is extensive, including expanding preservation duration, evaluating extended-criteria donors, and using donor hearts retrieved following cDCD.

In lung transplants, *Ex-vivo* lung perfusion (EVLP) enables the precise assessment of lungs from DCD donors and extended-criteria donors. EVLP mimics the environment of the lungs inside the body. In addition, it enhances the management of logistical issues by extending preservation time safely [56] and provides a platform for advanced molecular diagnosis [69] and injured lung graft repair [56, 70]. The donated lungs are put inside a clear plastic dome attached to a ventilator and filtration system. While in the dome, the lungs are maintained at a constant temperature and treated with a specialized solution containing nutrients and oxygen. Once the lungs are flushed out and ventilated, the retrieval team will reevaluate them. They will examine their blood vessel pressure, tissue elasticity, oxygen capacity, and other investigative medical procedures.

Three EVLP protocols are used worldwide, including Lund, Toronto, and the Organ Care System Lung [70]. The Lund and Toronto protocols are similar. The former is the original protocol, while the latter was adapted from it. The Toronto protocol is now the most used [71]. The Toronto protocol modified the EVLP technology to include an optimal lung protective strategy. This strategy involves low tidal volume ventilation and a low flow rate in combination with a centrifuge pump. Compared with the initial technique that did not result in a stable preservation period longer than 60 minutes, the Toronto protocol has achieved an extended period of stable perfusion of more than 12 hours [72, 73]. The third protocol, the Organ Care System Lung, includes using a transportable device that uniquely removes the need to keep lungs in static cold storage before transplant, thus effectively reducing the cold ischemic time [74]. It uses a blood-based perfusate with a modified perfusion rate and different pumps. It addresses issues regarding cold ischemic storage by maintaining the organ in a normothermic and physiologically functioning state throughout transportation. A prospective, single-arm, multicenter trial evaluating OCS Lung for lungs from extended-criteria donors and DCD (EXPAND trial) showed an 87% donor lung utilization rate with excellent post-transplant clinical outcomes [71]. Hence, techniques for repairing and restoring organs can significantly enhance outcomes for DCD recipients. This can allow organs currently deemed unsuitable for transplant to be safely used after repair and reconditioning.

2.6.1 Normothermic machine perfusion (NMP)

Several temperatures have been evaluated for *ex-vivo* machine perfusion, including normothermic machine perfusion (NMP) at 35–38°C and hypothermic machine perfusion (HMP) at 0–8°C [75]. Sub- normothermic machine perfusion (SNMP) at 20–34°C has also been explored in some studies [76]. Normothermic machine perfusion (NMP) aims to preserve *ex-vivo* organ viability by mimicking the natural environment, including body temperature, oxygen, and nutrient provision, supporting tissue metabolism, and removing toxic metabolic waste. It utilizes CPB technology with extracorporeal membrane oxygenation to perfuse organs using a warm, oxygenated, plasma-free red cell-based solution [77]. This keeps an organ in a near-physiological state while restoring function *ex vivo*. In addition, NMP allows for a more straightforward organ assessment during the perfusion period. NMP holds promise in reducing the sequelae of ischemia–reperfusion injury, extending organ preservation times, and assessing donor organ quality before transplantation. The TransMedics OCS system uses normothermic technology. Hypothermic machine perfusion (0–8°C) is based on the concept that oxidative energy production by mitochondrial electron transport is sustained at low temperatures. In contrast to warm graft reperfusion in NMP, HMP technology uses cardioplegia and hypothermia to induce cardiac arrest, thereby reducing metabolic demand during perfusion [78]. During this process, the heart is perfused with a cold solution (8°C) enriched with nutrients and hormones. This cardioplegia solution also includes red blood cells, which restore the depleted ATP levels within myocardial cells, as supported by preclinical studies [79]. Existing data suggest that HMP technology has decreased rates of delayed graft function and improved outcomes in the case of marginal donors relative to SCS in kidney transplants [80]. However, no difference in primary non-function was seen in livers preserved *via* HMP compared to SCS. Compared with NMP, HMP is less complex and requires lower cost because it does not require oxygen carriers or all supplements necessary to maintain optimal organ metabolism [81]. In addition, different parameters of organ assessment, such as flow rate and mitochondria oxidative function metabolites, can be measured using HMP technology [81]. The outcomes of some preclinical studies investigating hypothermic oxygenated perfusion have been encouraging. Successful heart preservation for up to 48 hours has been reported [68]. The XVIVO® Heart Preservation System (XVIVO Inc., Gothenburg, Sweden) uses hypothermic technology and is currently undergoing testing in a phase II clinical trial [73]. It must be noted that *ex-situ* machine perfusion techniques incur additional costs, but these must be weighed against the potential benefits of improved organ function post-transplant. One challenge in using OCS is transporting the heart from facilities. OCS transportation is more complex than SCS, which may require upgraded cars and airplanes. Additionally, the OCS machine must be plugged into an outlet and connected to a wireless service during transport [82].

2.6.2 Normothermic regional perfusion

Normothermic regional perfusion (NRP) refers to *in-situ* perfusion of a region of the donor's body with extracorporeal organ support (ECOS) excluding the brain or brain stem. Using ECOS in DCD allows circulation to be re-established after cardiac cessation, and a mandatory "hands-off" period is observed before organ procurement is started. Depending on the target organs, the re-established circulation will be limited to a specific body area. NRP could be either isolated to the abdominal area (A-NRP) or include both the thorax and abdomen (TA-NRP). To maintain regional perfusion, the arch vessels, including the cerebral arteries, are clamped and vented to prevent brain perfusion. The aorta and right atrium are then cannulated to initiate circulatory support after the sternotomy and pericardiotomy. TA-NRP allows for *in-situ* assessment of the DCD donor heart. The Royal Papworth Hospital group pioneered it. They used this technique to provide a structural and functional evaluation of the donor's heart without relying on OCS Heart lactate profiles [83].

The general principle of TA-NRP relies on peripheral or central cannulations to establish a bypass circuit where donor blood is oxygenated and re-circulated following the declaration of death [83]. Clamping the aortic arch vessels prevents the recommencement of oxygenated cerebral circulation. The cardiac function is then evaluated with Swan-Ganz and trans-esophageal echocardiogram after it has been weaned off bypass. If the evaluation is satisfactory, the heart can be considered suitable for transplant and is then explanted in the usual fashion and transported to the donor using either NMP or traditional SCS [83, 84]. The reported outcome of the Papworth experience is encouraging, with comparable short-term survival between the DCD and DBD cohorts. The 1-year survival was 86% in the DCD-DPP group and 100% in the DCD-NRP arm. The survival was 96% in the DBD group. The use of ECMO was reported at 12% [84].

2.7 Challenges and limitations of DCD in heart and lung transplant

There are shared challenges that impact both controlled and uncontrolled DCD, while some challenges are unique to individual programs. Factors common to both programs include prolonged warm ischemic time and ethical challenges, while factors peculiar to cDCD include the inability to predict the time of death following WLST. Challenges peculiar to uDCD include low donor utilization and organizational aspects, including limited confidence in such programs (particularly on transplantation outcomes),

2.7.1 Warm ischemic time (WIT)

There is no current consensus definition of WIT or its related concept of functional WIT (fWIT) in clinical settings despite the physiologic significance of this concept. For example, donation WIT (DWIT), used in Australia, refers to the time from WLST to reperfusion [39]. In contrast, functional warm ischemic time (FWIT) is used in the United Kingdom. fWIT refers to the time from donor systolic pressure < 50 mm Hg to reperfusion [83]. FWIT used in Australian clinical setting is the systolic blood pressure of 90 mm Hg [18].

During DCD, donor grafts experience two phases of WIT that subject donor grafts to significant ischemic injury, which has been associated with impaired graft function in preclinical models [85]. The first occurs after WLST due to worsening hypoxia and hypoperfusion. In contrast, the second occurs after cardiac arrest (CA) and the mandatory stand-off period to confirm permanent cessation of circulation. It is important to note that DCD grafts also experience a period of cold ischemia following cold flush, the duration of which depends on the procurement method.

Immediately after death is confirmed, one of two technical approaches to procure the donor's heart involves the Direct procurement and perfusion (DPP) and thoracoabdominal NRP strategies (TA-NRP). The latter entails cannulation to ensure extracorporeal-driven circulation and *in-situ* reanimation of the heart. The Papworth group compared these strategies and determined that the median interval from CA to blood perfusion is 22 minutes (range: 21–25) for DPP and 14 minutes (range: 11–15) for TA-NRP ($p < .001$) [84]. It must be noted that not all jurisdictions permit the use of TA-NRP.

Most heart transplant programs set a maximum acceptable WIT of 30 minutes, based on data from a porcine model, since investigating the maximum tolerable WIT in humans is challenging [86]. However, limiting warm ischemia time (WIT) to 30 minutes may prevent viable heart donation, as prolonged donation WIT (DWIT) (time from withdrawal of life-sustaining therapy to blood reperfusion) of more than 60 minutes has not affected recipient outcomes [87]. Sánchez-Cámara et al. reported that the time after CA is the critical component in warm ischemia, and the time to restore circulation should not exceed 10 minutes [36]. However, Gerosa et al. reported a successful transplant with a prolonged functional ischemic time (43 minutes) due to a mandatory stand-down period of 20 minutes for the confirmation of circulatory death in Italy [88]. They used the Paragonix SherpaPak Cardiac Transport System (SCTS) to transport the donor heart.

In lung transplants, most institutions consider WIT below 60 minutes acceptable in DCD transplants even though 30–90 minutes would usually be tolerable [89]. The cooling process is primarily divided into topical cooling and antegrade perfusion. Topical cooling involves putting the preservation solution (Perfadex) into the thoracic cavity, while antegrade cooling involves perfusing the pulmonary artery (PA) with Perfadex. Infusion of Perfadex through PA is the gold-standard cooling method. Following completion of antegrade perfusion through the PA, the pulmonary veins are retrogradely flushed to enable the Perfadex to be transmitted to the parenchyma, which the earlier antegrade flush could not reach [90].

2.7.2 Ethical considerations controlled cDCD

The challenges policymakers face for DCD programs differ from those faced historically. However, some solutions are based on national or state-specific interpretations of the relevant ethical and legal frameworks rather than internationally applicable clinical research. DCD raises several unique ethical concerns since it involves terminating the care of dying patients to obtain quality donor organs. The dead donor rule states that "the retrieval of organs for transplantation should not cause the donor's death" [91]. This first ethical concern is when and how death is determined. To ensure that circulatory death meets both the criteria of permanent cessation of functions, invasive confirmatory tests such as intra-arterial monitoring should be used to verify that the donor fulfills the first requirement [17]. Second, there is a need for permanent cessation of respiration and circulation, which requires a mandatory observation period, depending on the institutional policy [17]. All states in the US have adopted a version of the Uniform Determination of Death Act (UDDA). This act defines circulatory death as the irreversible cessation of circulatory and respiratory functions. The word "irreversible," which implies that function could never resume, has been replaced with "permanent," suggesting that function will not spontaneously resume in the consensus UDDA interpretation [92]. The second ethical consideration is the potential conflicts of interest for physicians in managing the withdrawal of life support for a patient with potential organ donation. The withdrawing life-sustaining treatment is ethically acceptable when further treatments are considered futile. However, end-of-life care should not be suspended for organ procurement. Thus, it is vital to establish that decisions to withdraw treatment are separated from the fact that the patient is a potential organ donor. Because of these concerns, there should be institutional policies governing donation after circulatory death, which the physicians involved in organ procurement should strictly adhere to, as well as specific and clear clinical criteria for identifying prospective donors whose organs are reasonably likely to be suitable for transplantation. Physicians who participate in retrieving organs under a protocol of donation after circulatory death should ensure that the decision to withdraw life-sustaining treatment is made before and independent of any offer of the opportunity to donate organs unless the patient or surrogate decision-maker spontaneously raises organ donation. Also, the assignments of each healthcare team member must be well defined to prevent the risk of a conflict of interest between the interests of the potential DCD donor and the interests of the recipient. Finally, the physician who declares a patient dead must not play a role in the transplant process and the care of the organ recipient [17].

Thirdly, Informed consent from the donor or their surrogates is crucial during the transplantation process. The informed consent process should include organ procurement and transplantation risks and benefits. The potential recipient, donor, or surrogate decision-maker should know the most current information about the outcomes of the proposed organ transplants in DCD programs. This will help both parties to make informed decisions about accepting or refusing organs from DCD donors. The donor and their relatives should know the detailed plan and the extent to which the DCD protocol modifies the course of death. Also, informed consent should include premortem interventions that are not beneficial to the patient but preserve organs to improve the opportunity for successful transplantation. For instance, using ECMO (extracorporeal membrane oxygenation) increases the quality of organ transplants and can provide cardiorespiratory support to individuals with reversible cardiorespiratory failure [93, 94]. This has the potential to artificially replace the circulatory functions if established too quickly and can return circulation to the brain and restore consciousness, thus interfering with the determination of death. A potential modification is to prevent perfusion of the brain or organs above the diaphragm [22]. Care should be taken to ensure that death determination is not compromised. Other examples of premortem interventions include premortem heparinization, which has the potential to hasten death in DCD donors who have traumatic brain injury and are particularly susceptible to bleeding. Premortem heparinization is based on the report that thromboembolisms are found in 38% of donors, which can impact transplantation outcomes [95]. Cardiac catheterization and premortem cannulation of major vessels to expedite the application of postmortem extracorporeal circulatory support and reduce warm ischemia are other invasive procedures that are beneficial but provide no inherent benefit to the still-living donor. The minimum premortem interventions should be utilized to facilitate successful organ transplants. It must be noted that consent practices differ in different countries; in Spain [96] and Chile [32], the *opt-out* model is practiced [32]. The opt-out model assumes that everybody is a donor if they have documented their wish not to donate. In contrast, countries like Canada, Australia, and the United States have *opt-in* (explicit) consent methods [32]. The opt-in system allows individuals to register their legally binding decision to be a donor, which the family or surrogate decision-maker cannot overturn. Another critical issue regarding consent is the timing of the permission from family members. Reports in the literature are conflicting. While some authors advocate for family involvement after the suitability of the organs has been determined, others suggest that early family involvement, even before investigations for organ evaluation, is essential and considered suitable for donation [97, 98]. Finally, Serological testing in itself is of ethical interest due to the potential of uncovering sexually acquired infections like Hepatitis B or Hepatitis C and Human Acquired Immunodeficiency Virus (HIV), which were in many cases unknown to the donor's family members by the donor's choice [99].

2.7.3 Prediction tools for donor selection

Another challenge encountered in the DCD programs is the inability to predict death, which affects the precise success of a donation. Not all potential donors after circulatory death progress to death within a timeframe suitable for organ procurement. Following WLST, some potential donors may remain hemodynamically stable or experience a prolonged agonal phase that can result in prohibitive ischemic organ damage. Consequently, many tools have been developed to predict the time from WLST to death in the DCD donor population. No existing tool has been created or validated exclusively for potential heart and lung DCD donors who generally have medical criteria different from other DCD organs. Predictive tools are essential since the transplant team must be on-site and ready during WLST, particularly if the retrieval team is not local. Significant costs are incurred if donor progression to death is prolonged. Also, the latter can impact effective organ utilization. Hence, the importance of an accurate tool for selecting DCD heart and lung donors cannot be overemphasized.

2.7.4 Ethical considerations uncontrolled DCD

The first ethical dilemma in uDCD is the EMS team's determination of death and activation of the uDCD pathway. The uDCD donation pathway can be considered part of the out-of-hospital cardiac arrest resuscitation bundle. EMS team must align with national and international guidance on aCPR to avoid premature termination of resuscitation in favor of organ donation [100]. Given that the determination of irreversible circulatory death and the transition to organ donation in uDCD settings is time-sensitive, it is crucial to follow a precise protocol while shifting from resuscitative activities to organ donation. Thus, the cessation of aCPR must be independent of any organ donation consideration. Most programs require additional death confirmation by the hospital care team independent of the EMS and the donor and transplant teams, reassess the irreversibility of the CA, and determine death [101]. This is the reason why death determination only occurs in the hospital after the transfer of the potential donor. Though this will result in continuing aCPR and mechanical ventilation beyond futility during transfer, it will also allow time to determine the patient's position and that of their legal representatives toward posthumous donation. If post-Morten CPR is reinstated, potential donors remain monitored while being transferred to the hospital, which enables the identification of any return of spontaneous circulation.

A further crucial ethical consideration in uDCD is the timing of *in-situ* organ preservation after death but before consent from relatives has been obtained. From the pathologic standpoint, the crucial factor that affects uDCD organ donation is ischemia perfusion injury. Organs from uncontrolled DCD donors are exposed to a more significant duration of warm ischemia than those from comparable DBD donors and cDCD. Thus, the ischemia-reperfusion phenomenon affects organ function in the uDCD donor, distinguishing it from donors after brain death (BD) and cDCD donors. Potential uDCD donors are exposed to prolonged periods of low flow and at least two no-flow periods (that of the CA and that of the no-touch period) [102]. Though 5 minutes "no-touch periods" are acceptable in most European countries, Italy requires a no-touch period of at least 20 minutes [24]. The "ischemia-reperfusion clock" starts with the time of witnessed cardiac arrest. Some authors have reported that shorter periods of ischemia do not cause reperfusion injury. Instead, they can lead to ischemic preconditioning, which provides protection and reduces injury [103]. *In-vivo* and *ex-vivo* machine perfusions are the only existing measures to counteract the harmful effect of reperfusion injury. To be effective, early use of these machine perfusion techniques is required. Their early usage has the potential to cause distress to the family of the potential donor. Some countries, like Spain, a leading nation in uDCD, have a consent framework that supports postmortem interventions, including organ preservation, without the requirement of family consent [32]. In addition, using ECMO (extracorporeal membrane oxygenation) helps to increase the quality of the organs to be transplanted [94]. However, some authors argue that it can interfere with the end-of-life care of the potential donor, as well as damage bodily integrity with the potential risk of inducing pain since ECMO cannulation can be done premortem [104]. Regardless, the use of ECMO is becoming widespread because it has not been found to harm the potential donor patient in any way and does not invalidate the determination of death [94].

2.7.5 Organizational factors

For uDCD programs to function, there is a need for an appropriate regulatory framework and organizational capacity or technical expertise. While international consensus would likely assist in developing national uDCD programs, the need to clarify nation-specific ethical or legislative issues will remain the same. Successful uDCD programs will, therefore, continue to rely on a national regulatory framework establishing the legality and moral acceptability of fundamental aspects of the procedure, as well as on societal and professional consensus [105]. In addition, uDCD pathways require the effective collaboration of the EMS and Emergency department, which has access to 24-hour ECMO facilities. With an early alert by the EMS, the ECMO team will be available. A transplant coordinator should also be available to discuss death and donation with the family of the potential donor. Because these events are time-sensitive, having a clear policy and protocol to regulate uDCD programs is important.

2.7.6 Donor utilization

Donor utilization and the number of organs recovered and transplanted per donor are less effective and lower when compared with cDCD and DBD [26] In 2016, a European study that evaluated the effectiveness of the different deceased donation pathways found that 75% of uDCD donors utilized their organs, compared with 91% in cDCD and 93% in DBD [26]. In addition, the number of organs transplanted per donor was lower for uDCD. The urgency of the uDCD procedures may also contribute to the low utilization rate. This is because the organs harvested depend on the availability of a specific organ retrieval team in the donor hospital. The utilization of *in-situ* preservation strategies can provide time for dedicated recovery teams from other centers to reach the donor hospital; however, this will require the availability of an experienced ECMO team.

2.8 Future

2.8.1 Peri-transplant graft treatment

The next frontier in translating research into improved clinical outcomes is optimizing DCD organs for transplantation. DCD and ECD donors have the potential to significantly expand the donor pool and increase access to organ transplantation. Although greatly needed, these organs are known to be particularly susceptible to ischemia-reperfusion injury (IRI), the innate immune-driven tissue damage during cadaver-organ harvesting. Reperfusion injury can result in suboptimal organ transplant experience with a high incidence of primary graft dysfunction, early allograft dysfunction, and late rejections [106]. Donor organ rejuvenation in the peri-transplant period to improve their quality by mitigating IRI stress and promoting tissue regeneration *via* specific molecular signaling pathways (e.g., antioxidant) [107]. Hence, improving donor organ quality and targeting peri-transplant tissue IRI through a better understanding of the molecular and cellular events triggered by IRI is essential to save lives, benefit patient outcomes, and enhance the overall success of transplantation.

2.8.2 Prediction tools for organ donor selection

For optimal resource utilization, predicting which patients will or will not expire within 60 minutes after the withdrawal of care would be beneficial. Not all potential DCD donors progress to death within the period suitable for graft procurement. Some potential organ donors may remain hemodynamically stable after withdrawal of life-sustaining therapy, while some may experience a prolonged agonal phase resulting in ischemic organ damage. Given that the donation process is terminated in the former group while the latter reduces the suitability of the organs, DCD donor

Predictive tool for suitability of cardiac death donation	
The University of Wisconsin Donation after Cardiac Death Evaluation Tool [109]	83.7% of the time within 60 minutes and 74.4% within 120 minutes.
UNOS DCD consensus committee criteria [110]	
0	29%
1	52%
2	65%
3	82%

Table 4.
Predictive tool for suitability of cardiac death donation.

selection remains a challenge. Also, assembling the transplant team without successful progression to death has cost implications. Results in the literature show that the clinical judgment of the intensivist can predict death within 60 and 120 minutes with a sensitivity of 73 and 89 percent, respectively, and a specificity of 56 and 25 percent, respectively [108]. Some validated scores have been developed to better predict the probability of the potential donor's death within 60 minutes of withdrawal of life support, with different degrees of accuracy. Since the best predictive tools are inaccurate 30 percent of the time, some transplant programs are not using any predictive tools but instead pursuing DCD if the patient has an organ that is deemed transplantable (**Table 4**). No score for potential heart and lung donors has been validated to predict death after WLST. Developing a prediction tool to predict death accurately will enhance DCD practice worldwide.

Author details

Chinedu Okoli[1]*, Obieze Nwanna-Nzewunwa[2] and Suresh Keshavamurthy[2]

1 Department of General Surgery, Maine Medical Center, Portland, Maine, USA

2 Department of Cardiovascular and Thoracic Surgery, University of Texas Southwestern Medical Center, Dallas, USA

*Address all correspondence to: chinedu.okoli@mainehealth.org

References

[1] UNOS Data and Transplant Statistics. Organ Donation Data. Available from: https://unos.org/data [Accessed: June 21, 2024]

[2] Paradis NA, Halperin HR, Kern KB, Wenzel V, Chamberlain DA, editors. Cardiac Arrest: The Science and Practice of Resuscitation Medicine. Cambridge: Cambridge University Press; 2007

[3] Kacmarek RM. The mechanical ventilator: Past, present, and future. Respiratory Care. 2011;**56**(8):1170-1180

[4] Smith M, Dominguez-Gil B, Greer DM, Manara AR, Souter MJ. Organ donation after circulatory death: Current status and future potential. Intensive Care Medicine. 2019;**45**(3):310-321

[5] Spears W, Mian A, Greer D. Brain death: A clinical overview. Journal of Intensive Care. 2022;**10**(1):16

[6] Starr R, Tadi P, Pfleghaar N. Brain Death [Internet]. Treasure Island (FL): StatPearls Publishing; 2024. Available from: https://www.ncbi.nlm.nih.gov/books/NBK538159/ [Accessed: March 21, 2024]

[7] Dalle Ave AL, Bernat JL. Donation after brain circulation determination of death. BMC Medical Ethics. 2017;**18**(1):15

[8] Venuta F, Van Raemdonck D. History of lung transplantation. Journal of Thoracic Disease. 2017;**9**(12):5458-5471

[9] Hatami S, Conway J, Freed DH, Urschel S. Thoracic organ donation after circulatory determination of death. Transplantation Reports. 2023;**8**(1):100125

[10] World Health Organization. Global Observatory on Donation and Transplantation. World Health Organization; 2017

[11] Siddiqi HK, Trahanas J, Xu M, Wells Q, Farber-Eger E, Pasrija C, et al. Outcomes of heart transplant donation after circulatory death. Journal of the American College of Cardiology. 2023;**82**(15):1512-1520

[12] Schaapherder A, Wijermars LGM, de Vries DK, de Vries APJ, Bemelman FJ, van de Wetering J, et al. Equivalent long-term transplantation outcomes for kidneys donated after brain death and cardiac death: Conclusions from a Nationwide evaluation. EClinicalMedicine. 2018;**4-5**:25-31

[13] Doppenberg JB, Nijhoff MF, Engelse MA, de Koning EJP. Clinical use of donation after circulatory death pancreas for islet transplantation. American Journal of Transplantation. 2021;**21**(9):3077-3087

[14] Van Raemdonck DE, Keshavjee S, Levvey B, Cherikh WS, Snell G, Erasmus ME, et al. 5-year results from the ISHLT DCD lung transplant registry confirm excellent recipient survival from donation after circulatory death donors. The Journal of Heart and Lung Transplantation. 2019;**38**(4):S103

[15] Curtis RMK, Manara AR, Madden S, Brown C, Duncalf S, Harvey D, et al. Validation of the factors influencing family consent for organ donation in the UK. Anaesthesia. 2021;**76**(12):1625-1634

[16] Bernat JL, D'Alessandro AM, Port FK, Bleck TP, Heard SO, Medina J, et al. Report of a national conference

on donation after cardiac death. American Journal of Transplantation. 2006;**6**(2):281-291

[17] Reich DJ, Mulligan DC, Abt PL, Pruett TL, Abecassis MMI, D'Alessandro A, et al. ASTS recommended practice guidelines for controlled donation after cardiac death organ procurement and transplantation. American Journal of Transplantation. 2009;**9**(9):2004-2011

[18] Niederberger P, Farine E, Raillard M, Dornbierer M, Freed DH, Large SR, et al. Heart transplantation with donation after circulatory death. Circulation. Heart Failure. Apr 2019;**12**(4):e005517

[19] Kootstra G, Daemen JH, Oomen AP. Categories of non-heart-beating donors. Transplantation Proceedings. 1995;**27**(5):2893-2894

[20] Manara AR, Murphy PG, O'Callaghan G. Donation after circulatory death. British Journal of Anaesthesia. 2012;**108**:i108-i121

[21] Joshi Y, Villanueva J, Gao L, Hwang B, Zhao C, Doyle A, et al. Donation after circulatory death: A new frontier. Current Cardiology Reports. 2022;**24**(12):1973-1981

[22] Bernat JL. Controversies in defining and determining death in critical care. Nature Reviews. Neurology. 2013;**9**(3):164-173

[23] Institute of Medicine (US) Committee on Non-Heart-Beating Transplantation II: The Scientific and Ethical Basis for Practice and Protocols. Non-Heart-Beating Organ Transplantation. Washington, D.C.: National Academies Press; 2000

[24] Musso V, Righi I, Damarco F, Mazzucco A, Zanella A, Vivona L, et al. Lung donation after circulatory death. Current Challenges in Thoracic Surgery. 2023;**5**:9-9

[25] Zorko DJ, Shemie J, Hornby L, Singh G, Matheson S, Sandarage R, et al. Autoresuscitation after circulatory arrest: An updated systematic review. Canadian Journal of Anaesthesia. 2023;**70**(4):699-712

[26] Lomero M, Gardiner D, Coll E, Haase-Kromwijk B, Procaccio F, Immer F, et al. Donation after circulatory death today: An updated overview of the European landscape. Transplant International. 2020;**33**(1):76-88

[27] Choudhury RA, Prins K, Moore HB, Yoeli D, Kam A, Nydam TL. Uncontrolled deceased cardiac donation: An unutilized source for organ transplantation in the United States. Clinical Transplantation. 2019;**33**(3):e13474

[28] Gräsner JT, Lefering R, Koster RW, Masterson S, Böttiger BW, Herlitz J, et al. EuReCa ONE-27 nations, ONE Europe, ONE registry: A prospective one month analysis of out-of-hospital cardiac arrest outcomes in 27 countries in Europe. Resuscitation. 2016;**105**:188-195

[29] Coll E, Miñambres E, Sánchez-Fructuoso A, Fondevila C, Campo-Cañaveral de la Cruz JL, Domínguez-Gil B. Uncontrolled donation after circulatory death: A unique opportunity. Transplantation. 2020;**104**(8):1542-1552

[30] Monsieurs KG, Nolan JP, Bossaert LL, Greif R, Maconochie IK, Nikolaou NI, et al. European resuscitation council guidelines for resuscitation 2015. Resuscitation. 2015;**95**:1-80

[31] Link MS, Berkow LC, Kudenchuk PJ, Halperin HR, Hess EP, Moitra VK, et al. Part 7: Adult advanced cardiovascular life

support. Circulation. 2015;**132**(18_suppl. 2):S444-S464

[32] Pérez, Castro P, Salas SP. Ethical issues of organ donation after circulatory death: Considerations for a successful implementation in Chile. Developing World Bioethics. 2022;**22**(4):259-266

[33] Healey A, Watanabe Y, Mills C, Stoncius M, Lavery S, Johnson K, et al. Initial lung transplantation experience with uncontrolled donation after cardiac death in North America. American Journal of Transplantation. 2020;**20**(6):1574-1581

[34] Domínguez-Gil B, Duranteau J, Mateos A, Núñez JR, Cheisson G, Corral E, et al. Uncontrolled donation after circulatory death: European practices and recommendations for the development and optimization of an effective programme. Transplant International. 2016;**29**(8):842-859

[35] Streit S, Johnston-Webber C, Mah J, Prionas A, Wharton G, Casanova D, et al. Ten lessons from the Spanish model of organ donation and transplantation. Transplant International. 2023;**36**:11009

[36] Sánchez-Cámara S, Asensio-López MC, Royo-Villanova M, Soler F, Jara-Rubio R, Garrido-Peñalver JF, et al. Critical warm ischemia time point for cardiac donation after circulatory death. American Journal of Transplantation. 2022;**22**(5):1321-1328

[37] Pettit SJ, Petrie MC. Transplantation of hearts donated after circulatory-determined death. Circulation. Heart Failure. Apr 2019;**12**(4):e005991

[38] Boucek MM, Mashburn C, Dunn SM, Frizell R, Edwards L, Pietra B, et al. Pediatric heart transplantation after declaration of cardiocirculatory death. The New England Journal of Medicine. 2008;**359**(7):709-714

[39] Dhital KK, Iyer A, Connellan M, Chew HC, Gao L, Doyle A, et al. Adult heart transplantation with distant procurement and *ex-vivo* preservation of donor hearts after circulatory death: A case series. Lancet. 2015;**385**(9987):2585-2591

[40] Ardehali A, Esmailian F, Deng M, Soltesz E, Hsich E, Naka Y, et al. *Ex-vivo* perfusion of donor hearts for human heart transplantation (PROCEED II): A prospective, open-label, multicentre, randomised non-inferiority trial. Lancet. 2015;**385**(9987):2577-2584

[41] Dugbartey GJ. Therapeutic benefits of nitric oxide in lung transplantation. Biomedicine & Pharmacotherapy. 2023;**167**:115549

[42] Krutsinger D, Reed RM, Blevins A, Puri V, De Oliveira NC, Zych B, et al. Lung transplantation from donation after cardiocirculatory death: A systematic review and meta-analysis. The Journal of Heart and Lung Transplantation. 2015;**34**(5):675-684

[43] Palleschi A, Rosso L, Musso V, Rimessi A, Bonitta G, Nosotti M. Lung transplantation from donation after controlled cardiocirculatory death. Systematic review and meta-analysis. Transplantation Reviews (Orlando, Fla.). 2020;**34**(1):100513

[44] Bobba CM, Whitson BA, Henn MC, Mokadam NA, Keller BC, Rosenheck J, et al. Trends in donation after circulatory death in lung transplantation in the United States: Impact of era. Transplant International. 2022;**35**:10172

[45] Sabashnikov A, Patil NP, Popov AF, Soresi S, Zych B,

Weymann A, et al. Long-term results after lung transplantation using organs from circulatory death donors: A propensity score-matched analysis. European Journal of Cardio-Thoracic Surgery. 2016;**49**(1):46-53

[46] Hulme W, Allen J, Manara AR, Murphy PG, Gardiner D, Poppitt E. Factors influencing the family consent rate for organ donation in the UK. Anaesthesia. 2016;**71**(9):1053-1063

[47] Jones JM, Kracalik I, Levi ME, Bowman JS, Berger JJ, Bixler D, et al. Assessing solid organ donors and monitoring transplant recipients for human immunodeficiency virus, hepatitis B virus, and hepatitis C virus infection - U.S. Public Health Service guideline, 2020. MMWR - Recommendations and Reports. 2020;**69**(4):1-16

[48] Cao Y, Shahrestani S, Chew HC, Crawford M, Macdonald PS, Laurence J, et al. Donation after circulatory death for liver transplantation: A meta-analysis on the location of life support withdrawal affecting outcomes. Transplantation. 2016;**100**(7):1513-1524

[49] Hessheimer AJ, Polak W, Antoine C, Dondero Pozzo F, Maluf D, Monbaliu D, et al. Regulations and procurement surgery in DCD liver transplantation: Expert consensus guidance from the international liver transplantation society. Transplantation. 2021;**105**(5):945-951

[50] Croome KP, Barbas AS, Whitson B, Zarrinpar A, Taner T, Lo D, et al. American Society of Transplant Surgeons recommendations on best practices in donation after circulatory death organ procurement. American Journal of Transplantation. 2023;**23**(2):171-179

[51] Recommendations for nonheartbeating organ donation. Critical Care Medicine. 2001;**29**(9):1826-1831

[52] Ngai J, Jankowska A. Donation after circulatory death heart transplants: Doing more and waiting less. Journal of Cardiothoracic and Vascular Anesthesia. 2023;**37**(12):2409-2412

[53] Nicholson ML, Hosgood SA. Renal transplantation after *ex vivo* normothermic perfusion: The first clinical study. American Journal of Transplantation. 2013;**13**(5):1246-1252

[54] Michel SG, LaMuraglia Ii GM, Madariaga MLL, Anderson LM. Innovative cold storage of donor organs using the Paragonix Sherpa Pak ™ devices. Heart Lung Vessel. 2015;7(3):246-255

[55] Ruaengsri CM, Bethencourt D, Koyano T, Shudo Y. Heart Preservation Techniques for Transplantation. London, UK: IntechOpen; 2024

[56] Yeung JC, Krueger T, Yasufuku K, de Perrot M, Pierre AF, Waddell TK, et al. Outcomes after transplantation of lungs preserved for more than 12 h: A retrospective study. The Lancet Respiratory Medicine. 2017;**5**(2):119-124

[57] Snell GI, Rabinov M, Griffiths A, Williams T, Ugoni A, Salamonsson R, et al. Pulmonary allograft ischemic time: An important predictor of survival after lung transplantation. The Journal of Heart and Lung Transplantation. 1996;**15**(2):160-168

[58] Gammie JS, Stukus DR, Pham SM, Hattler BG, McGrath MF, McCurry KR, et al. Effect of ischemic time on survival in clinical lung transplantation. The Annals of Thoracic Surgery. 1999;**68**(6):2015-2019

[59] Hartwig M, Bush E, Langer N, Haney J. Report of the GUARDIAN-LUNG registry: An analysis of advanced hypothermic preservation on lung

transplantation. The Journal of Heart and Lung Transplantation. 2022;**41**(4):S37

[60] Lautner LJ, Freed DH, Nagendran J, Acker JP. Current techniques and the future of lung preservation. Cryobiology. Jun 2020;**94**:1-8

[61] Metcalfe MS, Butterworth PC, White SA, Saunders RN, Murphy GJ, Taub N, et al. A case-control comparison of the results of renal transplantation from heart-beating and non-heart-beating donors. Transplantation. 2001;**71**(11):1556-1559

[62] McLaren AJ, Friend PJ. Trends in organ preservation. Transplant International. 2003;**16**(10):701-708

[63] Tong CKW, Khush KK. New approaches to donor selection and preparation in heart transplantation. Current Treatment Options in Cardiovascular Medicine. 2021;**23**(5):28

[64] Radakovic D, Karimli S, Penov K, Schade I, Hamouda K, Bening C, et al. First clinical experience with the novel cold storage SherpaPakTM system for donor heart transportation. Journal of Thoracic Disease. 2020;**12**(12):7227-7235

[65] Qin G, Jernryd V, Sjöberg T, Steen S, Nilsson J. Machine perfusion for human heart preservation: A systematic review. Transplant International. 2022;**35**:10258

[66] Pahuja M, Case BC, Molina EJ, Waksman R. Overview of the FDA's circulatory system devices panel virtual meeting on the TransMedics organ care system (OCS) heart – portable extracorporeal heart perfusion and monitoring system. American Heart Journal. 2022;**247**:90-99

[67] Schroder JN, D'Alessandro D, Esmailian F, Boeve T, Tang P, Liao K, et al. Successful utilization of extended criteria donor (ECD) hearts for transplantation - results of the OCS™ heart expand trial to evaluate the effectiveness and safety of the OCS heart system to preserve and assess ECD hearts for transplantation. The Journal of Heart and Lung Transplantation. 2019;**38**(4):S42

[68] Ughetto A, Roubille F, Molina A, Battistella P, Gaudard P, Demaria R, et al. Heart graft preservation technics and limits: An update and perspectives. Frontiers in Cardiovascular Medicine. 6 Nov 2023;**10**:1248606

[69] Machuca TN, Cypel M, Yeung JC, Bonato R, Zamel R, Chen M, et al. Protein expression profiling predicts graft performance in clinical ex vivo lung perfusion. Annals of Surgery. 2015;**261**(3):591-597

[70] Nakajima D, Date H. Ex vivo lung perfusion in lung transplantation. General Thoracic and Cardiovascular Surgery. 2021;**69**(4):625-630

[71] Loor G, Warnecke G, Villavicencio MA, Smith MA, Kukreja J, Ardehali A, et al. Portable normothermic ex-vivo lung perfusion, ventilation, and functional assessment with the organ care system on donor lung use for transplantation from extended-criteria donors (EXPAND): A single-arm, pivotal trial. The Lancet Respiratory Medicine. 2019;**7**(11):975-984

[72] Cypel M, Yeung JC, Hirayama S, Rubacha M, Fischer S, Anraku M, et al. Technique for prolonged normothermic *ex vivo* lung perfusion. The Journal of Heart and Lung Transplantation. 2008;**27**(12):1319-1325

[73] Erasmus ME, Fernhout MH, Elstrodt JM, Rakhorst G. Normothermic ex vivo lung perfusion of non-heart-beating donor lungs in pigs: From pretransplant function analysis towards

a 6-h machine preservation. Transplant International. 2006;**19**(7):589-593

[74] Schmack B, Weymann A, Mohite P, Garcia Saez D, Zych B, Sabashnikov A, et al. Contemporary review of the organ care system in lung transplantation: Potential advantages of a portable ex-vivo lung perfusion system. Expert Review of Medical Devices. 2016;**13**(11):1035-1041

[75] Jing L, Yao L, Zhao M, Ping PL, Liu M. Organ preservation: From the past to the future. Acta Pharmacologica Sinica. 2018;**39**(5):845-857

[76] Rojas-Pena A, Bartlett RH. Ex situ organ preservation. Transplantation. 2018;**102**(4):554-556

[77] Hosgood SA, Callaghan CJ, Wilson CH, Smith L, Mullings J, Mehew J, et al. Normothermic machine perfusion versus static cold storage in donation after circulatory death kidney transplantation: A randomized controlled trial. Nature Medicine. 2023;**29**(6):1511-1519

[78] Nilsson J, Jernryd V, Qin G, Paskevicius A, Metzsch C, Sjöberg T, et al. A nonrandomized open-label phase 2 trial of nonischemic heart preservation for human heart transplantation. Nature Communications. 2020;**11**(1):2976

[79] Wyss RK, Méndez Carmona N, Arnold M, Segiser A, Mueller M, Dutkowski P, et al. Hypothermic, oxygenated perfusion (HOPE) provides cardioprotection via succinate oxidation prior to normothermic perfusion in a rat model of donation after circulatory death (DCD). American Journal of Transplantation. 2021;**21**(3):1003-1011

[80] Bellini MI, Nozdrin M, Yiu J, Papalois V. Machine perfusion for abdominal organ preservation: A systematic review of kidney and liver human grafts. Journal of Clinical Medicine. Aug 15 2019;**8**(8):1221

[81] Muller X, Schlegel A, Kron P, Eshmuminov D, Würdinger M, Meierhofer D, et al. Novel real-time prediction of liver graft function during hypothermic oxygenated machine perfusion before liver transplantation. Annals of Surgery. 2019;**270**(5):783-790

[82] Sunjaya AF, Sunjaya AP. Combating donor organ shortage: Organ care system prolonging organ storage time and improving the outcome of heart transplantations. Cardiovascular Therapeutics. 2019;**2019**:1-7

[83] Messer S, Cernic S, Page A, Berman M, Kaul P, Colah S, et al. A 5-year single-center early experience of heart transplantation from donation after circulatory-determined death donors. The Journal of Heart and Lung Transplantation. 2020;**39**(12):1463-1475

[84] Messer S, Page A, Axell R, Berman M, Hernández-Sánchez J, Colah S, et al. Outcome after heart transplantation from donation after circulatory-determined death donors. The Journal of Heart and Lung Transplantation. 2017;**36**(12):1311-1318

[85] Kearns MJ, Miller SD, Cheung A, Bashir J, Wong S, Seidman MA, et al. A rodent model of cardiac donation after circulatory death and novel biomarkers of cardiac viability during ex vivo heart perfusion. Transplantation. 2017;**101**(8):e231-e239

[86] Ayer A, Schroder JN, Casalinova S, Doberne JW, Bryner BS, Patel CB, et al. The future of heart procurement with donation after circulatory death: Current practice and opportunities for advancement. The Journal of

Heart and Lung Transplantation. 2022;**41**(10):1385-1390

[87] Chew HC, Iyer A, Connellan M, Scheuer S, Villanueva J, Gao L, et al. Outcomes of donation after circulatory death heart transplantation in Australia. Journal of the American College of Cardiology. 2019;**73**(12):1447-1459

[88] Gerosa G, Zanatta P, Angelini A, Fedrigo M, Bianco R, Pittarello D, et al. Overcoming the boundaries of heart warm ischemia in donation after circulatory death: The Padua Case. ASAIO Journal. 9 Feb 2024:10-97

[89] Oto T, Levvey B, McEgan R, Davies A, Pilcher D, Williams T, et al. A practical approach to clinical lung transplantation from a Maastricht category III donor with cardiac death. The Journal of Heart and Lung Transplantation. 2007;**26**(2):196-199

[90] Hyun S, Haam S. Donation after circulatory death in lung transplantation. Journal of Chest Surgery. 2022;**55**(4):283-287

[91] Potter J. Imminent death donation: Ethical and practical policy considerations. Journal of Law, Medicine & Ethics. 2018;**46**(2):524-537

[92] Nikas NT, Bordlee DC, Moreira M. Determination of death and the dead donor rule: A survey of the current law on brain death. Journal of Medicine and Philosophy. 2016;**41**(3):237-256

[93] Hogen R, Sedra AH, Motamed A, Emamaullee J. The evolving role of ECMO in liver transplantation. Current Opinion in Organ Transplantation. 2021;**26**(3):333-338

[94] Gravel MT, Arenas JD, Chenault R, Magee JC, Rudich S, Maraschio M, et al. Kidney transplantation from organ donors following cardiopulmonary death using extracorporeal membrane oxygenation support. Annals of Transplantation. 2004;**9**(1):57-58

[95] Oto T, Rabinov M, Griffiths AP, Whitford H, Levvey BJ, Esmore DS, et al. Unexpected donor pulmonary embolism affects early outcomes after lung transplantation: A major mechanism of primary graft failure? The Journal of Thoracic and Cardiovascular Surgery. 2005;**130**(5):1446.e1-1446.e9

[96] Dalal AR. Philosophy of organ donation: Review of ethical facets. World Journal of Transplantation. 2015;**5**(2):44-51

[97] Graftieaux JP, Bollaert PE, Haddad L, Kentish-Barnes N, Nitenberg G, Robert R, et al. Contribution of the ethics committee of the French society of intensive care medicine to a scenario for the implementation of organ donation after Maastricht III-type cardiac death in France. Annales Françaises d'Anesthèsie et de Rèanimation. 2014;**33**(2):128-134

[98] Overby KJ, Weinstein MS, Fiester A. Addressing consent issues in donation after circulatory determination of death. The American Journal of Bioethics. 2015;**15**(8):3-9

[99] Leichliter JS, Copen C, Dittus PJ. Confidentiality issues and use of sexually transmitted disease services among sexually experienced persons aged 15-25 years — United States, 2013-2015. MMWR. Morbidity and Mortality Weekly Report. 2017;**66**(9):237-241

[100] Soar J, Nolan JP, Böttiger BW, Perkins GD, Lott C, Carli P, et al. European resuscitation council guidelines for resuscitation 2015:

Section 3. Adult advanced life support. Resuscitation. 2015;**95**:100-147

[101] Haase B, Bos M, Boffa C, Lewis P, Rudge C, Valero R, et al. Ethical, legal, and societal issues and recommendations for controlled and uncontrolled DCD. Transplant International. 2016;**29**(7):771-779

[102] Lazzeri C, Peris A. Uncontrolled donation after circulatory death: A by-product of the controlled? A narrative review. European Journal of Transplantation. 2023;**1**(2):136-142

[103] Becker LB. New concepts in reactive oxygen species and cardiovascular reperfusion physiology. Cardiovascular Research. 2004;**61**(3):461-470

[104] Dalle Ave AL, Shaw DM, Bernat JL. Ethical issues in the use of extracorporeal membrane oxygenation in controlled donation after circulatory determination of death. American Journal of Transplantation. 2016;**16**(8):2293-2299

[105] Domínguez-Gil B, Haase-Kromwijk B, Van Leiden H, Neuberger J, Coene L, Morel P, et al. Current situation of donation after circulatory death in European countries. Transplant International. 2011;**24**(7):676-686

[106] O'Neill S, Roebuck A, Khoo E, Wigmore SJ, Harrison EM. A meta-analysis and meta-regression of outcomes including biliary complications in donation after cardiac death liver transplantation. Transplant International. 2014;**27**(11):1159-1174

[107] Kojima H, Nakamura K, Kupiec-Weglinski JW. Therapeutic targets for liver regeneration after acute severe injury: A preclinical overview. Expert Opinion on Therapeutic Targets. 2020;**24**(1):13-24

[108] Wind J, Snoeijs MGJ, Brugman CA, Vervelde J, Zwaveling J, van Mook WN, et al. Prediction of time of death after withdrawal of life-sustaining treatment in potential donors after cardiac death*. Critical Care Medicine. 2012;**40**(3):766-769

[109] Lewis J, Peltier J, Nelson H, Snyder W, Schneider K, Steinberger D, et al. Development of the University of Wisconsin Donation after cardiac death evaluation tool. Progress in Transplantation. 2003;**13**(4):265-273

[110] DeVita MA, Brooks MM, Zawistowski C, Rudich S, Daly B, Chaitin E. Donors after cardiac death: Validation of identification criteria (DVIC) study for predictors of rapid death. American Journal of Transplantation. Feb 2008;**8**(2):432-441

Chapter 4

ICU Care of Solid Organ Transplant Donors and Recipients

Sohel Mohamed Gamal Ahmed, Abdelrahman Balal, Sujith Madambikattil Prabhakaran, Zia Mahmood Awan, Mogahed Ismail Hassan Hussein, Siddhartha Banerjee and Wael Khalaf

Abstract

The intensive care unit (ICU) is crucial to solid organ transplant donor and recipient treatment, guaranteeing optimum organ procurement and transplant survival. Before retrieval, donors need specialist care to maintain organ function, whereas recipients typically need ICU-level management for rejection, infections, or organ malfunction. Improving treatment and results requires understanding these groups' physiological and ethical needs. This chapter covers clinical procedures, ethical frameworks, and best practises for solid organ transplant donors and recipients in ICU treatment. To maximise transplant success, it optimises donor organ function and manages potential recipient complications. A multidisciplinary evaluation of literature, clinical guidelines, and case studies identified ICU transplant donor and recipient management best practices. The main areas of attention include haemodynamic stability, immunosuppressive treatment management, infection control, and donor consent and allocation ethics. ICU treatment improves donor organ viability by optimising haemodynamic support, oxygenation, and metabolic stability, reducing graft failure and improving organ quality. Early detection and treatment of rejection, infection, and organ malfunction lowers recipient morbidity and death. Ethics and family-centered communication in donor management and interdisciplinary recipient care were also stressed in this review. Effective ICU care for solid organ transplant donors and recipients needs sophisticated clinical treatments, ethical awareness, and teamwork. Clinicians may improve organ procurement, transplant results, and donor and recipient care by following evidence-based practices. This chapter emphasises the ICU's crucial role in transplant care and offers practical ideas to improve clinical and ethical outcomes.

Keywords: intensive care, solid organ transplant, pre-donation optimisation, post-transplant care, complications

1. Introduction

Solid organ transplantation is a life-saving medical procedure involving the surgical transfer of organs such as the kidney, liver, heart, lungs and pancreas from donors to recipients. It is a cornerstone of modern medicine, offering patients with end-stage organ failure a second chance at life and significantly improving their long-term outcomes. Advances in surgical techniques, immunosuppressive therapies and critical care medicine have made transplantation a viable and effective treatment option, with expanding indications across various patient populations.

Solid organ transplantation relies on the coordinated efforts of healthcare teams, including intensive care (ICU) specialists, to ensure the optimal care of both donors and recipients. For transplant recipients, the ICU plays a pivotal role in managing perioperative complications, such as hemodynamic instability, infections and graft rejection. For donors, particularly brain-dead donors, meticulous ICU management is essential to preserve organ function, minimise ischemic damage and maximise the viability of the donated organs.

ICU teams play a critical role in balancing these complexities to ensure successful outcomes. The care provided in the ICU is integral to the success of solid organ transplantation. The stakes are particularly high due to the finite availability of donor organs and the risks associated with organ rejection or recipient morbidity.

The ICU care of solid organ transplant donors and recipients represents a vital and highly specialised area of critical care medicine. This chapter will delve into the principles and practices that guide ICU management, highlighting strategies to optimise recipient outcomes and ensure ethical and effective donor management. By addressing the challenges inherent in transplantation, ICU teams contribute to the success of this transformative medical intervention.

2. Organ donation: ICU management of brain-dead donors

2.1 History of brain stem testing

The neurological examination techniques that have advanced from the nineteenth century and early twentieth century helped physicians to have a systematic assessment of brain stem functions, and it is this development that laid the foundation for modern brain stem testing. Computed tomography (CT) and magnetic resonance imaging (MRI) revolutionised the diagnosis and assessment of brain stem lesions and injuries.

In 1959, the concept of brain death/death by neurologic criteria (BD/DNC) was first described. Later, in 1968, the Harvard Brain Death Criteria defined the importance of irreversible loss of brainstem function, which was emphasised by Minnesota criteria in 1971 [1]. The Uniform Determination of Death Act established a legal basis for neurologically determining death in the US, and adult guidelines were published in 1995 and revised in 2010 [2].

2.2 Criteria for brainstem testing

The Uniform Determination of Death Act (UDDA), the legal foundation for the declaration of BD/DNC in the United States, is declared when there is irreversible cessation of all functions of the entire brain, including the brainstem [2]. The criteria for brain stem death testing typically include the following:

2.3 Prerequisites for determination of brain death or death by neurological criteria

2.3.1 Unresponsive coma

Clinicians should ascertain that a patient has sustained a catastrophic and irreversible coma caused by an identifiable mechanism. Neuroimaging must be consistent with the mechanism and severity of brain injury. After medical or surgical interventions to treat elevated intracranial pressure, it is recommended to wait a sufficient amount of time to ensure there is no recovery of brain function. This observation period must be based on the pathophysiology of the brain injury [3].

2.3.2 Exclusion of confounding factors

Before determining brain death, a few confounding factors shall be excluded, such as metabolic derangements and drug or substance intoxication that causes CNS depressants and muscle relaxants. If drug intoxication is suspected, ensure drug levels are within the normal range. If not, consider waiting five half-life of the drug metabolism. Exclude severe metabolic, acid-base, electrolyte and endocrine derangements. Maintain Systolic BP $\geq$ 100 mm Hg and mean arterial pressure (MAP) $\geq$75 mmHg and avoid hypothermia, maintaining core temperature $\geq$ 36°C.

2.4 Performing neurological examination for brain stem reflexes

Neurological examinations are used to determine the absence of cranial nerve (CN) reflexes. Pupillary light reflex (CN II & III), corneal reflex (CN V & VII) and trigeminal nerve testing by painful stimulus over supraorbital nerve (CN V & VII), are employed. In addition to these, the vesibulo-ocular reflex -using ice cold water installation into both ears (CN III, IV, VI & VIII), the gag reflex (CN IX & X), and the cough reflex (CN X) are also examined

Apnea test: This test must be carried out only after brainstem reflexes have been tested. Absence of respiratory movements after disconnection from the ventilator for sufficient duration (8–10 minutes) to have PaCO2 rise above threshold (>60 mmHg) or 20% above baseline for stimulating respiration is considered a positive apnea test.

Most international regulatory bodies do not mandate performing ancillary tests. These tests are only indicated in special circumstances, such as inability to correct metabolic derangement, severe facial injury, when in doubt regarding origin of movements (i.e. motor vs spinal reflexes), and if apnea test is not feasible

2.5 Acceptable ancillary tests

Four-vessel catheter angiography is the gold standard [3]. Other tests are a Radionuclide cerebral blood flow scan and a Transcranial Doppler ultrasonography (in adults only).

3. Pathophysiological changes and management of brain death

A range of organ dysfunction and physiological changes may occur in many systems, including hypotension, catecholamine surge leading to hypertension, tachycardia, cardiac arrhythmias and neurogenic myocardial dysfunction [4]. Pulmonary oedema, ventilator-induced lung injury and infections are the pulmonary complications. Diabetes insipidus, hypoglycemia and acute kidney injury can occur. Disseminated intravascular coagulation metabolic and electrolyte disturbances must also be anticipated and managed accordingly.

The endocrine changes that occur in brain death are as follows. An increase and then a fall in catecholamines can occur. Cortisol and anti-diuretic hormone levels reduce, and the hypothalamic pituitary thyroid axis alters. Thyroid hormone replacement remains controversial as there is not much evidence that it can benefit the quality of organs, but so far, no harm has been reported. Levothyroxine infusion can be administered in refractory shock. It would be reasonable to manage hyperglycemia with insulin.

Hemodynamic instability is managed using advanced hemodynamic monitoring devices. Maintain adequate organ perfusion by targeting normal cardiac output and blood pressure. Keep in eubalance, Hydration, electrolyte correction and temperature management to optimise the maintenance of a healthy organ. Vasopressin is used as the first line of vasopressor in diabetes insipidus patients.

Brain death causes diffuse vascular and metabolic cellular injury, leading to organ failure and, eventually, cardiovascular death. This occurs in two phases:

1. Early phase: Massive sympathetic outflow (autonomic storm) causes bradycardia, and hypertension (Cushing's reflex), with adrenaline levels rising 750 times and noradrenaline 400 times.

2. Secondary phase: A significant reduction in sympathetic outflow leads to decreased cardiac output, vasodilatation and impaired autoregulation.

Cardiovascular effects include bradyarrhythmias, later tachycardia, multifocal ventricular ectopics and ischemic changes. Kidney function is compromised due to poor renal perfusion, while the liver can usually tolerate hypotension due to its reserve. Pituitary dysfunction causes diabetes insipidus; there is a marked reduction in thyroid hormone and cortisol levels. Coagulation is disrupted by the catecholamine storm, leading to consumption coagulopathy.

4. General post-operative ICU care of solid organ transplant recipients

4.1 Pain management post solid organ transplant

Appropriate perioperative pain management is crucial for enhancing the patient's experience, optimising post-operative results and facilitating functional recovery after surgery. Poorly managed pain may exacerbate the body's stress response to the surgical procedure and prolong the recovery period, leading to both physical and psychological distress. Effective post-operative pain control is a multidisciplinary process, and it should be individualised to each patient's needs, using a multimodal approach that follows Enhanced Recovery After Surgery guidelines [5]. Opioids are crucial in pain management, but nonopioid analgesics like APAP, neuropathic pain agents and epidural and local anaesthetics can enhance analgesia and reduce opioid requirements [6].

Liver transplantation (LT) is one of the most extensive abdominal surgery, requiring adequate analgesia to prevent pathophysiological consequences. Factors such as increased plasma levels of endogenous neuropeptides and the initial large doses of steroids may contribute to pain relief [7]. However, the likelihood of perioperative hemodynamic and coagulation changes presents challenges in recommending an optimal analgesic regimen for all patients. Intravenous patient-controlled opioid-based analgesia, with morphine and fentanyl, is the most commonly used analgesic in liver and renal transplants [8]. However, there is increasing concern about opioids due to their adverse effects [8]. Thoracic epidural analgesia is considered the golden standard in major open abdominal surgeries but is controversial due to post-operative coagulopathy and the risk of epidural hematoma [8]. The safety of thoracic epidural analgesia (TEA) in liver resections depends on appropriate timing and individual skill. Intrathecal morphine (ITM) is effective post-operative pain control. However, its use is limited due to adverse side effects [8].

Paracetamol has been commonly used as part of multimodal analgesia, either alone or as an adjunct to opioids for managing mild-to-moderate pain. It is metabolised in the liver to N-acetyl-p-benzoquinone imine (NAPQI), which can cause hepatotoxicity. Studies show increased NAPQI production in the first 10 days post-liver transplant, suggesting avoiding it until liver function stabilises [9]. In renal transplant recipients, no studies exist, but it should be safe for patients with normal liver function. Post-operative pain management is crucial for early recovery after kidney transplant surgery, but options are limited due to comorbidities, altered drug pharmacokinetics and contraindications to nephrotoxic NSAIDs [10].

In summary, Opioid use in abdominal organ transplant recipients affects short- and long-term outcomes. Nonopioid management strategies should be considered post-operatively, especially for opioid-using patients. However, evidence is limited, and further research is needed.

4.2 Nutritional support and management

Assessment of the nutritional status and nutritional support in organ transplant recipients can improve outcomes, especially so during the pretransplant stage. Nutritional assessment should consider physical state, medical history, anthropometric measurements and laboratory data. Malnutrition can compromise post-transplant survival, and severe obesity can decrease graft function and survival [11].

Adequate nutrition is needed during the acute post-transplant phase to prevent infection, promote wound healing, support metabolic demands and mediate the immune response [11]. Subjective global assessment (SGA) is a reliable method, while other tests like DEXA and dilution techniques are often restricted for research purposes [11]. Solid organ transplant patients face unique challenges due to chronic disease, transplant-specific complications and immunosuppressant medications. Common transplant challenges affect nutrition therapy, necessitating consideration of malnutrition, metabolic aberrations and organ dysfunction in developing a nutrition care plan [12]. The ESPEN Guidelines advocate initiating early normal oral intake or enteral nutrition following heart, lung, liver, pancreas or kidney transplantation. While enteral or parenteral support may be necessary in certain complex cases, oral nutrition is preferential [13].

Nutritional care post-transplant concentrates on recovery, wound healing, mobilisation, correcting anaemia and managing acute complications. Maintaining a neutral or positive nitrogen balance demands a high-protein, high-calorie diet, especially for those with malnutrition or frailty before transplantation [14]. Supplements are commonly needed to counter phosphate and magnesium losses induced by immunosuppressants. Dysglycaemia is common in the first weeks after transplantation, and postsurgical inflammation and high-dose immunosuppressive medications promote insulin resistance [14]. Close collaboration between physicians and dietitians is essential, and understanding changes in blood sugar levels is important for advising food intake and diabetes medication timing [14].

The formula of 25 kcal/kg ideal body weight provides an approximate estimate of daily energy requirements. Under severe stress conditions, requirements may approach 30 kcal/kg ideal body weight, and a protein intake of 1.5 g/kg ideal body weight is generally effective in limiting nitrogen losses [15]. In the acute phase of critical severe illness, it is recommended not to provide more than 20–25 kcal/kg daily [15]. Appropriate and timely nutrition intervention becomes increasingly important in some situations, such as encephalopathy and acute kidney failure. Early post-operative enteral nutrition support is beneficial in decreasing mortality and morbidity in gastrointestinal surgery and liver transplantation (LT) [16]. Studies have shown that early initiation of enteral nutrition can lower the incidence of infectious complications [17]. Parenteral nutrition should only be used when EN is not feasible. If the patient is well-nourished before the surgery, parenteral nutrition should be delayed for 5–7 days other than initiating it immediately, except when enteral nutrition is not available [18]. Special nutritional agents have been shown to improve outcomes in specific critically ill patients, including post-LT. However, each agent may have different effects on patient outcomes, making it difficult to make a consistent and definite conclusion due to the disparity of literature [15].

5. Complications in ICU care of transplant recipients

5.1 Acute rejection

Allograft rejection is a significant challenge to successful solid organ transplantation, affecting graft survival and patient outcomes [19]. Allorecognition, the recognition of donor-derived antigens by recipient T cells, triggers graft rejection, leading to effector cells infiltrating the graft and causing tissue damage [20]. Advancements in immunosuppressive therapy have significantly improved short-term outcomes, with graft half-life significantly increasing in patients who avoid acute rejection in the first year post-transplantation [21]. The main types of rejection of transplanted organs are hyperacute, acute and chronic, based on their underlying mechanisms and timelines. Acute cellular rejection is the predominant mechanism in the absence of pre-existing antibodies against the donor.

Hyperacute rejection is a severe form of rejection that occurs within minutes of transplantation and affects vascularised grafts. It is characterised by blood vessel thrombosis leading to graft death. Hyperacute rejection occurs due to pre-existing anti-donor antibodies that recognise antigens in the donor org [22]. These antibodies trigger complement activation and endothelial cells to release Von Willebrand factor, leading to platelet adhesion, aggregation, intravascular thrombosis and graft loss [22]. Nowadays, this form of rejection is primarily prevented by checking for ABO compatibility and excluding the presence of anti-donor HLA antibodies through crossmatching techniques between donor cells and recipient.

Acute rejection is an immune response against the graft and occurs within 1 week to several months post-transplantation. It occurs when the recipient's immune system recognises the transplanted organ as foreign, leading to an immune response that damages the graft [23]. This is achieved by activating the innate system, which releases molecules from damaged cells during graft ischemia-perfusion injury. This process allows the maturation of APCs, particularly dendritic cells, which activate the adaptive immune system, causing a lymphocytic infiltrate in the tissue [24]. Antibody-mediated rejection (ABMR) is characterised by the development of *de novo* donor-specific antibodies (DSAs). In contrast, T-cell-mediated rejection (TCMR) occurs when the recipient's T cells are activated against allogeneic graft peptides [23, 24].

Diagnosis of acute rejection involves clinical assessment of signs and symptoms, laboratory studies to assess organ function and histopathologic inflammatory changes on tissue biopsy [25]. Acute rejection is managed with immunosuppressive treatment, but continuous biochemical follow-up and detection of *de novo* DSAs are necessary for differential diagnosis and correct management [24].

5.2 Graft dysfunction

Graft dysfunction is the impaired function of a transplanted organ, which can occur at various times after the transplant and may have several underlying reasons [26].

5.2.1 Lung transplant patients

Primary graft dysfunction is an acute lung injury that occurs within the first 72 hours after lung transplantation. It is the leading cause of early mortality in lung transplant recipients, characterised by pulmonary oedema, diffuse alveolar damage, progressive hypoxemia and radiographic pulmonary infiltrates [27]. The severity of PGD is based on the ARDS definition and is similarly graded by a P/F ratio ranging from grade 0 to 3. It is assessed at four time points, starting at the time of reperfusion of the second lung and then at 24, 48 and 72 hours [27]. Treatments for PGD are mainly supportive and guided by approaches used for ARDS patients, such as lung-protective ventilation strategies, avoidance of fluid overload, inhaled nitric oxide or prostacyclin and extracorporeal membrane oxygenation (ECMO) support.

5.2.2 Liver transplant patients

Early allograft dysfunction (EAD) describes grafts with marginal function early after liver transplantation, ranging from mild transient biochemical derangement to acute liver failure, potentially leading to graft loss [28]. EAD is a severe form of ischemia/reperfusion injury to the liver graft, often linked to damage from reactive oxygen species [29]. Another feared post-operative complication is primary graft failure (PGF), manifested by hepatic coma, renal dysfunction, coagulopathy, jaundice and hypoglycemia. Several markers of hepatocellular damage and synthetic impairment, such as INR, bilirubin, ALT, and AST during the first week after transplantation, are used to evaluate graft dysfunction [30]. Treatment is supportive care focused on organ failure management and potential retransplantation consideration, especially in cases of PGF [28].

5.2.3 Renal transplant patients

Delayed graft function (DGF) is generally defined as the need for dialysis treatment within the first week after kidney transplantation, low or absent urine output immediately after transplantation or failure of serum creatinine to decline by more than 25% within 24 hours of transplant. Persistent dysfunction without timely intervention may lead to irreversible loss of allograft function. Early allograft dysfunction can occur due to various causes, such as acute rejection, vascular thrombosis, urinary obstruction and medication toxicity [31]. Clinical evaluation of DGF includes measuring serum creatinine concentration and associated eGFR and Doppler ultrasonography to assess for vascular and urological complications [31].

6. Infection risk and prophylaxis

Infection risk and prophylaxis are critical aspects of managing transplanted patients, who face a heightened risk of infections due to immunosuppression, surgical exposure and the potential reactivation of latent infections [32]. Tailored strategies are necessary to mitigate morbidity and mortality while minimising the risk of graft rejection and drug-related toxicities.

Transplanted patients encounter distinct phases of infection risk. In the early post-transplant period (0–1 month), infections commonly stem from surgical procedures, hospital-acquired sources or donor-derived pathogens [33]. Gram-positive cocci (*Staphylococcus spp.*), gram-negative bacteria (*Pseudomonas spp.*, *Klebsiella spp.*) and fungi (*Candida*) are frequent pathogens, leading to complications like wound infections, UTIs or pneumonia. The intermediate period (1–6 months) is marked by the reactivation of latent infections and opportunistic pathogens, such as viruses (*CMV, BK virus, EBV, HSV and VZV*), fungi (*Aspergillus, Cryptococcus*), and protozoa (*Toxoplasma*), causing conditions like cytomegalovirus disease, invasive fungal infections or polyomavirus-associated nephropathy. Beyond 6 months, during the late post-transplant phase, community-acquired or latent infections predominate. Respiratory viruses (*influenza, RSV*), opportunistic pathogens in patients with prolonged immunosuppression and chronic viral infections (*HBV, HCV* and *HIV*) become more relevant.

Prophylactic measures are crucial for reducing infection risks. Antibacterial prophylaxis often involves TMP-SMX for preventing *Pneumocystis jirovecii* pneumonia (PCP), toxoplasmosis and UTIs, with alternatives like dapsone, atovaquone or pentamidine for sulfa-allergic patients [34]. This is generally administered 6–12 months post-transplant or longer in high-risk cases. Viral prophylaxis depends on risk stratification, such as valganciclovir or ganciclovir for CMV, particularly in high-risk D+/R– patients [35], and acyclovir or valacyclovir for HSV and VZV during the initial post-transplant period [36]. HBV management includes pre-transplant vaccination for seronegative individuals and post-transplant prophylaxis with entecavir or tenofovir for HBV-positive cases [37], while HCV is addressed with direct-acting antivirals, either pre- or post-transplant [38]. Fungal prophylaxis targets pathogens like *Candida* with fluconazole and *Aspergillus* with voriconazole or posaconazole, especially in lung or heart transplant recipients, with TMP-SMX covering *Pneumocystis jirovecii*. Protozoal infections like *Toxoplasma gondii* are also managed with TMP-SMX in at-risk patients [39].

Immunisation is another cornerstone of infection prevention. Pre-transplant vaccinations should be administered before initiating immunosuppression, including pneumococcal, influenza, HBV, Tdap, and, where appropriate, MMR and varicella. Post-transplant vaccinations are limited to inactivated vaccines, given after immunosuppression stabilises, usually 3–6 months post-transplant, with live vaccines avoided unless deemed safe [40].

Long-term care and monitoring focus on surveillance for latent infections like CMV, BK virus or TB, alongside regular assessment of graft function, as infections may present subtly, such as a rise in creatinine in cases of BK virus nephropathy. Patient education is vital to ensure early reporting of symptoms like fever, malaise or wound redness and adherence to prophylaxis and hygiene measures. Adopting proactive approaches to prophylaxis, monitoring and immunisation can minimise infection risks, leading to improved outcomes.

6.1 Early recognition and management of sepsis

Sepsis management in transplant patients is particularly challenging due to immunosuppression, which blunts typical inflammatory responses, masking symptoms like fever. Atypical presentations, such as lethargy, confusion or unexplained organ dysfunction, are common [41]. Early recognition relies on subtle clinical and laboratory indicators, including vital signs, elevated CRP or procalcitonin and organ dysfunction markers like lactate or creatinine. Risk factors for sepsis include recent transplantation, intensive immunosuppression, invasive devices and viral reactivations like CMV or EBV.

Management begins with early identification using qSOFA or SOFA criteria, prompt administration of broad-spectrum antibiotics targeting likely pathogens (e.g., *Pseudomonas*, *Candida*), fluid resuscitation and source control, such as removing infected catheters. Immunosuppressive therapy may need temporary adjustment to balance infection control with graft rejection risks. Adjunctive measures include organ support, such as vasopressors for hemodynamic stability and renal replacement therapy for acute kidney injury. Preventive strategies are essential, including antimicrobial prophylaxis, immunisations, strict infection control measures and regular monitoring.

6.2 Immunosuppressive therapy

Immunosuppressive therapy aims to prevent graft rejection while minimising adverse effects like infections, malignancies or metabolic complications [42]. Induction therapy involves high-dose immunosuppressants, such as ATG or IL-2 receptor antagonists, at the time of transplantation to suppress early immune responses. Maintenance therapy uses a combination of calcineurin inhibitors (CNIs), antimetabolites, corticosteroids or mTOR inhibitors for long-term graft preservation. In cases of acute rejection, rescue therapy with high-dose corticosteroids or antibody therapies is employed. Regular monitoring of drug levels and organ function is necessary to mitigate risks like nephrotoxicity, hypertension or infections.

6.3 Cardiovascular complication

Cardiovascular complications post-transplant are influenced by pre-existing conditions, immunosuppressive drugs, and sedentary lifestyles, including hypertension, dyslipidemia, arrhythmias, coronary artery disease (CAD) and heart failure. Hypertension, often linked to CNIs, is managed with ACE inhibitors, while statins address dyslipidemia. Arrhythmias stemming from electrolyte imbalances or surgical scarring require antiarrhythmic medications or pacemaker implantation. CAD and transplant vasculopathy necessitate annual screenings and aggressive risk reduction. Lifestyle interventions, such as low-sodium diets, exercise and smoking cessation, are critical alongside pharmacologic therapy with cardioprotective agents and regular monitoring.

6.4 Pulmonary complications

Pulmonary complications, both infectious and noninfectious, are significant in transplant patients. Bacterial infections like *Pseudomonas aeruginosa* and *S. aureus*, fungal infections like *Aspergillus* and *Pneumocystis jirovecii* and viral infections like CMV and respiratory viruses are managed with tailored antibiotic, antifungal and antiviral regimens. Noninfectious complications include primary graft dysfunction, chronic lung allograft dysfunction (CLAD), drug-induced pulmonary toxicity, pulmonary hypertension and pulmonary oedema or embolism. Regular pulmonary function tests, imaging and prophylactic strategies like TMP-SMX and antifungals help prevent and monitor these conditions.

By addressing these risks comprehensively through prophylaxis, monitoring and patient education, the outcomes for transplant recipients can be significantly improved.

7. Special considerations for specific organ transplants

7.1 Dialysis after renal transplant

Compared to individuals on dialysis, kidney transplant recipients exhibit improved survival outcomes, enhanced quality of life and reduced healthcare resource utilisation [43]. Despite advancements in immunosuppressive therapies, patient management and the growing utilisation of living donors, a return to dialysis following transplant failure remains a common outcome. Approximately one-third of cadaveric kidney transplant recipients experience graft loss within 5 years post-transplantation [44]. Patients who require dialysis after transplant failure have higher mortality rates, yet they may benefit from a repeat transplantation procedure; however, only 15% of these patients will ultimately receive an additional transplant [45]. Continued immunosuppression to maintain residual graft function has been identified as a potential contributing factor for increased mortality, likely due to the associated risks of cardiovascular complications, infectious diseases and increased malignancy risk. However, continued low-dose immunosuppression has been proposed to provide a survival advantage for patients reverting to peritoneal dialysis after transplant failure [46].

Dialysis required within the first post-operative week after kidney transplantation is defined as delayed graft function, irrespective of the underlying cause of kidney dysfunction. Delayed graft function has been independently linked to approximately two- to threefold higher risks of patient mortality, graft failure and death-censored graft failure [47]. The optimal timing for initiating dialysis following graft failure remains unclear. Thus, clinicians must rely on the indications used for the general population of CKD patients, guided by their clinical presentation and biochemical parameters such as fluid overload refractory to diuretic therapy, severe hyperkalemia, severe metabolic acidosis and over manifestations of uremia [48].

The optimal dialysis choice in the post-operative period after kidney transplantation has been well studied. Haemodialysis is usually the preferred modality in the post-transplant setting due to worries about potential peritoneal disruption during surgery and increased infectious risk. The best management of peritoneal dialysis catheters after kidney transplantation remains controversial. Numerous transplant facilities have adopted keeping the PD catheter in place for no less than 12 weeks post-op, only removing it provided graft function is satisfactory. This method aims to maintain the option to transition back to peritoneal dialysis should the transplant fail [49].

Some experts advise the removal of the peritoneal dialysis catheter during transplantation to lower peritonitis risk [50]. However, peritoneal dialysis can be a viable alternative for selected patients with delayed graft function after kidney transplantation [51]. Lastly, excessive fluid removal should be prevented to avoid potential ischemic injury to the transplanted kidney.

7.2 Urinary output monitoring and complications

Immediate graft function refers to urine output and declining serum creatinine levels immediately after renal transplantation. It should be 100% for living donor kidney transplants, but for deceased donor kidneys, it will be influenced by the functioning of the donor organ at the time of procurement and the cold ischemia time [52]. Delayed graft function is common in kidney transplantation from deceased donors. In such cases, oliguria or even anuria may be tolerated, provided the patient's blood pressure remains adequate [53].

Post-operative poor graft function manifested as oliguria or anuria should prompt immediate evaluation. Complications such as vascular thrombosis, ureteral obstruction or acute rejection require urgent identification and management to prevent further deterioration of renal function. Absent or diminished urine output associated with increasing serum creatinine levels may indicate significant graft dysfunction or failure [54].

Moreover, the evaluation of volume status is essential. Hypovolemic oliguric transplant patients may benefit dramatically from volume resuscitation, while those who are overloaded could respond well to diuretics. The transplant recipient's condition dictates the precise approach, so discerning the appropriate remedy necessitates astute assessment and monitoring. Polyuria is frequent in the early post-operative period in living donor transplants. This should be closely monitored, and overall fluid status should be managed carefully to avoid dehydration [52].

A sudden decrease in urine output following adequate drainage necessitates prompt evaluation of the Foley catheter. Initially, a catheter examination is warranted to check for kinks obstructing urine flow. Should this fail to resolve the issue, catheter irrigation may clear potential clots inhibiting passage. If irrigation proves ineffective at improving output, catheter replacement should occur under the guidance of the transplant surgeon. When interventions with the Foley catheter do not restore the urine output, urgent notification of the transplant surgeon is critical, given the possibility of life-threatening complications such as vascular thrombosis [52].

8. Liver transplantation

Liver transplantation (LT) stands as a crucial intervention for patients with end-stage liver disease, acute liver failure or severe metabolic liver disorders. This chapter aims to provide a brief overview of the essential aspects of ICU management following liver transplantation, encompassing monitoring, early identification of complications and therapeutic interventions.

8.1 Hemodynamic monitoring

Hemodynamic monitoring is a cornerstone of post-operative care in liver transplant recipients. In the immediate post-operative period, continuous hemodynamic monitoring is vital. Orthotopic liver transplantation (OLT) is associated with significant hemodynamic instability [55]. Hemodynamic disturbance can be managed using the standard thermodilution technique by using a pulmonary artery catheter (PAC) or measuring cardiac output (CO) by pulse contour analysis technique [55]. Until now, no consensus exists on the type of hemodynamic monitoring in liver transplants.

The goals of fluid resuscitation are to maintain perfusion, prevent organ dysfunction and optimise urine output. Crystalloids are the primary choice, with colloids or blood products used as necessary. Avoid chloride-rich solutions to prevent acidosis. It is generally recommended for rational use of transfusion as there has been an association between blood transfusion and increased morbidity/mortality [56, 57].

Regular arterial blood gas (ABG) analysis is integral to hemodynamic monitoring, providing vital information regarding the patient's acid-base balance, strong ion difference, base deficit and so forth.

8.2 Respiratory management

Given the complexity of liver transplantation, patients are at risk for various respiratory complications that necessitate vigilant monitoring and timely intervention. Ventilating a patient in post-operative period, strategies like lung-protective ventilation with low tidal volumes and appropriate PEEP reduce lung injury [58]. Extubation is encouraged early if the patient is stable, using non-invasive ventilation (NIV) or high-flow nasal cannula as bridges. In order to prevent pulmonary complications and improve oxygenation, the use of incentive spirometry, appropriate positioning and early mobilisation is recommended.

8.2.1 Special situations

Hepatopulmonary Syndromes (HPS) and Porto pulmonary hypertension are the complications that exist in this group of patients. A certain group of HPS patients remains hypoxic due to this condition even 6–12 months after transplantation. In these groups of patients, careful monitoring of oxygenation and early extubation facilitated with NIV and high FiO2 support could be an option [59].

8.3 Graft function monitoring

Monitoring and management of liver graft function is critical in the immediate post-operative period following liver transplantation. Multiple factors, including those related to the donor, recipient and the graft itself, contribute to predicting post-operative graft function. Key parameters for graft function monitoring are liver enzymes (ALT and AST indicate hepatocyte integrity; ALP and GGT signal cholestasis), bilirubin Levels (rising levels may indicate complications), coagulation tests, imaging and biopsy. Early identification and supportive care are vital for ischemia-reperfusion injuries or primary non-function. Tailored regimens prevent rejection while minimising infections and side effects.

8.4 Acute rejection

Acute rejection typically occurs within the first few weeks following transplant and can manifest with fever, malaise or jaundice. Elevated liver enzymes and bilirubin levels may be present. Management of acute rejection is being done with steroid therapy and, in some cases (Antibody-mediated rejection), with IVIG.

8.5 Renal dysfunction and management

Follow up with serum creatinine, BUN and urine output to look for any acute kidney injury. Early intervention with fluid management, medication adjustment or renal replacement therapy (RRT) prevents complications. Treat prerenal causes like dehydration promptly. Adjusting nephrotoxic medications is an important area in dealing with renal failure.

8.6 Coagulation and bleeding

Management: Liver transplantation is associated with coagulopathy due to the decreased production of clotting factors and fibrinolysis. Coagulation status must be carefully monitored using standard laboratory tests, such as PT/INR, and more advanced techniques, like point-of-care viscoelastic tests like thromboelastography (TEG) or rotational thromboelastometry (ROTEM). Restrict blood products to minimise risks like sepsis and/or rejection [56, 57].

8.7 Immunosuppression

Immunosuppression was achieved with calcineurin inhibitors (e.g., Tacrolimus), antiproliferative agents (e.g., Mycophenolate Mofetil) and steroids. Acute rejection should promptly be recognised by elevated liver enzymes and managed with high-dose steroids or additional immunosuppressive agents.

8.8 Infection prevention and management

Preoperative hepatocellular dysfunction in cirrhotic patients predisposes an increased risk of infections, including spontaneous bacterial peritonitis (SBP), cholangitis, pneumonia, urinary tract infections (UTIs) and catheter-related bloodstream infections [60]. Immunosuppression and preoperative liver disease heighten infection risks, necessitating stringent empirical prophylaxis. Pre-transplant vaccinations, strict aseptic techniques, and minimising invasive device use are critical for preventing infections in the post-transplant phase.

8.9 Neurologic monitoring

Neurological complications are not so uncommon after LT, with a 15–30% incidence rate. In recipients from living donors, major neurologic complications in the immediate post-operative period include altered mental status, seizures, hepatic encephalopathy, CNI neurotoxicity, cerebrovascular complications, central nervous system infections and central pontine myelinolysis (CPM) [61].

8.10 Nutritional management

It has been observed that in patients with ESLD, malnutrition is a major problem due to the disease process, and it deteriorates with the progression of liver failure and affects the patients' outcomes [62]. A tailored approach to nutritional care is essential to meet the unique needs of these patients during the recovery phase.

The management of patients following liver transplantation in the intensive care unit (ICU) is multifaceted and requires a comprehensive, multidisciplinary approach. Effective post-transplant care is essential not only for preventing acute and chronic rejection but also for ensuring overall patient safety and promoting optimal recovery.

9. ICU management of the heart transplant recipient

Managing heart transplant recipients is a delicate, ongoing balancing act requiring constant vigilance. While complications like graft failure, arrhythmias and renal dysfunction are common, timely recognition and intervention can often mitigate their impact, improving both survival and quality of life [63]. The success of a heart transplant is not defined solely by the surgery itself but by the meticulous care that follows—an intricate orchestration of monitoring, intervention and adaptation to each patient's unique needs.

Hemodynamic monitoring is critical in the post-transplant period. Even minor fluctuations in preload or afterload can jeopardise graft function. Continuous monitoring of systemic and pulmonary artery pressures and central venous pressure (CVP) provides essential insight into the cardiovascular status. Intermittent measures like pulmonary capillary wedge pressure (PCWP) and cardiac output (CO) offer a fuller picture [64]. Reperfusion injury often leads to both systolic and diastolic dysfunction, making echocardiography vital, especially when instability arises. Detecting complications such as right ventricular (RV) failure early—marked by impaired systolic function and paradoxical septal movement—can make all the difference [65].

Arrhythmias, due to the denervated nature of the transplanted heart, are common, with sinus bradycardia and supraventricular arrhythmias often requiring atrial pacing [66]. A heart rate of 90–110 beats per minute is crucial for optimal cardiac output, particularly with the diastolic dysfunction characteristic of a transplanted heart. Inotropic agents like isoproterenol, dopamine and milrinone are used to support both chronotropic and inotropic function in the early post-operative phase, gradually tapering off as the patient stabilises [64]. Norepinephrine is introduced to maintain adequate mean arterial pressure, though its potential to worsen RV failure is mitigated by current evidence suggesting minimal impact on pulmonary vasoconstriction [67]. In severe cases of RV failure, therapies like inhaled nitric oxide or prostacyclin may be used to induce selective pulmonary vasodilation, reducing RV afterload. If these fail, mechanical circulatory support becomes necessary [68].

Graft failure, particularly early primary graft dysfunction (PGD), remains a leading cause of mortality, especially in the first year. PGD may present as left ventricular (LV), RV or biventricular dysfunction, with isolated RV failure being the most serious and significant risk factor for mortality [69]. RV failure often stems from pre-existing pulmonary vascular resistance (PVR) or donor-recipient size mismatch. Other factors, like cardiopulmonary bypass or blood transfusions, can exacerbate PVR. Immediate intervention is crucial when RV failure is suspected—marked by elevated CVP or a mismatch between CVP and PCWP/LAP. Management involves careful monitoring of filling pressures and maintaining a balanced intraventricular state, which can be tracked with echocardiography and by adjusting hemodynamic values to optimise flow and oxygenation.

Immunosuppression is crucial to preventing graft rejection but comes with its own challenges, notably increased susceptibility to infections and malignancies. Around half of heart transplant recipients receive induction therapy, often with anti-thymocyte or anti-lymphocyte globulins or interleukin-2 receptor antagonists, which has been linked to improved long-term survival [70]. However, CNIs can be nephrotoxic, especially in patients with pre-existing renal dysfunction. To minimise this risk, induction therapy may be used to delay CNI exposure. An everolimus-based regimen, which eliminates CNIs early, has been shown to preserve kidney function and reduce the need for renal replacement therapy, ultimately improving both survival and quality of life [71].

Renal dysfunction, particularly acute kidney injury (AKI), complicates up to 50% of heart transplants, with many requiring dialysis [72]. Contributing factors include reduced renal oxygen delivery during surgery, RV failure and nephrotoxic medications like calcineurin inhibitors (CNI). Early recognition and intervention are essential to prevent progression to dialysis dependence [73]. The infusion of low-dose atrial natriuretic peptide (ANP) has shown promise in improving renal blood flow and reducing the need for dialysis, offering a valuable tool in managing post-transplant renal dysfunction [74].

In the end, the success of a heart transplant depends on more than just the surgery—it requires continuous, tailored care. Every complication, from graft failure to renal dysfunction, demands quick identification and intervention, often in the form of a finely tuned balance of medications, monitoring and support. Through careful management, the challenges of heart transplantation can be navigated, leading to better outcomes for recipients.

10. ICU management of the lung transplant recipient

In managing post-lung transplant patients, the ICU team must balance the myriad physiological challenges the patient faces. With careful monitoring, strategic interventions and a deep understanding of the complex interplay of respiratory and cardiovascular function, the risks associated with transplantation can be mitigated, optimising outcomes for these critically ill patients.

In the hours and days following a lung transplant, the challenges of hemodynamic support are immense. Reperfusion injury, pulmonary hypertension and systemic inflammation often contribute to hemodynamic instability, so careful monitoring is of vital importance [75]. The pulmonary artery catheter (PAC), which tracks pulmonary artery pressures, cardiac output and pulmonary capillary wedge pressure, becomes an essential tool. These metrics are vital for detecting graft dysfunction, right ventricular failure and fluid management needs.

Fluid management requires a delicate balance. Hypovolemia can compromise perfusion, while fluid overload risks pulmonary oedema. Crystalloids are typically used in early post-op, while colloids like albumin help manage oedema. Goal-directed therapy ensures perfusion while preventing overload, but diuretics like furosemide must be used cautiously to avoid kidney injury [76].

For more severe hemodynamic instability, vasopressors like norepinephrine are essential to maintain blood pressure, with vasopressin sometimes added to reduce norepinephrine needs. Inotropes such as dobutamine and milrinone support right ventricular function, improving contractility and reducing pulmonary pressures [77]. In cases of severe pulmonary hypertension, inhaled nitric oxide and medications like sildenafil can help lower pulmonary vascular resistance and improve right ventricular performance [78].

Right ventricular failure is a significant concern post-transplant, especially for those with pre-existing pulmonary hypertension. In less severe cases, inotropes are used to support heart function. However, when failure is more pronounced, veno-arterial ECMO offers life-saving circulatory support, buying time for recovery [79].

Ventilatory management is equally critical. Most patients require mechanical ventilation early on, with strategies designed to protect the lung graft. Low tidal volumes, careful monitoring of peak pressures and the use of PEEP and FiO2 help optimise oxygenation without causing graft injury. Volume-controlled ventilation (VCV) or pressure-controlled ventilation (PCV) is chosen based on the patient's needs, particularly in cases of low lung compliance or graft dysfunction [80]. The goal is early extubation to avoid the complications of prolonged ventilation. However, extubation must be timed carefully based on good oxygenation, hemodynamic stability and respiratory drive. When extubation is delayed, non-invasive ventilation (NIV) can provide support without the risks of extended mechanical ventilation.

Primary graft dysfunction (PGD) is a common complication, occurring in up to 30% of recipients [75]. Managing PGD involves lung-protective strategies, including high PEEP, prone positioning and the use of inhaled nitric oxide. In severe cases, ECMO may be required to provide respiratory support until the graft stabilises [81]. Preventing ventilator-associated pneumonia (VAP) is another priority; early extubation, head-of-bed elevation and vigilant oral care help reduce the risk.

Beyond respiratory and hemodynamic support, special considerations complicate recovery. Renal dysfunction, often due to nephrotoxic immunosuppressive drugs or surgical stress, must be managed with care. Close monitoring of renal function and electrolytes and early intervention with renal replacement therapy, if needed, are essential [82]. Neurological complications, such as delirium and stroke, are common and must be addressed with early detection and appropriate interventions [83]. Immunosuppressive therapy is critical in preventing acute rejection, yet it must be carefully managed to avoid infection or drug toxicity. A typical regimen includes calcineurin inhibitors, antimetabolites and corticosteroids, with adjustments based on monitoring for nephrotoxicity, neurotoxicity and bone marrow suppression [84]. Despite these precautions, infections remain a significant risk. Bacterial pneumonia, particularly from *Pseudomonas aeruginosa*, is common early on, as are viral and fungal infections. Prophylaxis, early detection and timely treatment are crucial to reducing infection-related morbidity and mortality [85].

11. Pancreas transplantation

11.1 ICU management of pancreas transplant recipients

The management of pancreas transplant patients in the intensive care unit (ICU) requires a multidisciplinary approach to ensure graft survival, prevent complications and support patient recovery. Pancreas transplantation is primarily performed for patients with Type 1 diabetes and select cases of Type 2 diabetes to restore glycemic control and improve quality of life. ICU care is critical in the immediate post-operative period to manage surgical, immunological and systemic challenges [86]. Key post-operative concerns include hemodynamic stability, graft function monitoring, infection control, immunosuppression management and management of any complication that might arise from surgery (e.g., bleeding, leaks at anastomosis sites, vascular thrombosis, etc.) or because of rejection (e.g., hyperglycemia or elevated pancreatic enzymes).

Pancreas transplant patients often undergo simultaneous kidney-pancreas transplantation, which increases surgical complexity. Close monitoring of fluid status, blood pressure and perfusion is essential to avoid graft thrombosis, a significant cause of early graft loss. Vasopressors may be required, but excessive use can compromise graft perfusion. Early assessment of graft function is crucial. Serum glucose levels often normalise rapidly post-transplant, but persistent hyperglycemia or signs of pancreatitis may indicate graft dysfunction. Monitoring amylase, lipase and C-peptide levels can help detect complications [87]. Immunosuppression increases the risk of bacterial, fungal and viral infections. ICU protocols must include infection prevention strategies, including aseptic techniques, prophylactic antimicrobials and vigilant monitoring for fever, leukocytosis or other signs of infection. Patients require lifelong immunosuppression to prevent rejection. In the ICU, therapeutic drug monitoring of agents like tacrolimus or mycophenolate mofetil is necessary to maintain adequate levels while minimising toxicity [88].

ICU care should include comprehensive supportive care, including glycemic control (if needed), adequate pain management, deep vein thrombosis (DVT) prevention and early mobilisation. Nutritional support should avoid hyperglycemia-inducing solutions; enteral feeding is preferred to preserve gut integrity.

12. Ethical issues and communication with relatives

In the ICU, ethical issues and effective communication with family members are paramount. Families of potential donors often face emotionally charged decisions under significant stress, raising concerns about informed consent, respect for autonomy and maintaining trust. Ethical challenges include ensuring that the withdrawal of life-sustaining treatment is independent of the decision to donate organs and avoiding perceptions of conflict of interest. Clear, compassionate and transparent communication is essential to address family concerns, explain the donation process and navigate potential misconceptions or cultural sensitivities. Ethical guidelines also emphasise the need to respect the donor's prior wishes while balancing the emotional needs of the family. Clinicians must foster a supportive environment, ensuring that families have the time and information needed to make an informed decision without undue pressure. This approach not only upholds ethical standards but also supports the dignity of both the donor and their loved ones during a challenging time.

13. Long-term care and ICU discharge considerations

13.1 Criteria for ICU discharge for solid organ transplant patients

Discharging solid organ transplant patients from the ICU is a critical step that requires careful assessment to ensure their stability and continued recovery. A key criterion is the stability of graft function and the patient's overall clinical condition. The transplanted organ's function should demonstrate consistent and acceptable physiological parameters, such as stable renal function in kidney transplant recipients or normalised liver enzymes in liver transplant patients. Vital signs must remain within normal limits without the need for intensive monitoring or vasoactive drugs. Signs of rejection, infection or other complications should be addressed and under control before considering discharge [88].

Another essential component is the involvement of a multidisciplinary team in the decision-making process. Collaboration between transplant coordinators, intensivists, surgeons and allied health professionals, such as physical therapists, ensures comprehensive care. Transplant coordinators facilitate the transition to ward care by organising follow-up protocols, while physical therapy is essential for assessing mobility and initiating early rehabilitation to promote recovery. This team-based approach ensures continuity of care and minimises the risk of missed complications during the transition.

13.2 Post-ICU follow-up care

13.2.1 Transition to ward care and long-term immunosuppression management

Once stabilised in the ICU, transplant patients transition to ward care, where the focus shifts to long-term recovery and management. A critical element is long-term immunosuppression management, which prevents graft rejection. Close monitoring of immunosuppressive drug levels, kidney and liver function and infection markers is vital to prevent rejection and opportunistic infections. Protocols for immunosuppression often include a combination of calcineurin inhibitors, antiproliferative agents and corticosteroids tailored to individual patient needs.

13.2.2 Outpatient follow-up protocols

Effective post-discharge care involves robust outpatient follow-up. Transplant recipients typically undergo regular clinic visits to monitor graft function, adjust immunosuppressive therapy and manage complications. These visits often include blood tests, imaging and consultations with transplant specialists. Early detection of complications like chronic rejection or infection significantly improves long-term outcomes [88].

13.2.3 Psychological and social support

Solid organ transplant recipients frequently experience psychological stress due to fear of rejection, infection or financial burden. Offering psychological and social support is integral to improving quality of life and adherence to treatment. Transplant recipients benefit from counselling, peer support groups and social work services to address emotional and practical challenges [89]. Additionally, addressing these issues early promotes adherence to medications and follow-up care, improving graft and patient survival.

Author details

Sohel Mohamed Gamal Ahmed[1*], Abdelrahman Balal[1],
Sujith Madambikattil Prabhakaran[2], Zia Mahmood Awan[1],
Mogahed Ismail Hassan Hussein[1], Siddhartha Banerjee[1] and Wael Khalaf[1]

1 Hamad Medical Corporation, Qatar University College of Medicine, Doha, Qatar

2 Qatar University, Doha, Qatar

*Address all correspondence to: sohelm@yahoo.com

References

[1] A definition of irreversible coma: Report of the ad hoc committee of the Harvard Medical School to examine the definition of brain death. JAMA. 1968;**205**(6):337-340. DOI: 10.1001/jama.1968.03140320031009

[2] Spears W, Mian A, Greer D. Brain death: A clinical overview. Journal of Intensive Care. 2022;**10**(1):16. DOI: 10.1186/s40560-022-00609-4

[3] Greer DM et al. Pediatric and adult brain death/death by neurologic criteria consensus guideline. Neurology. 2023;**101**(24):1112-1132. DOI: 10.1212/WNL.0000000000207740

[4] Yoshikawa MH, Rabelo NN, Welling LC, Telles JPM, Figueiredo EG. Brain death and management of the potential donor. Neurological Sciences: Official Journal of the Italian Neurological Society and of the Italian Society of Clinical Neurophysiology. 2021;**42**(9):3541-3552. DOI: 10.1007/s10072-021-05360-6

[5] Joliat G-R et al. Guidelines for perioperative care for liver surgery: Enhanced recovery after surgery (ERAS) society recommendations 2022. World Journal of Surgery. 2023;**47**(1):11-34. DOI: 10.1007/s00268-022-06732-5

[6] Kutzler HL et al. A systematic review of opioid use and multimodal strategies in solid organ transplant recipients and living donors. The Journal of Human Pharmacology and Drug Therapy. 2023;**43**(6):514-551. DOI: 10.1002/phar.2808

[7] Feltracco P et al. Pain control after liver transplantation surgery. Transplantation Proceedings. 2014;**46**(7):2300-2307. DOI: 10.1016/j.transproceed.2014.07.023

[8] Tufegdzic B, Lobo C, Kumar A. Postoperative pain management after abdominal transplantations. Current Opinion in Anaesthesiology. 2024;**37**(5):504-512. DOI: 10.1097/ACO.0000000000001389

[9] Park JM et al. Transiently altered acetaminophen metabolism after liver transplantation. Clinical Pharmacology and Therapeutics. 2003;**73**(6):545-553. DOI: 10.1016/S0009-9236(03)00062-6

[10] Sridharan K, Shah S. Use of non-steroidal anti-inflammatory drugs in renal transplant patients: A retrospective study. The International Journal of Risk and Safety in Medicine. 2023;**34**(4):379-386. DOI: 10.3233/JRS-220065

[11] Hasse JM. Nutrition assessment and support of organ transplant recipients. JPEN Journal of Parenteral and Enteral Nutrition. 2001;**25**(3):120-131. DOI: 10.1177/0148607101025003120

[12] Hahn M, Wood A, Hasse JM. Nutrition support management of organ transplant recipients in the acute posttransplant phase. Nutrition in Clinical Practice. 2024;**39**(1):45-58. DOI: 10.1002/ncp.11104

[13] Weimann A et al. ESPEN guidelines on enteral nutrition: Surgery including organ transplantation. Clinical Nutrition. 2006;**25**(2):224-244. DOI: 10.1016/j.clnu.2006.01.015

[14] Stoler ST, Chan M, Chadban SJ. Nutrition in the management of kidney transplant recipients. Journal of Renal Nutrition. 2023;**33**(Suppl. 6):S67-S72. DOI: 10.1053/j.jrn.2023.07.001

[15] Zhang Q-K, Wang M-L. The management of perioperative nutrition

in patients with end stage liver disease undergoing liver transplantation. Hepatobiliary Surgery and Nutrition, 2015;**4**(5). Article 5. DOI: 10.3978/j.issn.2304-3881.2014.09.14

[16] Sekido H et al. Impact of early enteral nutrition after liver transplantation for acute hepatic failure: Report of four cases. Transplantation Proceedings. 2003;**35**(1):369-371. DOI: 10.1016/s0041-1345(02)03989-1

[17] Ikegami T et al. Bacterial sepsis after living donor liver transplantation: The impact of early enteral nutrition. Journal of the American College of Surgeons. 2012;**214**(3):288-295. DOI: 10.1016/j.jamcollsurg.2011.12.001

[18] McClave SA et al. Guidelines for the provision and assessment of nutrition support therapy in the adult critically ill patient: society of critical care medicine (SCCM) and American Society for Parenteral and Enteral Nutrition (A.S.P.E.N.). JPEN Journal of Parenteral and Enteral Nutrition. 2009;**33**(3):277-316. DOI: 10.1177/0148607109335234

[19] Cozzi E, Colpo A, De Silvestro G. The mechanisms of rejection in solid organ transplantation. Transfusion and Apheresis Science. 2017;**56**(4):498-505. DOI: 10.1016/j.transci.2017.07.005

[20] Ingulli E. Mechanism of cellular rejection in transplantation. Pediatric Nephrology Berlin Germany. 2010;**25**(1):61. DOI: 10.1007/s00467-008-1020-x

[21] Vincenti F. A decade of progress in kidney transplantation. Transplantation. 2004;**77**(9):S52. DOI: 10.1097/01.TP.0000126928.15055.DC

[22] Wood KJ, Goto R. Mechanisms of rejection: Current perspectives. Transplantation. 2012;**93**(1):1. DOI: 10.1097/TP.0b013e31823cab44

[23] Moreau A, Varey E, Anegon I, Cuturi M-C. Effector mechanisms of rejection. Cold Spring Harbor Perspectives in Medicine. 2013;**3**(11):a015461. DOI: 10.1101/cshperspect.a015461

[24] Fernández DM, Delgado MD, Amador FR. Transplant immunology I: Mechanisms of rejection in solid organ transplants. Journal of Stem Cell Research and Therapy. 2022;**7**(1):22-24. DOI: 10.15406/jsrt.2022.07.00152

[25] Justiz Vaillant AA, Misra S, Fitzgerald BM. Acute transplantation rejection. In: StatPearls. Treasure Island (FL): StatPearls Publishing; 2024. Available from: http://www.ncbi.nlm.nih.gov/books/NBK535410/ [Accessed: July 28, 2024]

[26] Sawinski D, Goral S. 39 - Diagnosis and therapy of graft dysfunction. In: Himmelfarb J, Ikizler TA, editors. Chronic Kidney Disease, Dialysis, and Transplantation. 4th ed. Philadelphia: Elsevier; 2019. pp. 605-620.e4. DOI: 10.1016/B978-0-323-52978-5.00039-2

[27] Suzuki Y, Cantu E, Christie JD. Primary graft dysfunction. Seminars in Respiratory and Critical Care Medicine. 2013;**34**(3):305-319. DOI: 10.1055/s-0033-1348474

[28] Kok B, Dong V, Karvellas CJ. Graft dysfunction and management in liver transplantation. Critical Care Clinics. 2019;**35**(1):117-133. DOI: 10.1016/j.ccc.2018.08.002

[29] Deschenes M. Early allograft dysfunction: Causes, recognition, and management. Liver Transplant. official publication of the American Association for the Study of Liver Diseases and the International Liver Transplant Society.

2013;**19**(Suppl. 2):S6-S8. DOI: 10.1002/lt.23746

[30] Olthoff KM et al. Validation of a current definition of early allograft dysfunction in liver transplant recipients and analysis of risk factors. Liver Transplant. official publication of the American Association for the Study of Liver Diseases and the International Liver Transplant Society. 2010;**16**(8):943-949. DOI: 10.1002/lt.22091

[31] Goldberg RJ, Weng FL, Kandula P. Acute and chronic allograft dysfunction in kidney transplant recipients. The Medical Clinics of North America. 2016;**100**(3):487-503. DOI: 10.1016/j.mcna.2016.01.002

[32] Fishman JA. Infection in solid-organ transplant recipients. The New England Journal of Medicine. 2007;**357**(25):2601-2614. DOI: 10.1056/NEJMra064928

[33] Pagalilauan GL, Limaye AP. Infections in transplant patients. The Medical Clinics of North America. 2013;**97**(4):581-600. DOI: 10.1016/j.mcna.2013.03.002

[34] Haseeb A et al. Trimethoprim-sulfamethoxazole (bactrim) dose optimisation in pneumocystis jirovecii pneumonia (PCP) management: A systematic review. International Journal of Environmental Research and Public Health. 2022;**19**(5):2833. DOI: 10.3390/ijerph19052833

[35] Humar A, Snydman D, the A. I. D. C. of Practice. Cytomegalovirus in solid organ transplant recipients. American Journal of Transplantation. 2009;**9**(s4):S78-S86. DOI: 10.1111/j.1600-6143.2009.02897.x

[36] Zuckerman RA, Limaye AP. Varicella zoster virus (VZV) and herpes simplex virus (HSV) in solid organ transplant patients. American Journal of Transplantation. 2013;**13**(s3):55-66. DOI: 10.1111/ajt.12003

[37] Lee YB et al. Efficacy of entecavir-tenofovir combination therapy for chronic hepatitis B patients with multidrug-resistant strains. Antimicrobial Agents and Chemotherapy. 2014;**58**(11):6710-6716. DOI: 10.1128/AAC.03845-14

[38] Bethea E et al. Immediate administration of antiviral therapy after transplantation of hepatitis C-infected livers into uninfected recipients: Implications for therapeutic planning. American Journal of Transplantation. 2020;**20**(6):1619-1628. DOI: 10.1111/ajt.15768

[39] Shoham S, Marr KA. Invasive fungal infections in solid organ transplant recipients. Future Microbiology. 2012;**7**(5):639-655. DOI: 10.2217/fmb.12.28

[40] Gangappa S et al. Immune responsiveness and protective immunity after transplantation. Transplant International. 2008;**21**(4):293-303. DOI: 10.1111/j.1432-2277.2007.00631.x

[41] Bafi AT, Tomotani DYV, de Freitas FGR. Sepsis in solid-organ transplant patients. Shock Augusta Ga. 2017;**47**(1S Suppl. 1):12-16. DOI: 10.1097/SHK.0000000000000700

[42] Claeys E, Vermeire K. Immunosuppressive drugs in organ transplantation to prevent allograft rejection: Mode of action and side effects. Journal of Immunological Sciences. 2019;**3**(4):14-21

[43] Strohmaier S et al. Survival benefit of first single-organ deceased donor kidney transplantation compared

with long-term dialysis across ages in transplant-eligible patients with kidney failure. JAMA Network Open. 2022;**5**(10):e2234971. DOI: 10.1001/jamanetworkopen.2022.34971

[44] Gill JS, Abichandani R, Kausz AT, Pereira BJG. Mortality after kidney transplant failure: The impact of non-immunologic factors. Kidney International. 2002;**62**(5):1875-1883. DOI: 10.1046/j.1523-1755.2002.00640.x

[45] Ojo AO et al. Prognosis after primary renal transplant failure and the beneficial effects of repeat transplantation: Multivariate analyses from the United States renal data system: 1,2. Transplantation. 1998;**66**(12):1651. Available from: https://journals.lww.com/transplantjournal/fulltext/1998/12270/prognosis_after_primary_renal_transplant_failure.14.aspx [Accessed: December 10, 2024]

[46] Pham P-T, Everly M, Faravardeh A, Pham P-C. Management of patients with a failed kidney transplant: Dialysis reinitiation, immunosuppression weaning, and transplantectomy. World Journal of Nephrology. 2015;**4**(2):148-159. DOI: 10.5527/wjn.v4.i2.148

[47] Tapiawala SN et al. Delayed graft function and the risk for death with a functioning graft. Journal of the American Society of Nephrology. 2010;**21**(1):153-161. DOI: 10.1681/ASN.2009040412

[48] Messa P, Ponticelli C, Berardinelli L. Coming back to dialysis after kidney transplant failure. Nephrology, Dialysis, Transplantation. 2008;**23**(9):2738-2742. DOI: 10.1093/ndt/gfn313

[49] Solak Y, Atalay H, Polat I, Yeksan M. CAPD-related peritonitis after renal transplantation. Peritoneal Dialysis International. Journal of the International Society for Peritoneal Dialysis. 2010;**30**(6):596-599. DOI: 10.3747/pdi.2009.00169

[50] Warren J et al. Should peritoneal dialysis catheters be removed at the time of kidney transplantation? Canadian Urological Association Journal. 2012;**6**(5):376-378. DOI: 10.5489/cuaj.12112

[51] Thomson BKA et al. Peritoneal dialysis versus hemodialysis in patients with delayed graft function. Clinical Transplantation. 2013;**27**(6):E709-E714. DOI: 10.1111/ctr.12266

[52] Barone CP, Lightfoot ML, Barone GW. The postanesthesia care of an adult renal transplant recipient. Journal of Perianesthesia Nursing. 2003;**18**(1):32-41. DOI: 10.1053/jpan.2003.50002

[53] Van Den Hoogen MWF et al. Care for the organ transplant recipient on the intensive care unit. Journal of Critical Care. 2021;**64**:37-44. DOI: 10.1016/j.jcrc.2021.03.003

[54] Michael Cecka J, Shoskes DA, Gjertson DW. Clinical impact of delayed graft function for kidney transplantation. Transplantation Reviews. 2001;**15**(2):57-67. DOI: 10.1016/S0955-470X(05)80001-1

[55] Rudnick MR, Marchi LD, Plotkin JS. Hemodynamic monitoring during liver transplantation: A state of the art review. World Journal of Hepatology. 2015;**7**(10):1302-1311. DOI: 10.4254/wjh.v7.i10.1302

[56] Cywinski JB, Alster JM, Miller C, Vogt DP, Parker BM. Prediction of intraoperative transfusion requirements during orthotopic liver transplantation and the influence on postoperative patient

survival. Anesthesia and Analgesia. 2014;**118**(2):428. DOI: 10.1213/ANE.0b013e3182a76f19

[57] Dunn LK, Thiele RH, Ma JZ, Sawyer RG, Nemergut EC. Duration of red blood cell storage and outcomes following orthotopic liver transplantation. Liver Transplant. Official Publication of the American Association for the Study of Liver Diseases and the International Liver Transplant Society. 2012;**18**(4):475-481. DOI: 10.1002/lt.23379

[58] Tobin MJ, Jubran A. Chapter 58. Weaning from mechanical ventilation. In: Tobin MJ, editor. Principles and Practice of Mechanical Ventilation. 3rd ed. New York, NY: The McGraw-Hill Companies; 2013. Available from: accessmedicine.mhmedical.com/content.aspx?aid=57079614 [Accessed: December 10, 2024]

[59] Cosarderelioglu C, Cosar AM, Gurakar M, Dagher NN, Gurakar A. Hepatopulmonary syndrome and liver transplantation: A recent review of the literature. Journal of Clinical and Translational Hepatology. 2016;**4**(1):47-53. DOI: 10.14218/JCTH.2015.00044

[60] Fischer SA, Lu K, AST Infectious Diseases Community of Practice. Screening of donor and recipient in solid organ transplantation. American Journal of Transplantation. Official Journal of the American Society of Transplantation and the American Society of Transplant Surgeons. 2013;**13**(Suppl. 4):9-21. DOI: 10.1111/ajt.12094

[61] Shi B. Clinical-analysis-of-neurological-complications-following-liver-transplantation. Biomedical Research. 2017;**28**(6):2471-2474

[62] Mandell MS et al. A multicenter evaluation of safety of early extubation in liver transplant recipients. Liver Transplantation. 2007;**13**(11):1557-1563. DOI: 10.1002/lt.21263

[63] Velleca A et al. The International Society for Heart and Lung Transplantation (ISHLT) guidelines for the care of heart transplant recipients. The Journal of Heart and Lung Transplantation. The Official Publication of the International Society for Heart and Lung Transplantation. 2023;**42**(5):e1-e141. DOI: 10.1016/j.healun.2022.10.015

[64] Costanzo MR et al. The international society of heart and lung transplantation guidelines for the care of heart transplant recipients. The Journal of Heart and Lung Transplantation (JHLT), The Official Publication of the International Society for Heart and Lung Transplantation. 2010;**29**(8):914-956. DOI: 10.1016/j.healun.2010.05.034

[65] Segovia J et al. Primary graft failure in heart transplantation: A multivariate analysis. Transplantation Proceedings. 1998;**30**(5):1932. DOI: 10.1016/s0041-1345(98)00485-0

[66] von Scheidt W, Böhm M, Schneider B, Autenrieth G, Erdmann E. Cholinergic baroreflex vasodilatation: Defect in heart transplant recipients due to denervation of the ventricular baroreceptor. The American Journal of Cardiology. 1992;**69**(3):247-252. DOI: 10.1016/0002-9149(92)91314-t

[67] Redfors B, Bragadottir G, Sellgren J, Swärd K, Ricksten S-E. Effects of norepinephrine on renal perfusion, filtration and oxygenation in vasodilatory shock and acute kidney injury. Intensive Care Medicine. 2011;**37**(1):60-67. DOI: 10.1007/s00134-010-2057-4

[68] Takeda K et al. Improved outcomes from extracorporeal membrane oxygenation versus ventricular assist

device temporary support of primary graft dysfunction in heart transplant. The Journal of Heart and Lung Transplantation (JHLT), The Official Publication of the International Society for Heart and Lung Transplantation. 2017;**36**(6):650-656. DOI: 10.1016/j.healun.2016.12.006

[69] Kobashigawa J et al. Report from a consensus conference on primary graft dysfunction after cardiac transplantation. The Journal of Heart and Lung Transplantation (JHLT), The Official Publication of the International Society for Heart and Lung Transplantation. 2014;**33**(4):327-340. DOI: 10.1016/j.healun.2014.02.027

[70] Ansari D et al. Induction with anti-thymocyte globulin in heart transplantation is associated with better long-term survival compared with basiliximab. The Journal of Heart and Lung Transplantation (JHLT), The Official Publication of the International Society for Heart and Lung Transplantation. 2015;**34**(10):1283-1291. DOI: 10.1016/j.healun.2015.04.001

[71] Andreassen AK et al. Everolimus initiation with early calcineurin inhibitor withdrawal in de novo heart transplant recipients: Three-year results from the randomised schedule study. American Journal of Transplantation. Official Journal of the American Society of Transplantation and the American Society of Transplant Surgeons. 2016;**16**(4):1238-1247. DOI: 10.1111/ajt.13588

[72] Lannemyr L, Bragadottir G, Krumbholz V, Redfors B, Sellgren J, Ricksten S-E. Effects of cardiopulmonary bypass on renal perfusion, filtration, and oxygenation in patients undergoing cardiac surgery. Anesthesiology. 2017;**126**(2):205-213. DOI: 10.1097/ALN.0000000000001461

[73] Aneman A et al. Advances in critical care management of patients undergoing cardiac surgery. Intensive Care Medicine. 2018;**44**(6):799-810. DOI: 10.1007/s00134-018-5182-0

[74] Nigwekar SU, Kulkarni H, Thakar CV. Natriuretic peptides in the management of solid organ transplantation associated acute kidney injury: A systematic review and meta-analysis. International Journal of Nephrology. 2013;**2013**:949357. DOI: 10.1155/2013/949357

[75] Di Nardo M et al. Postoperative management of lung transplant recipients in the intensive care unit. Anesthesiology. 2022;**136**(3):482-499. DOI: 10.1097/ALN.0000000000004054

[76] Duan Q, Zhang Y, Yang D. Perioperative fluid management for lung transplantation is challenging. Heliyon. 2023;**9**(4):e14704. DOI: 10.1016/j.heliyon.2023.e14704

[77] Legrand M, Zarbock A. Ten tips to optimise vasopressors use in the critically ill patient with hypotension. Intensive Care Medicine. 2022;**48**(6):736-739. DOI: 10.1007/s00134-022-06708-y

[78] Saygili A, Canter B, Iriz E, et al. Use of sildenafil with inhaled nitric oxide in the management of severe pulmonary hypertension (Gazi Univ, Ankara, Turkey). Journal of Cardiothoracic and Vascular Anesthesia. 2004;**18**:775-776. Available from: https://www.researchgate.net/publication/244862026_Use_of_Sildenafil_With_Inhaled_Nitric_Oxide_in_the_Management_of_Severe_Pulmonary_HypertensionSaygili_A_Canter_B_Iriz_E_et_al_Gazi_Univ_Ankara_Turkey_J_Cardiothorac_Vasc_Anesth_18775-776_2004 [Accessed: December 10, 2024]

[79] Hoyler M, Ivascu NS. Postoperative right ventricular failure. In:

Cardiothoracic Critical Care. UK: Oxford University Press; 2020. pp. 121-128. DOI: 10.1093/med/9780190082482.003.0011

[80] Beer A et al. Mechanical ventilation after lung transplantation. An international survey of practices and preferences. Annals of the American Thoracic Society. 2014;**11**(4):546-553. DOI: 10.1513/AnnalsATS.201312-419OC

[81] Van Raemdonck D et al. Report of the ISHLT working group on primary lung graft dysfunction part IV: Prevention and treatment: A 2016 consensus group statement of the International Society for Heart and Lung Transplantation. The Journal of Heart and Lung Transplantation is The Official Publication of the International Society for Heart and Lung Transplantation. 2017;**36**(10):1121-1136. DOI: 10.1016/j.healun.2017.07.013

[82] Lertjitbanjong P et al. Acute kidney injury after lung transplantation: A systematic review and meta-analysis. Journal of Clinical Medicine. 2019;**8**(10):1713. DOI: 10.3390/jcm8101713

[83] Živković SA, Jumaa M, Barišić N, McCurry K. Neurologic complications following lung transplantation. Journal of the Neurological Sciences. 2009;**280**(1):90-93. DOI: 10.1016/j.jns.2009.02.308

[84] Yeung JC, Keshavjee S. Overview of clinical lung transplantation. Cold Spring Harbor Perspectives in Medicine. 2014;**4**(1):a015628. DOI: 10.1101/cshperspect.a015628

[85] Burguete SR, Maselli DJ, Fernandez JF, Levine SM. Lung transplant infection. Respirology (Carlton, Vic.). 2013;**18**(1):22-38. DOI: 10.1111/j.1440-1843.2012.02196.x

[86] Bindi ML et al. Pancreas transplantation: Problems and prospects in intensive care units. Minerva Anestesiologica. 2005;**71**(5):207-221

[87] White SA, Shaw JA, Sutherland DE. Pancreas transplantation. The Lancet. 2009;**373**(9677):1808-1817. DOI: 10.1016/S0140-6736(09)60609-7

[88] Poudel S, Gupta S, Saigal S. Basics and Art of Immunosuppression in Liver Transplantation. Journal of Clinical and Experimental Hepatology. May-Jun 2024;**14**(3):101345. DOI: 10.1016/j.jceh.2024.101345.

[89] Chisholm-Burns MA, Spivey CA, Graff Zivin J, Lee JK, Sredzinski E, Tolley EA. Improving outcomes of renal transplant recipients with behavioral adherence contracts: A randomised controlled trial. American Journal of Transplantation. Official Journal of the American Society of Transplantation and the American Society of Transplant Surgeons. 2013;**13**(9):2364-2373. DOI: 10.1111/ajt.12341

Chapter 5

Key Factors in Management of Donors and its Impact on Transplant Outcomes and Graft Survival

Katarina Tomulić Brusich, Ivana Acan and Saša Živković

Abstract

Cadaveric donors are often presented with several pathophysiological alterations in hemodynamics, hormone balance, body temperature, and lung function. Therefore, appropriate medical management of a potential organ donor can be very challenging. However, it is one of the main conditions that ensures the preservation and quality of organs. There are still many controversies and conflicting recommendations in the management of organ donors. In this chapter, we present the main factors that influence early graft survival and transplant outcome, including socio-economic and organizational factors, factors related to the demographics and genetics of the donor, and factors related to the direct donor preparation until the explantation procedure. The aim of this chapter is to cover all controversies and to abolish uncertainties in order to facilitate the management of potential donors.

Keywords: brain death, intensive care, donor hemodynamics, pathophysiological alteration, organ donation, graft function, acute rejection, graft survival, transplant outcome

1. Introduction

Transplantation provides life-saving treatment for patients suffering from end-stage organ failure. Over the last few decades, solid-organ transplantation has greatly evolved with changes in organ allocation, improvements in organ management, surgical techniques, and immunosuppression therapy. Both waitlist survival and post-transplant survival have shown steady improvements. For kidney transplants, this is largely due to better maintenance of dialysis and diabetes care. Survival among patients listed for liver transplantation has improved, most likely due to aggressive use of marginal allografts, while patients on the heart and/or lung transplant waiting list have shown improvements due to optimized listing behaviors, medical management, and improved mechanical devices [1].

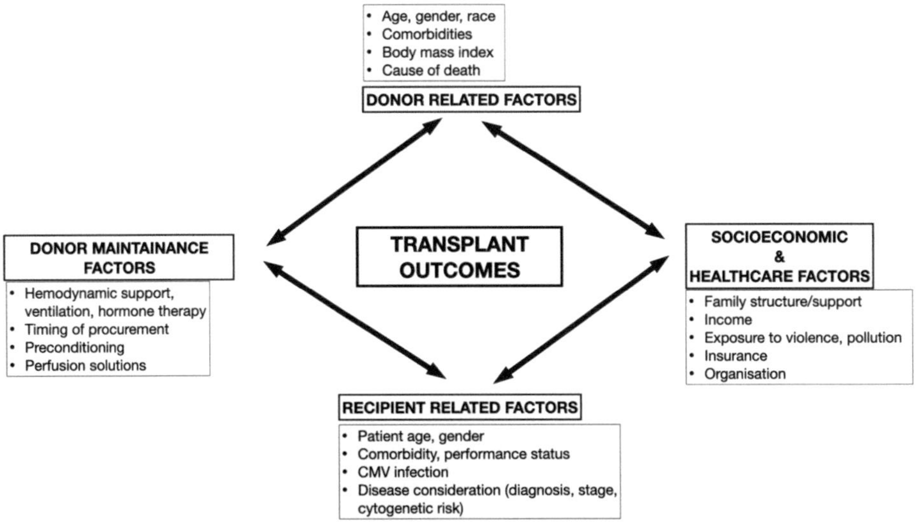

Figure 1.
Factors associated with transplant outcomes.

Many factors can influence the primary non-function or delayed function of grafts, which are associated with significant post-transplantation morbidity and mortality. This is especially true for marginal grafts used primarily in order to increase the donor pool, as they are prone to a higher degree of ischemia/reperfusion injury. Accordingly, a broad spectrum of strategies has been undertaken in order to reduce graft injury and to safely expand the donor pool [2]. However, before we can make any alterations in strategies, factors that influence graft survival and transplant outcome have to be well defined in order to determine which of them are modifiable.

In our opinion, they can be divided into four factors: donor-related factors, donor maintenance factors, socioeconomic and healthcare system organization factors, and recipient-related factors (**Figure 1**).

Many studies have shown progress in post-transplant survival in solid-organ transplants after donor maintenance protocol standardization and socioeconomic standards improvement. On the other hand, there is still a need to provide a more comprehensive perspective of transplant outcomes [3]. Likewise, we must focus on the identification of vulnerable populations and reveal specific risk factors for barriers along the pathway from end-stage organ disease to transplantation.

In this chapter, we will disregard recipient-related factors and focus on donor-related factors, donor maintenance, and socioeconomic factors in order to clarify the causes of poor outcomes in transplanted patients.

2. Donor-related factors

Recognition of donor-related factors associated with graft survival or outcome is essential for all transplant patients. These factors include [4]:

- Age
- Gender

- Race
- Comorbidities (poorly regulated hypertension or diabetes mellitus)
- Donor status: heartbeating vs. non-heartbeating
- Cause of donor death: cerebrovascular accident, hemorrhage, or trauma

2.1 Age

In the last few decades, there has been an increase in the donor age. There are two reasons that could explain this. Firstly, there is a change in the incidence of donor's cause of death. The number of donors that died from cerebrovascular accidents exceeded the deaths from head trauma. These donors are statistically older and have more comorbidities. The second reason for the increased donor age is the expansion of the screening criteria, which means that even older candidates are considered donors [5]. Therefore, it is crucial to determine the influence of the expansion criteria on graft survival in order to make better decisions in donor selection.

While the issue is still controversial, most authors report poorer long-term survival outcomes with organs from elderly donors. The impact of older donor age it is emphasized in younger recipients and patients with severe end-stage organ failure. Older donor age is generally accepted as a risk factor for renal graft failure, and it is important to match donor and recipient age to mitigate these disproportions [6].

In heart transplant patients, this donor-recipient age difference does not significantly impact long-term outcomes [7]. This is possibly due to donors' cut-off age. Traditionally, heart transplant donors are under 55 years old, whereas liver and kidney donors can be over 70 years old if the organ function is acceptable.

On the other hand, the younger age of the donor and recipient is reported as an important factor in graft rejection, especially in liver transplantation. Younger recipient age is the dominant risk factor for acute cellular rejection. Kueht *et al.* found that patients between 18 and 25 years of age have a three times higher risk for acute cellular rejection (ACR) compared to patients older than 40 years, whereas the recipients older than 70 years of age seem to be the most significant protective factor against rejection [8]. Likewise, a study conducted by Onaca *et al.* reported that patients older than 60 years show a higher incidence of ACR if their donors were less than 50 years old [9]. As patients grow older, their immune response gradually weakens while the grafts from younger donors seem to be more immunogenic. This may be the explanation for the listed immunological disproportion. For this reason, patients older than 60 years could be considered for a reduction in the immunosuppressive therapy dose in order to reduce the incidence of side effects and complications related to the treatment.

2.2 Gender

Gender plays a role in all stages of the organ transplantation process, including listing and matching organs by sex and size, graft survival, complications, and mortality. Gender-related differences in organ transplantation are related to several factors, mostly to biological and social characteristics [10]. Although the role of gender in solid-organ and bone marrow transplantations has been extensively studied, the impact of gender mismatch on transplant outcomes remains controversial [11]. Hypothetically, it could be due to anatomic, immune, hormone, and genetic differences between women and men.

A large number of studies have been published on the topic of gender incompatibility between donors and recipients and its influence on the outcome of transplantation. They indicate that gender incompatibility between donor and recipient is an independent risk factor for acute cellular rejection (ACR). In particular, this has been demonstrated in liver and heart transplant patients, where the female donor-male recipient combination revealed the worst graft survival [12, 13]. It has been assumed that this result is a consequence of several factors. The quality of the female donors is often reported as diminished due to the fact that female donors die more often from cerebrovascular causes and less often from trauma. Also, male recipients have undesirable characteristics, such as a high frequency of hepatocellular carcinoma.

Interestingly, in animal model studies, female rat livers have been shown to exhibit increased levels of acidosis during ischemia compared to male rat livers. This gender difference in the metabolic response of the liver to ischemia appears to be mediated by estrogen and could have a significant impact on transplant outcomes [14, 15]. A similar sex-dependent metabolic response was also found in myocardial function [16]. Therefore, it is possible that this gender difference could affect recipients after heart transplantation.

Analogous results were obtained in heart transplant patients, where the worst survival of male recipients receiving female hearts was noted, possibly due to higher rates of urgent transplantation and cardiac size mismatch [17]. Therefore, in our opinion, it is crucial to avoid cardiac donor-recipient mismatch, and the optimization of cardiac size should be considered essential for graft survival [18].

2.3 Race

Racial and ethnic disparities may pervade healthcare delivery and transplant surgery outcomes. It has been suggested that donor race may be a stronger risk factor for graft failure than donor comorbidities, such as a history of hypertension accounted with the recipients body mass index. Organs procured from African American donors may be independently associated with graft loss due to recurrent disease or acute rejection after renal transplantation [19, 20]. This is possibly due to undiagnosed glomerulonephritis influenced by donor hypertension, which is more frequently found among the African American population.

However, a study from Brown *et al.* reports no difference in recipient survival among Black race donors, although it was associated with a higher incidence of acute rejection and decreased graft survival [21]. This was additionally confirmed in the study by Sun *et al.*, which indicated that donor race is not associated with worse outcomes and that race-matching did not confer advantages [22].

The overall impression is that donor race should not be considered when determining the best characteristics for the kidney donor. Unequal access and quality of care are commonly associated with racial differences, as well as the variation among individual transplant centers and income disparities (which will be discussed later in this chapter).

2.4 Comorbidities

Due to the increasing number of patient on waiting list, it is logical to expand the criteria for organ acceptance. These donors tend to be older and have a higher prevalence of various comorbidities such as hypertension, diabetes mellitus, and obesity, which all can lead to systemic atherosclerosis predisposition [23]. The direct impact of these comorbidities on graft survival and transplant outcome is still insufficiently investigated.

Only recently, there have been studies on how donor comorbidities influence these outcomes. In the research by Martinez Insfran *et al.* among donors older than 75 years, there seems to be no impact on graft survival despite the higher prevalence of arterial hypertension and diabetes [24]. When analyzed separately, graft survival is influenced solely by the presence of peripheral vascular disease. However, patient survival, on the other hand, is influenced by the presence of all comorbidities. But despite this, survival after transplantation in the population with comorbidity is very good. This leads us to the conclusion that even patients with comorbidities should have access to transplantation and should be considered as transplant candidates.

As for obese donors, the high body mass index (BMI) was only associated with a significant increase in warm ischemia time. However, no significant association between cadaveric donor BMI and long-term clinical outcomes has not been confirmed in kidney transplant recipients [25]. Likewise, high donor BMI was not associated with graft and patient survival or long-term outcomes in patients undergoing liver transplantation [26]. High donor BMI was only associated with a higher chance of macrosteatosis liver, which, as a consequence, has a higher incidence of declined organs for transplantation.

2.5 Donor status: Heartbeating vs. non-heartbeating

Death in donors without a heartbeat is defined as an irreversible cessation of circulation and respiratory function, whereas brain death in donors with a heartbeat is determined according to neurologic criteria. Therefore, a non-heartbeating donor has had hypotension over an extended period of time after cardiac arrest, just before organ procurement. It is considered that the long-lasting lack of perfusion causes irreversible damage, resulting in poor short-term and long-term outcomes after transplantation [27].

There has been reported a higher incidence of delayed graft function among renal transplant recipients retrieved from donors without a heartbeat. However, there seems to be no difference in long-term outcomes between heartbeating vs. non-heartbeating donors [28]. Likewise, data retrieved among liver transplant recipients with liver retrieved from non-heartbeating donors support the fact that this kind of donor status does not impact graft loss or patient survival [29]. Thus, in appropriately selected patients, the outcomes for non-heartbeating donors are similar to those using liver from heartbeating donors, with no significant differences in complication rate, patient survival, or transplanted liver survival. Ultimately, these non-heartbeating donors represent a potential treatment option in organ shortage, but the timing and organization of the procurement have to be very swift.

2.6 Donor cause of death (DCOD)

Donor cause of death (DCOD) has been described to influence allograft survival. Stroke, head trauma, and anoxia are the most frequent causes of DCOD, accounting for 97% of cadaveric solid-organ donors. Most studies associate stroke DCOD with worse graft survival across all organs. DCOD directly influences the incidence of graft rejection. DCOD by head trauma and stroke was associated with a significantly higher rejection rate compared to anoxia DCOD [30].

Unlike previous studies, a report by Ganesh *et al*. associates DCOD and post-transplantation survival, but it was not maintained after adjustment for confounding variables [31]. It seems that donors that died of vascular accidents and brain tumors were significantly older, compared to post-traumatic donors. Post-traumatic donors were younger, more likely to be male, and taller than donors from other groups, with a lower body mass index. All these factors combined (age, sex, and size) are potentially advantageous for the outcome in the trauma group and can lead to improved survival. DCOD therefore should not influence donor organ acceptance or donor-recipient matching and does not identify marginal donors.

Because of the long waiting list for transplantation, any adequately maintained brain-dead patient with acceptable organ function should be positively considered as organ donor. Donor age, gender, racial or ethnic background should never be a single exclusionary criterion. Donors with significant comorbidities should not be discouraged, but graft and patient survival analyses should account for their presence.

Since these factors are not modifiable, we cannot directly influence them. However, knowing the limitations of potential donor (age, gender mismatch, and comorbidities), we can predict clinical implications and can help in future patients' care management.

3. Donor maintenance

3.1 Donor maintenance

Cadaveric donors are often presented with several pathophysiological alterations in hemodynamics, hormone balance, body temperature, and lung function. Due to systemic inflammatory response, an up-regulation of pro-inflammatory mediators occurs, which can have a negative impact on the graft survival after transplantation. Therefore, appropriate medical management of a potential organ donor can be very challenging.

Organ donor management strategies already exist, and their aim is to reestablish a normal physiological balance. In most cases, this state is extremely difficult to achieve, especially in the long term. Management difficulties have risen to a higher level with the introduction of marginal donors of advanced age. Nevertheless, current guidelines for critical care management for potential organ donors should focus on a multimodal strategy consisting of preserving peripheral organ function [32].

Basically, the management of potential organ donors is similar to the management of critically ill patients. The main goal of that treatment is to achieve hemodynamic stability as well as the homeostasis establishment of endocrine and metabolic disturbances [33].

Table 1 summarizes how to manage the potential organ donor, parameter management, and goals [34].

As we can see, a tailor-made approach that strives to optimize each donor organ is pursued. It ensures graft quality that can possibly lead to an enlargement of the donor pool and improved outcomes after transplantation [35, 36]. One of the first conditions that has to be met is the achievement of hemodynamic stability with timely resuscitation using balanced isotonic crystalloid solutions in combination with vasoactive and hormone therapy. As for additional donor maintenance

Monitoring
• Admission in ICU • Central vein access • Invasive arterial pressure • Continuous monitoring of electrocardiogram, peripheral oxygen saturation (SpO2), urinary output, and temperature
Hemodynamic support
• Maintain mean arterial blood pressure between 60 and 80 mmHg • Central venous pressure (CVP) 4–10 mmHg (for lung donors 4–8 mmHg) • Diuresis 1–3 ml/kg/h (>100 ml/h) • Fluid resuscitation: initial infusion of 20–30 mL/kg of warm crystalloid solution for 30 min. If CVP < 4 mmHg, the volume infusion can be increased • Vasopressors: Vasopressin in bolus, followed by a dose of 0.5–2.4 U/h or Noradrenaline (norepinephrine) 0.1–2 mcg/kg/ min • Brady and tachyarrhythmia should be treated following the protocols of the American Heart Association. Do not use atropine for bradyarrhythmia treatment – consider a temporary transcutaneous pacemaker (4)
Temperature control
• Maintain body temperature between 36 and 37.5°C • Identify hypothermia as early as possible: central measurements in the tympanic membrane, nasopharynx, and esophagus • In hypothermia, warming blankets should be provided to the patient
Ventilation
• Tidal volume of 6 to 8 mL/kg of ideal body weight • FiO2 adjusted to obtain PaO2 ≥ 90 mmHg, PEEP 8–10, and Plato pressure < 30 cm H2O
Nutritional support
• Caloric intake equivalent to 70–85% of baseline energy expenditure • Contraindicated in conditions of severe hemodynamic instability
Hormone therapy
• Capillary blood glucose measured every 6 h • Persistent blood glucose levels above 180 mg/dL must be controlled following the institutional protocols. • pH should be kept between 7.35 and 7.45 • Serum sodium between 130 and 150 mEq/L and urine output between 0.5 and 4 mL/kg/h • In the presence of hypernatremia, it should be corrected with 0.45% saline solution or 5% glucose solution • Disturbances in other electrolytes (such as calcium, phosphorus, magnesium, and potassium) must also be monitored every 6 h • 15 mg/kg/day of methylprednisolone after the diagnosis • T3 replacement if the patient is unstable and under dopamine administration at doses higher than 10 μg/kg/min or with an ejection fraction of less than 45%
Transfusion
• Blood transfusion if hemoglobin levels <7 g/dL. When the hemoglobin level is between 7 and 10 g/dL, the blood transfusion should be performed exclusively if the resuscitation measures are not achieving the mean arterial pressure (MAP) goals • The hematocrit should be kept >30% • Cryoprecipitate transfusion if the fibrinogen value is <100 mg/dL and disseminated intravascular coagulation is suspected • The platelet transfusion is recommended when the platelet account is <80,000/mm3

Table 1.
Management of the potential organ donor [34].

measures, mild therapeutic hypothermia of the donor has shown some positive effects regarding the reduction of delayed graft function, especially in renal transplant recipients [37].

Hormonal replacement therapy for brain-dead donors remains controversial. Corticosteroids have anti-inflammatory properties and its use is endorsed in donor management due to the fact that in several studies they contribute to more effective lung transplantation and reduced post-transplant liver dysfunction [38]. However, the latest trials on acute liver rejection reported conflicting results. They demonstrated that steroid pretreatment does not impact long-term graft survival [39]. It is considered that corticosteroid administration in donors significantly reduces antioxidant levels in transplanted liver and can have an impact on episodes of acute cellular rejection and graft survival [40].

Intravenous levothyroxine is widely used in donor care. Some observational data suggest that more organs can be retrieved from donors who receive hormonal supplements [41]. However, data concerning its impact on graft survival are contradicting and have been mostly studied among heart transplant patients. On one hand, there are studies that suggest that pre-transplantation thyroid hormone supplementation of donors and recipients is associated with improved long-term survival after heart transplantation [42]. Whereas, in other studies, intravenous levothyroxine supplementation did not result in significantly more hearts (or the other organs) transplanted per donor, nor it led to vasopressor reduction and discontinuation or ejection fraction augmentation [43]. The major limitation of thyroid hormone use is time. Unlike vasopressors or inotropes, hormones need time to reach their full effect after they go through the process of genomic transcription and protein synthesis. It is a relatively slow process, but ultimately, they have the potential to modify myocardium and vasculature and, therefore, may contribute to long-term survival by primary graft dysfunction reduction [44]. However, over time, most of the potential donors tend to be hemodynamically unstable, making procurement a priority and denying hormones full potential development.

Also, as an essential part of donor management, donors are assessed clinical for infections. Bacteremia or sepsis are not contraindicated, in case adequate antibiotics have been timely administered prior to procurement. The rate of infection transmission is very low, occurring in less than 1% of solid-organ transplant recipients. Certain infections are still contraindicated in organ donation, although there has also been progress in this field. In order to expand the donor pool, organs from HIV-positive donors have been successfully transplanted to HIV-positive recipients. Successful use of organs from hepatitis C-positive donors due to new antiviral agents against hepatitis C has been reported [45].

As already mentioned, early events during transplantation may determine the outcome of the recipient. Variety of immune responses are activated after brain death, which can additionally aggravate ischemia-reperfusion injury in early transplantation period, and may compromise graft and recipient survival. Experimental studies show that simvastatin administered to the organ donor damps down inflammation and reduces biomarkers of myocardial injury after heart transplantation [46]. It's considered vasculoprotective and therefore it could serve as an inexpensive adjunct therapy in multiorgan donation. Similar findings and results were obtained in patients after liver transplantation. Donor simvastatin was considered safe and has potential to significantly improve early graft and patient survival after liver transplantation [47]. Statin administration is still not part of the donor maintenance protocol due to the fact that further research is mandatory.

To conclude, poor donor clinical and hemodynamic status may impact on delayed graft function (DGF) occurrence. In one single-center study, authors managed to extrapolate donor maintenance-related variables associated with DGF and listed them as blood pressure, use of high-dose vasopressors, urine output, and blood glucose [48]. However, none of the available predictive models does not include in the final formula variables reflecting donor maintenance.

3.2 Timing of procurement

By assuring the appropriate management of the potential donor, we can benefit many patients with end-stage disease. The longer the delay until the organ removal, the worse the inflammatory response and the outcomes of the transplantation. Therefore, the majority of transplant centers aim to procure as fast as possible [49].

There are no guidelines on the safe duration of donor management before procurement. There is shortage of literature regarding this topic in terms of large randomized trials. Research is limited to single-center retrospective studies examining the relationship between donor brain death duration and outcomes after transplantation, with conflicting results.

Earlier belief advocated fast organ procurement in order to avoid donor hemodynamic instability occurrence, which can ultimately lead to worse outcomes due to compromised perfusion. However, it has now been proposed that by maintaining organ perfusion, the organs can recover and be better prepared for cold ischemia as the autonomous and cytokine storm seems to "cool down" in the hours following brain death. This finding may have an impact on organ procurement in the future, where it may be safer to improve donor management prior to organ retrieval than to simply rush into the procurement [50].

This is supported by recent studies that have shown improved long-term outcomes and graft survival in renal, liver, and pancreas transplant recipients after longer donor procurement time and graft survival with longer procurement interval in renal, liver and pancreas transplant patients [51–53].

We also must emphasize significant differences in procurement intervals between Europe and the United States, which arise from organization of procurement schedule and the type of consent for organ donation. In the United States, procurement is mostly scheduled during office hours, due to their organization system and payment. As for the consent model for organ procurement the US system operates under a model of expressed consent, while European countries have relied on a method of presumed consent. Neither of these methods has shown superiority in increasing the donor pool [53].

3.3 Cold and warm ischemia time

It has long been known that warm ischemia time (WIT – the time from organ removal from cold storage to achieving organ perfusion following vessel anastomosis) and cold ischemia time (CIT – time that organ remains in the cold storage prior to transplantation) are important factors affecting organ transplantation outcomes. Both prolonged WIT and CIT are independently associated with post-transplant graft failure [54]. Each additional hour of CIT increases the risk of graft failure and mortality [55], whereas prolonged WIT is associated with delayed graft function, increased graft failure, and mortality after transplantation [56].

Similar conclusions tend to be demonstrated in studies focused on in-house transplantation with minimal duration of cold ischemia. Studies reported reduced incidence of delayed graft function after in-house donor kidney transplantation. However, there has not been significant difference for long-term graft function compared to imported organs [57].

Minimizing both warm and cold ischemic injury is the area of focus for the international transplant community because they are modifiable, and their amelioration can reduce organ injury and improve outcomes after transplantation.

In times when it is not possible to reduce CIT, due to the necessity for long-traveling organ transport in order to match donor and recipient immunological status, improved preservation solutions and mechanical graft support should be considered. Likewise, enhanced collaboration between organ procurement organizations, transplant centers, and optimized transportation systems is important for long-distance organ transport optimization [58].

3.4 Perfusion solutions and machine perfusion techniques

Procured organs are routinely preserved in a solution whose goal is to prevent cell swelling, acidosis, and oxygen radical formation. The most widely used solutions for organ preservation under hypothermic settings are the University of Wisconsin (UW) and Histamine Tryptophan Ketoglutarate (HTK) solutions, respectively.

Recent laboratory-based studies have explored the benefits of the preservation of fluid additives. Effects of volatile anesthetics or hydrogen sulfide (H2S) added to preservation solutions have been found to decrease oxidative stress, apoptosis, inflammation, and mitochondrial dysfunction in ischemic rodent kidneys [59]. Immune inhibitors added to preservation solutions inhibit complement activation, which lead to organ quality and function improvement by lowering inflammatory and pro-fibrotic gene expression in laboratory studies. Likewise, recent studies provide data on the reduction of immunosuppressive medication doses with mesenchymal stem cell application [60]. However, it will take time to bridge the gap between research and clinical practice.

In experimental models, a variety of settings regarding machine perfusion techniques has been proposed. In contrast to static cold storage, hypothermic pumping has been shown in laboratory models to improve ATP levels and reduce endothelial damage and swelling. Normothermic pumping allows the maintenance of cellular and metabolic processes at normal physiological rates. It has been considered that it reduces the injury associated with cold ischemia, reducing delayed graft function and ischemia-reperfusion rates. It has also been proposed that it restores ATP levels and increases blood flow and oxygenation. Likewise, normothermic pumping has been used in preclinical studies of immune inhibitors (mesenchymal stem cells, complement inhibitors, anesthetics) in order to find an agent that can offer protection from ischemia-reperfusion injury. Subnormothermic machine perfusion similarly avoids cold ischemia but it reduces the need for oxygen carriers, leading ultimately to increased urine production, improved creatine clearance and improved blood flow [61–63].

In combination with targeted perfusion solutions, an advanced machine perfusion method offers means of functional maintenance, restoration, and assessment while reducing damage associated with static cold storage and ultimately improving transplant outcomes [61].

3.5 Preconditioning

Ischemia/reperfusion (I/R) injury is an inevitable part of every transplant that significantly contributes to graft dysfunction, which is closely related to increased morbidity and mortality [64]. Given extremely limited donor resources, it is important to mitigate I/R injury and improve graft function.

Pre-, post-, and remote conditioning are protective strategies against I/R injury, which can be applied in the transplant setting. With ischemic preconditioning, the transplanted organ is conditioned with a brief ischemic period followed by reperfusion prior to sustained ischemia. Ischemic post-conditioning consists of intermittent sequential interruptions of blood flow in the early phase of reperfusion, whereas remote ischemic conditioning involves the implementation of brief and repetitive cycles of I/R in the extremities, inducing systemic protection against I/R injuries in distant organs [65, 66]. The potential mechanism involves slow, intermittent oxygenation through controlled reperfusion in order to reduce the burst production of oxygen free radicals, increase antioxidant activity, suppress neutrophil accumulation, and modulate the apoptotic cascade.

In addition to mechanical preconditioning, there is also a pharmacological post-conditioning. A variety of drugs have been selected and investigated (milrinone, diazoxide, sevoflurane, adenosine, ginsenoside Rb1, recombinant human erythropoietin) [66, 67]. Through different action mechanisms, they all more or less demonstrated a positive effect on I/R injury reduction.

These strategies hold the potential to reduce graft injury and to safely expand the donor pool. Both experimental and clinical studies have demonstrated its protective effects against I/R injury in various target organs such as the heart and kidney. However, despite convincing experimental data, clinical studies are required to show whether biochemical and histological improvements afforded by conditioning can be translated to a substantial clinical benefit.

4. Socioeconomic factors

As already mentioned, multiple factors determine patient and graft survival. Besides donor characteristics, characteristics related to surgery, post-transplant complications, and immunosuppressive drug intake, socioeconomic variables have also been reported to influence transplantation outcomes [68]. Lower socioeconomic status has been associated with worse health outcomes in general. More specifically, it is related to increased incidence and progression of chronic diseases, inadequate renal replacement therapy, and reduced chances of having access to transplantation. Lower economic status is usually associated with limited access to information about the health system and life quality, which ultimately leads to worse outcomes after transplantation.

4.1 Education level

Lower socioeconomic and educational status of the patients has been linked with late application for transplantation and with poor compliance in the post-transplantation period, especially regarding medical treatment. Insufficient patient compliance both decreases the quality of life and shortens the life span due to rejection and graft loss [68]. For instance, in the United States, patient incompliance has been held responsible for 50% of late acute rejection and for 25% of the deaths following liver transplantation [69].

In Europe, the research conducted by Gruttadauria *et al.* revealed a significant correlation between education and socioeconomic status, where high educational level decreased post-liver transplantation deaths [70]. This is also related to the health-related knowledge. The lack of it is associated with difficulties in understanding the favorable effects of physical activity, balanced diet, and adherence to treatment [71].

4.2 Income level

In the United States, lower income was identified as a factor related to poor graft and patient survival [68]. This factor persisted even in the first 3 years after transplantation, regardless of the fact that the health system made the availability of immunosuppressive therapy possible. Recipients off welfare had twice the chance of success than subjects on welfare. Additionally, patients with monthly incomes over $3000 were four times more likely to have successful transplants.

4.3 Employment status

Employment is a widely recognized component of quality of life. Employment status at the time of transplantation and in the post-transplant period has a strong and independent association with the graft and recipient survival. Full-time employment at the time of transplant and 1 year post-transplant is associated with a lower risk for graft failure and recipient mortality [72]. However, working overtime may be associated with an increased risk of graft dysfunction.

4.4 Marital status

Factors related to quality of life also have an impact on transplant outcomes. Among them, marital status and family support are considered to be important factors. Pre-transplant marital status is associated with positive outcomes for the graft, but unfortunately, it is not beneficial for the recipient's survival. This is particularly pronounced in male but not in female recipients [73]. Likewise, it has been proven that patients with children have a three times greater chance of survival than childless individuals. Family support is a major factor for successful outcomes after transplantation, and it is explained that in most cases, patients with children belong to more stable families [68].

4.5 Exposure to external factors (violence and pollution)

The characteristics of the places people inhabit influence many aspects of their health and well-being. The living environment does not only apply to geographic places, but it also includes an extent of neighborhood socioeconomic resources, which can be associated with adverse health outcomes. Living in a deprived neighborhood has been shown to be associated with risky health behaviors (alcohol and drug addiction), poor cardiovascular health, higher mortality, and greater depression [74]. In the study by Wadhwani *et al.*, neighborhood socioeconomic deprivation and black race were reported as important predictors of adverse outcomes after liver transplantation [75]. The reason for this may lay in the fact that neighborhood characteristics (violence, severe poverty, poor social cohesion) reduce the availability of the health system to the individual in the first place, as well as diminish one's ability to adhere to strict medication regimens after transplantation.

5. Healthcare factors

5.1 Health insurance

Access to health care is another key variable influencing transplant outcomes. There are differences in health care systems between countries, especially between the United States and European countries, that could influence results. In the United States, the presence of private health insurance significantly affected survival after transplantation. Those patients with private insurance have an advantage in the graft and recipient outcomes independent of racial differences [76]. Likewise, the presence of health insurance also influences patient compliance. For example, in the United States, the major medical insurance provides immunosuppressive medications for patients younger than 65 years who do not have a disability but only for the period of 3 years after transplantation. Beyond that, the provider does not extend coverage, which can be an important determinant of graft failure [68, 77]. In Europe, health insurance is mostly publicly financed and has no medication restrictions, which ensures better patient compliance with immunosuppressive drugs.

Therefore, if access to health care depends on socioeconomic status, patients with unfavorable social factors could be at a disadvantage and could have poorer outcomes after transplantation. Limitations in access to health care and medication have consequently a negative influence on adherence to treatment, as has been seen among the African American population. A policy change may contribute to improving graft survival and reducing health care spending. Studies suggest that patients of African origin have no difference in graft survival rates in healthcare systems that lack income-related barriers.

5.2 Transplant center organization

The outcomes of transplantation depend on numerous factors and vary between continents, countries, and between transplant centers. Likewise, despite multiple regulations, the variation between transplant centers in approaches to donor and recipient evaluations, health care and treatment delivery, communication, and frequency of follow-up were reported [78].

One of the major problems in the healthcare system organization is the lack of systematic postoperative patient monitoring. In the United States, studies conducted among patients after kidney transplantation demonstrate that 65% of kidney recipients do not have a dedicated transplant pharmacist in outpatient care, two-thirds do not see renal transplant recipients at least monthly during the first year, and only less than 30% has an established nephrology and transplant surgery collaboration [79].

Due to critical organ shortage in the United States, a new strategy has been proposed to increase the number and quality of organs recovered from deceased organ donors. Until recently, most of the organs retrieved from deceased donors have occurred in acute-care hospitals. However, donor maintenance requires intensive care treatment, which represents inconvenience because there is competition with living patients for intensive care unit beds and possible interference with previously planned operating room schedules. To address these issues, some organ procurement organizations have established dedicated organ recovery facilities (specialized donor care facilities or organ recovery centers). These new setting facilities accept potential organ donors from acute-care hospitals and provide advanced evaluation, diagnostic, and treatment management. Their aim is to ensure the best possible organ recovery

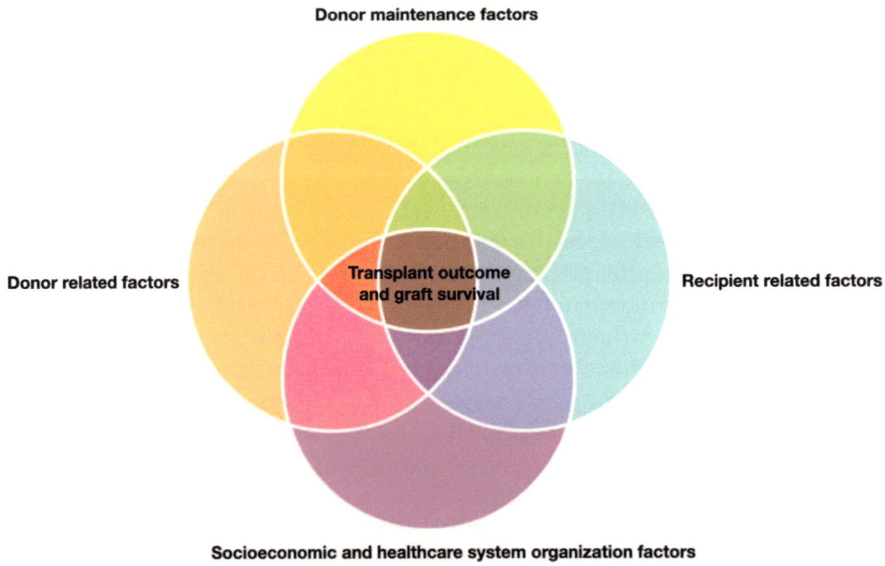

Figure 2.
Overlapping factors that influence transplant outcomes and graft survival.

for potential procurement. Already, single-facility evaluations have suggested improved organ donation outcomes and several practical advantages over hospital-based recovery [80].

6. Conclusion

In this chapter, we reviewed the impact of donor risk and socioeconomic factors on graft and/or recipient survival. Due to the fact that for many patients with end-stage organ diseases organ transplantation is the only feasible treatment, improving the brain death understanding and the potential donor management are important steps to save many future lives.

Most of these factors are modifiable but often overlapping and cumulative with other factors (**Figure 2**). Therefore, an exclusive reliance on donor factors or donor characteristics-based decision-making could result in unjustified rejection of organs for procurement.

Nevertheless, it is important to recognize those underlying factors in order to make improvements that could influence optimal transplant outcomes. We hope that some of these factors may become less important as our understanding and technology regarding transplant medicine advances.

Conflict of interest

The authors declare no conflict of interest.

Author details

Katarina Tomulić Brusich[1,2]*, Ivana Acan[3] and Saša Živković[3]

1 Department of Anesthesiology, Intensive Medicine and Pain Treatment, Clinical Hospital Centre Rijeka, Rijeka, Croatia

2 Faculty of Medicine, University of Rijeka, Rijeka, Croatia

3 Department of Anesthesiology and Surgical Intensive Care, University Medical Centre Ljubljana, Ljubljana, Slovenia

*Address all correspondence to: ktomulic@gmail.com

References

[1] Patrick G, Hickner B, Goli K. Trends in survival for adult organ transplantation. Annals of Surgery. 2024;**5**(1):e383. DOI: 10.1097/AS9.0000000000000383

[2] Mundt HM, Yard BA, Kramer BK. Optimized donor management and organ preservation before kidney transplantation. Transplant International. 2016;**29**:974-984

[3] Hameed AM, Hawthorne WJ, Pleass HC. Advances in organ preservation for transplantation. ANZ Journal of Surgery. 2017;**87**:976-980

[4] Swanson SJ, Hypolite IO, Agodoa LY, et al. Effect of donor factors on early graft survival in adult cadaveric renal transplantation. American Journal of Transplantation. 2002;**2**(1):68-75. DOI: 10.1034/j.1600-6143.2002.020112.x

[5] Barba Abad J, Tolosa Eizaguirre E, Rincón Mayans A, et al. Edad del donante y su influencia en la supervivencia del injerto [Influence of donor age on graft survival]. Actas Urologicas Españolas. 2010;**34**(8):719-725

[6] Waiser J, Schreiber M, Budde K, et al. Age-matching in renal transplantation. Nephrology, Dialysis, Transplantation. 2000;**15**(5):696-700. DOI: 10.1093/ndt/15.5.696

[7] Ram E, Lavee J, Kogan A, et al. Does donor-recipient age difference matter in outcome of heart transplantation? Clinical Transplantation. 2019;**33**(7):e13593. DOI: 10.1111/ctr.13593

[8] Kueht M, Cotton RT, Galvan NT, et al. Profiling immunologic risk for acute rejection in liver transplantation: Recipient age is an important risk factor. Transplantation Immunology. 2016;**38**:44-49

[9] Onaca N, Mckenna G, Testa G, et al. Lower incidence of acute cellular rejection in liver transplant recipients more than 60 years of age allows minimization of immunosuppression. Transplantation. 2012;**94**:132

[10] Walters SM, Richter EW, Lutzker T, et al. Perioperative considerations regarding sex in solid organ transplantation. Anesthesiology Clinics. 2020;**38**(2):297-310. DOI: 10.1016/j.anclin.2020.01.008

[11] Ge F, Huang T, Yuan S, et al. Gender issues in solid organ donation and transplantation. Annals of Transplantation. 2013;**18**:508-514. DOI: 10.12659/AOT.889323

[12] Rustgi VK, Marino G, Halpern MT, et al. Role of gender and race mismatch and graft failure in patients undergoing liver transplantation. Liver Transplantation. 2002;**8**:514-518

[13] Kaczmarek I, Meiser B, Beiras-Fernandez A, et al. Gender does matter: Gender-specific outcome analysis of 67,855 heart transplants. The Thoracic and Cardiovascular Surgeon. 2013;**61**:29-36

[14] Wittnich C, Belanger MP, Askin N, et al. Lower liver transplant success in females: Gender differences in metabolic response to global ischemia. Transplantation Proceedings. 2004;**36**:1485-1488

[15] Soric S, Belanger MP, Askin N, et al. Impact of female sex hormones on liver tissue lactic acidosis during ischemia. Transplantation. 2007;**84**:763-770

[16] Wittnich C, Tan L, Wallen J, et al. Sex differences in myocardial metabolism and cardiac function: An emerging concept. Pflügers Archiv. 2013;**465**:719-729

[17] Peled Y, Lavee J, Arad M, et al. The impact of gender mismatching on early and late outcomes following heart transplantation. ESC Heart Failure. 2017;**4**(1):31-39. DOI: 10.1002/ehf2.12107

[18] Ayesta A. Influence of sex-mismatch on prognosis after heart transplantation. Frontiers in Cardiovascular Medicine. 2021;**8**:617062. DOI: 10.3389/fcvm.2021.617062

[19] Shemesh E, Kleinman LC, Howell EA, et al. Racial and economic disparities in transplant outcomes: The not-so-hidden morbidities. Liver Transplantation. 2014;**20**:4-6

[20] Zhou YC, Cecka JM, Terasaki PI. Effect of race on kidney transplants. Clinical Transplants. 1990:447-459

[21] Brown KL, Doshi MD, Singh A, et al. Does donor race still make a difference in deceased-donor African-American renal allograft recipients? American Journal of Surgery. 2010;**199**:305-309

[22] Sun K, Singer P, Basalely A, et al. Influence of donor race and donor-recipient race-matching on pediatric kidney transplant outcomes. Transplantation Direct. 2022;**8**(6):e1324. DOI: 10.1097/TXD.0000000000001324

[23] Ojo AO, Leichtman AB, Punch JD, et al. Impact of pre-existing donor hypertension and diabetes mellitus on cadaveric renal transplant outcomes. American Journal of Kidney Diseases. 2000;**36**(1):153-159. DOI: 10.1053/ajkd.2000.8288

[24] Martinez Insfran L, Ramirez P, Cascales P, et al. Impact of the donor age and comorbidities on graft survival after liver transplant due to hepatocellular carcinoma. Experience in 100 consecutive cases. Transplantation. 2018;**102**:S863. DOI: 10.1097/01.tp.0000543940.12978.df

[25] Arshad A, Hodson J, Chappelow I, et al. The impact of donor body mass index on outcomes after deceased kidney transplantation - a national population-cohort study. Transplant International. 2018;**31**(10):1099-1109. DOI: 10.1111/tri.13263

[26] Takagi K, de Wilde RF, Polak WG, et al. The effect of donor body mass index on graft function in liver transplantation: A systematic review. Transplantation Reviews (Orlando, Fla.). 2020;**34**(4):100571. DOI: 10.1016/j.trre.2020.100571

[27] Kahan BD, Ponticelli C. Selection and operative approaches for donors: Non-heart-beating cadaveric donors. In: Kahan BD, Ponticelli C, editors. Principles and Practice of Renal Transplantation. London: Martin Dunitz; 2000. pp. 149-150

[28] Weber M, Dindo D, Demartines N, et al. Kidney transplantation from donors without a heartbeat. The New England Journal of Medicine. 2002;**347**(4):248-255. DOI: 10.1056/NEJMoa020274

[29] Trivedi PJ, Scalera I, Slaney E, et al. Clinical outcomes of donation after circulatory death liver transplantation in primary sclerosing cholangitis. Journal of Hepatology. 2017;**67**(5):957-965. DOI: 10.1016/j.jhep.2017.06.027

[30] Singhal AK, Sheng X, Drakos SG, et al. Impact of donor cause of death on transplant outcomes: UNOS registry analysis. Transplantation Proceedings.

2009;**41**(9):3539-3544. DOI: 10.1016/j.transproceed.2009.06.192

[31] Ganesh JS, Rogers CA, Banner NR, et al. Donor cause of death and medium-term survival after heart transplantation: A United Kingdom national study. The Journal of Thoracic and Cardiovascular Surgery. 2005;**129**(5):1153-1159. DOI: 10.1016/j.jtcvs.2004.09.029

[32] Mascia L, Mastromauro I, Viberti S, et al. Management to optimize organ procurement in brain dead donors. Minerva Anestesiologica. 2009;**75**(3):125-133

[33] Herrmann H, Suchodolski K, Logemann F. Management von Organspendern und Organempfängern - Spenderkonditionierung und Management der Organentnahme [Management of brain death organ donor]. Anästhesiologie, Intensivmedizin, Notfallmedizin, Schmerztherapie. 2012;**47**(3):188-196; quiz 197. German. DOI: 10.1055/s-0032-1307468

[34] Yoshikawa MH, Rabelo NN, Welling LC, et al. Brain death and management of the potential donor. Neurological Sciences. 2021;**42**(9):3541-3552. DOI: 10.1007/s10072-021-05360-6

[35] Kusumoto FM, Schoenfeld MH, Barrett C, et al. ACC/AHA/HRS guideline on the evaluation and Management of Patients with Bradycardia and Cardiac Conduction Delay: A report of the American College of Cardiology/American Heart Association task force on clinical practice guidelines and the Heart Rhythm Society. Circulation. 2018, 2019;**140**(8):e382-e482. DOI: 10.1161/CIR.0000000000000628

[36] van Zanden JE, Jager NM, Daha MR, et al. Complement therapeutics in the multi-organ donor: Do or Don't? Frontiers in Immunology. 2019;**10**:329. DOI: 10.3389/fimmu.2019.00329

[37] Patel MS, Abt PL. Current practices in deceased organ donor management. Current Opinion in Organ Transplantation. 2019;**24**(3):343-350. DOI: 10.1097/MOT.0000000000000638

[38] Kotsch K, Ulrich F, Reutzel-Selke A, et al. Methylprednisolone therapy in deceased donors reduces inflammation in the donor liver and improves outcome after liver transplantation: A prospective randomized controlled trial. Annals of Surgery. 2008;**248**(6):1042-1050

[39] Reindl-Schwaighofer R, Kainz A, Jelencsics K, et al. Steroid pretreatment of organ donors does not impact on early rejection and long-term kidney allograft survival: Results from a multicenter randomized, controlled trial. American Journal of Transplantation. 2019;**19**(6):1770-1776. DOI: 10.1111/ajt.15252

[40] Tomulic Brusich K, Škrtić A, Sobočan N, et al. Role of NRF2 and reactive aldehydes in acute cellular rejection in liver transplant recipients. Pathology, Research and Practice. 2023;**250**:154826. DOI: 10.1016/j.prp.2023.154826

[41] Dhar R, Marklin GF, Klinkenberg WD, et al. Intravenous levothyroxine for unstable brain-dead heart donors. The New England Journal of Medicine. 2023;**389**(22):2029-2038. DOI: 10.1056/NEJMoa2305969

[42] Holndonner-Kirst E, Nagy A, Czobor NR, et al. The impact of l-thyroxine treatment of donors and recipients on postoperative outcomes after heart transplantation. Journal of Cardiothoracic and Vascular Anesthesia.

2019;**33**(6):1629-1635. DOI: 10.1053/j.jvca.2018.10.024

[43] Novitzky D, Mi Z, Sun Q, Collins JF, et al. Thyroid hormone therapy in the management of 63,593 brain-dead organ donors: A retrospective analysis. Transplantation. 2014;**98**(10):1119-1127. DOI: 10.1097/TP.0000000000000187

[44] Lee R, Pedone E, Kwak J. Thyroid hormone supplementation in heart transplantation: Who's on first? Journal of Cardiothoracic and Vascular Anesthesia. 2024;**38**(6):1299-1301. DOI: 10.1053/j.jvca.2024.02.026

[45] Meyfroidt G, Gunst J, Martin-Loeches I, et al. Management of the brain-dead donor in the ICU: General and specific therapy to improve transplantable organ quality. Intensive Care Medicine. 2019;**45**(3):343-353. DOI: 10.1007/s00134-019-05551-y

[46] Nykänen AI, Holmström EJ, Tuuminen R, et al. Donor simvastatin treatment in heart transplantation. Circulation. 2019;**140**(8):627-640. DOI: 10.1161/CIRCULATIONAHA.119.039932

[47] Pagano D, Bosch J, Tuzzolino F, et al. Donor simvastatin treatment is safe and might improve outcomes after liver transplantation: A randomized clinical trial. Transplantation. 2022;**106**(12):2379-2390. DOI: 10.1097/TP.0000000000004220

[48] Costa SD, de Andrade LGM, Barroso FVC, et al. The impact of deceased donor maintenance on delayed kidney allograft function: A machine learning analysis. PLoS One. 2020;**15**(2):e0228597. DOI: 10.1371/journal.pone.0228597

[49] Pratschke J, Wilhelm MJ, Kusaka M, et al. Brain death and its influence on donor organ quality and outcome after transplantation. Transplantation. 1999;**67**(3):343-348. DOI:10.1097/00007890-199902150-00001

[50] Nijboer WN, Moers C, Leuvenink HG, et al. How important is the duration of the brain death period for the outcome in kidney transplantation? Transplant International. 2011;**24**(1):14-20. DOI: 10.1111/j.1432-2277.2010.01150.x

[51] Guner M, Pirat A, Zeyneloglu P, et al. Effect of the interval between organ donor brain death and organ harvesting on kidney graft function after transplantation. Transplantation Proceedings. 2007;**39**(4):837-841. DOI: 10.1016/J.TRANSPROCEED.2007.02.021

[52] Eerola V, Helanterä I, Åberg F, et al. Timing of organ procurement from brain-dead donors associates with short- and long-term outcomes after liver transplantation. Transplant International. 2022;**35**:10364. DOI: 10.3389/ti.2022.10364

[53] Eerola V, Sallinen V, Lempinen M, et al. Association of procurement time with pancreas transplant outcomes in brain-dead donors. Transplant International. 2023;**36**:11332. DOI: 10.3389/ti.2023.11332

[54] Foley ME, Vinson AJ, Skinner TAA, et al. The impact of combined warm and cold ischemia time on post-transplant outcomes. Canadian Journal of Kidney Health and Disease. 2023;**10**:20543581231178960. DOI: 10.1177/20543581231178960

[55] Debout A, Foucher Y, Trébern-Launay K, et al. Each additional hour of cold ischemia time significantly increases the risk of graft failure and mortality following renal

transplantation. Kidney International. 2015;**87**(2):343-349

[56] Tennankore KK, Kim SJ, Alwayn IP, Kiberd BA. Prolonged warm ischemia time is associated with graft failure and mortality after kidney transplantation. Kidney International. 2016;**89**(3):648-658

[57] Lim SY, Gwon JG, Kim MG, et al. Comparison of recipient outcomes after kidney transplantation: In-house versus imported deceased donors. Transplantation Proceedings. 2018;**50**(4):1025-1028. DOI: 10.1016/j.transproceed.2018.01.035

[58] Imaoka Y, Bozhilov KK, Bekki Y, et al. Breaking distance barriers in liver transplantation: Risk factors and outcomes of long-distance liver grafts. Surgery. 2024;**175**(2):513-521. DOI: 10.1016/j.surg.2023.09.052

[59] Motayagheni N, Phan S, Eshraghi C, et al. A review of anesthetic effects on renal function: Potential organ protection. American Journal of Nephrology. 2017;**46**:380-389

[60] Markel TA, Crafts TD, Jensen AR, et al. Human mesenchymal stromal cells decrease mortality after intestinal ischemia and reperfusion injury. The Journal of Surgical Research. 2015;**199**:56-66

[61] Soo E, Marsh C, Steiner R, et al. Optimizing organs for transplantation; advancements in perfusion and preservation methods. Transplantation Reviews (Orlando, Fla.). 2020;**34**(1):100514. DOI: 10.1016/j.trre.2019.100514

[62] Kaths JM, Paul A, Robinson LA, Selzner M. Ex vivo machine perfusion for renal graft preservation. Transplantation Reviews (Orlando, Fla.). 2018;**32**:1-9

[63] Matos ACC, Requiao Moura LR, Borrelli M, et al. Impact of machine perfusion after long static cold storage on delayed graft function incidence and duration and time to hospital discharge. Clinical Transplantation. 2018;**32**(1):13130. DOI: 10.1111/ctr.13130

[64] Selzner N, Boehnert M, Selzner M. Preconditioning, postconditioning, and remote conditioning in solid organ transplantation: Basic mechanisms and translational applications. Transplantation Reviews (Orlando, Fla.). 2012;**26**(2):115-124. DOI: 10.1016/j.trre.2011.07.003

[65] Zhang Y, Long Y, Li Y, et al. Remote ischemic conditioning may improve graft function following kidney transplantation: A systematic review and meta-analysis with trial sequential analysis. BMC Anesthesiology. 2024;**24**:168. DOI: 10.1186/s12871-024-02549-y

[66] Theodoraki K, Karmaniolou I, Tympa A, et al. Beyond preconditioning: Postconditioning as an alternative technique in the prevention of liver ischemia-reperfusion injury. Oxidative Medicine and Cellular Longevity. 2016;**2016**:8235921. DOI: 10.1155/2016/8235921

[67] Satoh K, Kume M, Abe Y, et al. Implication of protein kinase a for a hepato-protective mechanism of milrinone pretreatment. Journal of Surgical Research. 2009;**155**(1):32-39. DOI: 10.1016/j.jss.2008.07.004

[68] Ruppel P, Felipe CR, Medina-Pestana JO, et al. The influence of clinical, environmental, and socioeconomic factors on five-year patient survival after kidney transplantation. Jornal Brasileiro de Nefrologia. 2018;**40**(2):151-161. DOI: 10.1590/2175-8239-JBN-3865

[69] Onder AH, Bengi G, Ozbilgin M, et al. Analysis of socioeconomic status and other factors affecting patient-graft survival in patients undergoing liver transplantation. Hepatology Forum. 2020;**1**(1):25-36. DOI: 10.14744/hf.2020.0003

[70] Gruttadauria S, Grosso G, Mistretta A, et al. Impact of recipients' socio-economic status on patient and graft survival after liver transplantation: The IsMeTT experience. Digestive and Liver Disease. 2011;**43**(11):893-898. DOI: 10.1016/j.dld.2011.06.017

[71] Woodward RS, Page TF, Soares R, et al. Income-related disparities in kidney transplant graft failures are eliminated by Medicare's immunosuppression coverage. American Journal of Transplantation. 2008;**8**:2636-2646

[72] Petersen E, Baird BC, Barenbaum LL, et al. The impact of employment status on recipient and renal allograft survival. Clinical Transplantation. 2008;**22**(4):428-438. DOI: 10.1111/j.1399-0012.2008.00803.x

[73] Naiman N, Baird BC, Isaacs RB, et al. Role of pre-transplant marital status in renal transplant outcome. Clinical Transplantation. 2007;**21**(1):38-46. DOI: 10.1111/j.1399-0012.2006.00575.x

[74] Cullaro G, Ge J, Lee BP, et al. Association between neighborhood-based material deprivation and liver transplant waitlist registrants demographics and mortality. Clinical Transplantation. 2024;**38**(1):e15189. DOI: 10.1111/ctr.15189

[75] Wadhwani SI, Beck AF, Bucuvalas J, et al. Neighborhood socioeconomic deprivation is associated with worse patient and graft survival following pediatric liver transplantation. American Journal of Transplantation. 2020;**20**(6):1597-1605. DOI: 10.1111/ajt.15786

[76] Gondos A, Döhler B, Brenner H, et al. Kidney graft survival in Europe and the United States: Strikingly different long-term outcomes. Transplantation. 2013;**95**:267-274

[77] Goldfarb-Rumyantzev AS, Koford JK, Baird BC, et al. Role of socioeconomic status in kidney transplant outcome. Clinical Journal of the American Society of Nephrology. 2006;**1**(2):313-322. DOI: 10.2215/CJN.00630805

[78] Szymańska A, Mucha K, Kosieradzki M, et al. Organization of Post-Transplant Care and the 5-year outcomes of kidney transplantation. International Journal of Environmental Research and Public Health. 2022;**19**(4):2010. DOI: 10.3390/ijerph19042010

[79] Israni A, Dean CE, Salkowski N, et al. Variation in structure and delivery of care between kidney transplant centers in the United States. Transplantation. 2014;**98**:520-528. DOI: 10.1097/TP.0000000000000094

[80] Vail EA, Schaubel DE, Abt PL, et al. Organ transplantation outcomes of deceased organ donors in organ procurement organization-based recovery facilities versus acute-care hospitals. Progress in Transplantation. 2023;**33**(2):110-120. DOI: 10.1177/15269248231164176

Chapter 6

Professional and Emotional Challenges Nurses Experience while Caring for Brain-Dead Donors

Anja Meyer and Priya Walabh

Abstract

The research explores the professional and emotional challenges faced by nurses caring for brain-dead donors in South Africa. It highlights the importance of nurses in identifying organ donors and how their attitudes influence families' decisions on organ donation. Nurses experience mixed emotions, including sadness and hopelessness, anxiety, and fear, while caring for organ donors. It also mentions the cultural and religious barriers in South Africa regarding organ donation. The content covers the concepts of organ donation as the gift of life, the role of nurses in providing care, the challenges faced by nurses, and recommendations to improve the care provided to potential organ donors. Themes include the emotional experiences of nurses, mechanical care provided to donors, and continuous care provided to families. Overall, the chapter underlines the importance of education, assistance, and knowledge for nurses caring for potential organ donors. It recommends implementing training programs, support networks, and cultural sensitivity initiatives to improve the care provided and increase organ donation rates. The findings underscore the importance of embracing the notion that "every donor counts" to bridge the gap and save lives.

Keywords: brain death, caring, nurses, organ donor, professional and emotional challenges

1. Introduction

Before the early 1950s, organ failure was comparable to a death sentence and there was no other course of therapy available for patients experiencing end-stage organ failure. However, as time went on, organ transplantation became one of the medical miracles to save the lives of patients with organ failure. Organ transplantation became a widely accepted global practice and for several decades is the new norm to preserve lives and restore function [1, 2].

Unfortunately, organ scarcity remains a continuing concern, and it is known that the efficiency of a transplant program is dictated by the availability of organs, and as matters stand, there is no balance between demand and supply of organs in South Africa (SA). The global demand for organs vastly surpasses the availability of organ donors, as has been extensively documented. Organ donation and transplantation are still the best and most cost-effective medical solutions for end-stage organ failure [3, 4].

Nurses are typically the first to identify organ donors, as most professional nurses who have worked in a critical care unit are believed to have cared for a potential organ donor, who is by definition brain-dead. Therefore, their attitudes and knowledge about organ donation have a significant impact on a family to be included in organ donation as an end-of-life decision [5–7].

Research has shown that there is a wide range of sentiments among nurses regarding organ donation. Although most qualified nurses have a positive attitude toward organ donation and transplantation, nursing staff in China had a negative attitude, whereby only 33.4% of them said they would give their own organs. Only 32% of nurses in Serbia would donate their own organs, compared to 91% who would accept organ transplants. Nurses who work in intensive care units (ICUs) in transplant facilities in Sweden had a less favorable attitude toward organ donation. Brazil mandates that nurses participate in educational programs that challenge preconceived notions and encourage dissent. They elaborate that public opinions toward organ donation are influenced by religion, family values, and ideals [7–9].

In SA, the role of professional nurses toward families is of extreme importance, as they offer support to families regarding organ donation and transplantation. Therefore, potential development in the organ donation process is by transplant coordinators supporting professional nurses, who deal with the family in a precious manner during the organ donation process. Professional nurses are advised not to initiate conversations with families about organ donation, but rather timeous referral of potential donors is essential to allow the transplant coordinator time with the family and pursue the consenting process at the precise time [10, 11].

Nurses play a crucial role in the organ donation process and can influence family and community members' decision-making. Regrettably, the output of nurses in the organ donation process remains low. The main issue appears to be a lack of knowledge and awareness. Research demonstrates that the knowledge level linked to donation rates implies that teaching workshops on organ donation and transplantation need to be developed to fully utilize the potential of nurses in organ donation campaigns and the entire transplant process efficiently [12].

2. The gift of life

According to Ubuntu, individuals do not exist in isolation, but in relation to others. In organ donation, "Ubuntu" is a word that personifies all that organ donation represents. This is because of the recipient's life-changing experience by the family's selfless act of organ donation. The proverb of Ubuntu means a person does not live in isolation, "In Zulu: umuntu ngumuntu ngabantu/In Southern Sotho: motho ke motho ka batho". In translation, it means "a person is a person through other persons". The honorable theory of Ubuntu gives emphasis to the only way to develop one's humanness, which is to relate to others in a positive way. The Ubuntu values inspire individuals to place high moral value on respecting, caring, and recognizing the existence of fellow human beings [13–15].

Giving a part of oneself through organ donation is the most phenomenal gift a person can give another. Organ donation integrates the end of one life with the renewal of another. Organ transplantation is a unique technique where a patient can only get a healthy organ if a living donor or the family of a brain-dead donor consents to the gift of life. This occurs when a surgical operation is performed by means of transferring the organ from the donor to the patient with organ failure [16, 17].

To increase the donor pool, donor registration and discussions with patients, family, and friends about organ donation as an end-of-life care choice are recommended, as a significant percentage of families agree to organ donation when they are aware that their loved one has chosen to become a registered organ donor. Patients' families play a vital role in the organ donation procedure, and low consent rates from families remain a substantial hurdle. Some families are afraid to make that decision for their loved ones, but families that know what the deceased would have wanted found the process easier [5, 18, 19].

2.1 Nurses, the art of care

The American Nursing Association redefined nursing as follows: "Nursing integrates the art and science of caring and focuses on the protection, promotion and optimizing of health and human function, prevention of illness and injury, facilitates healing and alleviation of suffering through compassionate presence. Nursing is the diagnosis and the treatment of human responses and advocacy in the individuals, families, groups, communities, and populations in recognition of the connection of humanity". Nurses constitute a large percentage of the health-care workforce, and the success rate of organ donation is a result of their dedication, knowledge, and skills [6, 7, 9, 19].

While professional nurses care for a potential organ donor, Ubuntu remains the key guiding principle that drives people to see the existence of others in a holistic way. This idea creates a secure environment in which humans can seek comfort and feel safe in the presence of others. "I am because of you" is a strong remark made by the late Mr. Nelson Mandela to instill in himself the things he most desired for South Africa: peace, healing, and harmony. He became the epitome of Ubuntu, as it is known in South Africa. As a result, embodying the principle of Ubuntu through transplantation demonstrates that no one can exist in isolation. Patients expecting life-saving organs become dependent on the gift of life [7, 20].

2.2 The brain-dead donor

Brain death is an irreversible impairment of function of the entire brain and is defined by a catabolic storm, which can lead to a variety of challenges with organ viability. To care for brain-dead patients who could be potential organ donors is a complex activity, and the professional nurse's role stands out; they experience stress while spending time with the donor's family and managing the donor [21–23].

Nursing care for potential donors is a complex process that needs extensive mental preparation and skills. As a result, the professional nurse must be knowledgeable about brain death and its pathophysiological process as well as possess the abilities required to care for the brain-dead patient as a potential organ donor.

The professional nurse's perspective regarding brain death influences the successful outcome of organ donation. A constructive expansion of knowledge, skill, and understanding will foster a positive attitude toward organ donation [6, 23, 24].

Caring for brain-dead patients who could be potential organ donors is one of the most challenging duties for nurses, and the level of competency demonstrated while caring for a brain-dead patient has a direct impact on the outcome of organ viability and transplantation. To maintain the dignity of both organ donors and families during the donation process, it is critical to provide optimal nursing care, stay close to the patient, be available to relatives, and listen to their stories about their loved ones [24, 25].

2.3 Walk of honor: The time silence becomes tangible

Caring for a brain-dead patient is intense and emotionally draining. "The time to prepare the organ donor for the procurement procedure is a time the nurse experiences the most emotions as a silent supporter. It is when the nurse feels close to what a family feels when faced with this tragic situation". They will find themselves holding the donor's hand at times and even asking questions or have a last conversation. This is the time the nurse stands in the gap for the family and keeps on honoring their loved one [26].

An "Honor Walk" has grown into an increasingly common symbol of respect for organ donation. Prior to donation, the critical care team and other health-care personnel stand silently in the area leading to the operation room to honor the family's decision to donate their loved one's organs. The solemn end-of-life processions give you a sense of thankfulness toward a person you as the nurse did not even know [27].

"Being a part of the honor guard allowed me to take part in saying goodbye, which reminds me of the precious gift gave to others. I was thankful I was able to participate in the care of such a complex patient so early in my nursing career, and I have learned so much from that experience that I will take into my future practice." (**Figure 1**) [26, 28].

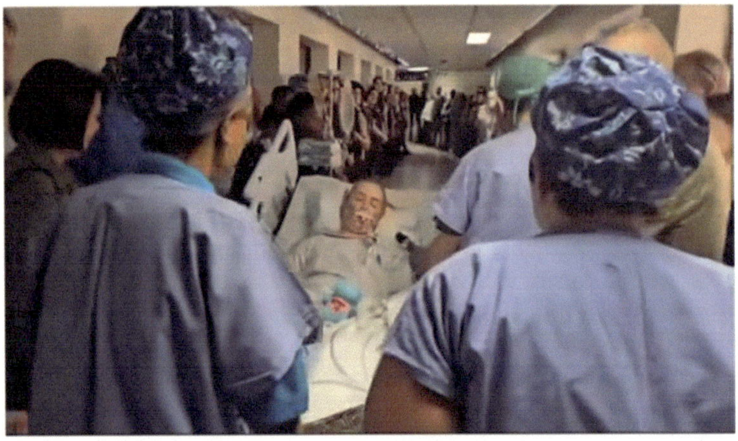

Figure 1.
Honor walk of a true hero, whose organs will save the lives of many.

2.4 The participants

Nurses from a government institution in Gauteng described their experiences caring for potential organ donors. The themes paint an accurate figure of the perspectives expressed by the participants. The researcher meticulously and verbatim transcribed all of the interviews to ensure that the significance of what the participants said was preserved. The chapter takes the reader on a wonderful trip through how professional nurses experienced conflicting feelings while caring for potential organ donors but ultimately felt gratified knowing there was hope when they shared their stories of assisting patients in receiving life-saving organs.

The essence of the professional nurses' experiences was captured through the data analysis process, which was done by engaging Giorgi's descriptive phenomenological data analysis process. A purposive sampling method was used. The sample consisted of seven (7) professional nurses with a diploma in Medical and Surgical Nursing Science: Critical Care Nursing (General) and an average of fifteen (15) years of nursing experience in an intensive care unit. Three (3) participants worked in a neurosurgery intensive care unit and four (4) in a trauma major critical care unit at the public hospital under investigation. There were two (2) male and five (5) female professional nurses, with a mean age of 45 years. Following seven (7) interviews, the researcher, supervisors, and independent coder confirmed data saturation, and no new information was discovered [29].

2.5 Identifying the gap: Themes and categories

2.5.1 Central theme

Despite their sadness and hopelessness, the participants continued to care for the potential organ donor holistically. Despite dealing with an emotional load of anxiety and fear while witnessing the family's reaction to hearing the devastating and heartbreaking news that their loved one was brain-dead, the professional nurses encountered a sense of purpose knowing that other people's lives could be saved through organ donation (**Table 1**).

Theme 1	Theme 2	Theme 3
• The participants experienced mixed emotions while caring for a potential organ donor.	• The participants experienced that the caring for potential organ donor was mechanical and involved caring for the family members.	• The participants experienced barriers in caring for the potential organ donors.

Table 1.
Themes of experiences of nurses caring for a brain-dead donor [30].

2.5.2 Theme 1: Navigating the emotional labyrinth of organ donation

The participants' employment conditions exposed them to death and dying at frequent intervals during their duties. They shared their mixed emotions of sadness and hopelessness that they experienced when they realized that nothing more could be done to save the potential organ donor's life. Observing the family's emotional suffering while caring for a potential organ donor caused them anxiety and fear. Participants felt fulfilled when providing holistic care, knowing their efforts could save another life. A few participants expressed their feelings as of sadness and hopelessness are expressed in the following quotes:

"It can become traumatic, more especially if you see the young kids who are more involved in accidents these days, so seeing such a young person lying there without anything that you can do and they cannot be woken up ... (sounding sad and lowering his voice)." (Participant D, male, 40 years).*

"Sadness comes when the very patient is diagnosed brain-dead because of the severity of the head injury ... you feel sad because you were hoping the patient will be healed and go home." (Participant C, female, 56 years).*

Caring for brain-dead patients is one of the most demanding responsibilities for nurses, and because of its intricacy, it is the most difficult component of nursing in an intensive care unit. One of the most difficult moral difficulties is determining the death of a person who still has a heartbeat, and many nurses have expressed concerns about brain death and organ donation in cultural and religious settings. As possible organ donors are admitted to the intensive care unit with the intention of repairing their condition, the professional nurse anticipates a miracle. According to the study results, caring for a brain-dead patient may cause nurses to feel sadness and hopelessness while caring for patients. Similarly, studies suggest that nurses experience anxiety after caring for a brain-dead patient, which may interfere with patient care and contribute to burnout [24, 29, 31, 32].

Because brain death can happen rapidly, most families do not have time to prepare for the unexpected death of a loved one. As a result, the professional nurse is responsible for caring for the mourning family during this process, and communication with the family is essential since they need to comprehend the cause of death. Anxiety and fear overwhelmed the participants as they witnessed the family's emotional turmoil while caring for a potential organ donor. The participants were filled with anxiety and fear as they witnessed the emotional distress of families who had been informed that their loved ones were brain-dead. The family of potential organ donors revealed a wide range of emotions, from complete denial and disbelief to knowing and accepting that their loved one was brain-dead [29, 31, 32].

The following quotes articulate the participants' feelings of anxiety, fear, and the families' emotional pain:

"I was really feeling scared to face them and tell them this sad news ... when they came I was shaking like a leaf ... (pause) ... and when they came in ... I was afraid to even say 'Good morning', you know ... as if they would see on my face ... written that their child is no more. It (experience) creates that feeling". (Participant F, female, 62 years).*

"It was very painful to see them cry like that because they had hoped that the person ... (long silence) ... Yeah, also you do not know how the family will react when hearing the devastating news ... Sometimes I think they ... look for someone to blame and since I am the first person to talk to them, they can blame me as a person who was looking after the patient ... but after some time you feel that you have done much to help them come to terms with the situation (sounding relieved)." (Participant G, male, 34 years).*

It is so critical to convey accurate details about brain death and ensure families comprehend the correct prognosis, since this may alleviate the family's misperceptions about the likelihood of their loved one still being alive. Not all families understand brain death since their loved one's body is warm to the touch, the heart is beating, and the person appears to be asleep despite being declared dead. This gives families hope for the patient's recovery, but it also makes nurses afraid and uncomfortable because families abuse them and cause them distress. This can be incredibly stressful for the nurse, instilling a sense of guilt and aggravating anxiety. Participants said that some families communicated their emotions in an aggressive and occasionally abusive manner, blaming the nursing personnel for their loved ones' deaths. Dealing with the possible organ donor's family was extremely stressful, and some relatives of brain-dead patients were disrespectful, angry, and confrontational to professional nurses [22, 33–35].

2.5.3 Theme 2: Transforming donor care - From mechanical to meaningful

Caring for a possible organ donor seems to be a mechanical process. This includes nursing behaviors such as ensuring the patient's hemodynamic stability, and as the treatment progressed, the participants developed a stronger sense of caring for the potential organ donor's family. As caring increased, the participants saw that it was more than only dualism; it also extended to being concerned for an unknown individual. Donor care aimed at optimizing organ function is crucial for increasing the number of patients who can benefit from each individual donor. Participants were responsible for the patient's hemodynamic stability, which included adequate respiration, a desirable perfusion pressure (MAP) of at least 60 mmHg, and urine output of at least 1 ml/kg/h. They also indicated that they did their best to look after potential organ donors and their families, treating them with dignity, respect, and professionalism. It is also important to honor the families, regardless of whether they approve of the donation [23, 36].

"I ensure my patient is clean and I nurse him with dignity. I continue to write observations, do arterial blood gases, obtain blood for electrolyte check and correct according to ward protocols ... (pause) ... Now, as a person you wouldn't work rough, you still respected them as a person, and you still respected the person for their relatives ... You just do the same thing and still have the same feelings (similar to those who are alive) ... (thinking) ... or even more now. Sympathy plus empathy." (Participant F, female, 62 years)*.

Participants discovered that care for potential organ donors and their families was comprehensive and consistent. The participants assisted bereaved families while caring for the potential organ donor, emphasizing the need for understanding and appreciating a patient's family as a whole. This is clear from the following quotes:

"It's the whole physical aspect as well as the family ... (thinking) ... Family I think is a big part of the holistic care since now you no longer nursing a human body alone but also you are nursing the family ..." (Participant B, female, 28 years).*

"I give holistic care and the factors that I involve ... Firstly ... (pause) .... I look at the emotional status more especially of the family ... and ensure that they are supported throughout .... Secondly, their psychological status ... and then after, their physical status. On the physical status then I also focus on ensuring that the patient's organs ... are ... viable at all times." (Participant E, female, 47 years).*

Nurses must provide excellent care and compassion to patients and their families while maintaining professional, continuous competence in nursing. The donor procedure involves both clinical management of the donor and interactions with the donor's family. Because the professional nurse is the primary source of communication and support to the patient's family on a daily basis, fulfilling the requirements of the family is part of the process of caring for a brain-dead patient. Although it can be challenging for participants to offer adequate support, providing emotional assistance and understanding the patient's condition is vital [2, 24, 37].

2.5.4 Theme 3: Cultural sensitivity in organ donation - A new frontier

Participants stated that they encountered difficulties in offering culturally sensitive treatment to potential organ donors and their families. These challenges developed as a result of most African families' cultural beliefs about and unfamiliarity with the occurrence of organ donation. Participants said that most African families are less familiar with the notion of organ donation than the majority of Caucasian homes. Participants became aware of the challenges that they faced as a result of their families' cultural beliefs. Many African families are unfamiliar with the cultural differences in organ donation. As a result, the participants became aware that ancestral traditions were given priority in African households, which meant that the deceased had to be buried with all of their organs.

The participants illustrated the cultural diversity barriers in the following quotations:

*"... (Moving her chair around) ... with the culture diversity it is very difficult especially with us Blacks because they would come up and tell you that 'No I cannot give you an organ what am I going to say to my ancestors when I die and you have taken this organ.'" (Participant A, female, 41 years) *.*

"Cultural beliefs differ, we as Blacks believe that when someone is dead, he or she will meet some other members of the family who died before him or her and if they (family) donated the organs, the ancestors will not be able to recognize him or her and the ancestors will be angry ... and we believe that the deceased person then brings darkness and evil spirit to the family ... (sternness in her voice) ..." (Participant C, female, 56 years).*

Organ donation and transplantation continue to provide many ethical, cultural, and religious issues and dilemmas on a personal and community level. Cultural variety also means that different civilizations respect one another's uniqueness. Numerous researchers have emphasized sociocultural barriers, such as religion and culture, which prevent Africans in South Africa from participating in organ donation as an end-of-life option. Religion and culture foster a sense of identity, and any action considered as divergent from a certain group's religion or culture is prohibited and viewed poorly. People's attitudes, opinions, and conduct are influenced by their cultural background and religious beliefs [3, 31, 38, 39].

Most Africans believe in life after death; however, this life is referred to as the ancestral world and necessitates a strong body and soul. To respect the ancestors, his or her body must be intact; otherwise, the ancestors will reject the person in the hereafter. Donating a deceased person's organs is thus prohibited in most African traditions, as it is believed that the person's spirit continues to wander and will not be accepted by ancestors. Cultural custodians must share an understanding that a person's existence does not end with physical death [1, 40].

*"... because he or she (family member) doesn't want to be responsible as the family will blame him or her to say 'You have just given the organs to ... other people that we do not even know' ... whereas White people ... like ... (clearing his throat) ... I mean they understand, they say 'Take the organs, our child will live on in someone else." (Participant D, male, 40 years) *.*

3. Close the gap: Recommendations in relation to each of the themes

The study presents recommendations for professional nurses caring for potential organ donors to ensure quality care. To provide effective and competent care to potential organ donors, the recommendations involve emotional support and education for nurses and communities. The data analysis has led to the following recommendations based on topics and categories (**Tables 2–5**) [30].

Recommendation	Description
Crafting the compassionate care curriculum	A workshop where empathy is the cornerstone. Transplant coordinators should develop a comprehensive awareness and in-service training program focusing on the nuanced care of brain-dead patients. This program would blend clinical expertise with emotional intelligence, transforming a challenging responsibility into a shared journey of understanding and compassion.
Building emotional fortitude through coping strategies	A toolkit designed for emotional resilience. Implement strategies like mindfulness practices, reflective journaling, or guided imagery exercises to help professional nurses manage their emotional responses. These tools will empower them to handle the responsibilities of caring for brain-dead patients with renewed strength and clarity.
Forming sanctuary support circles	Support circles led by experienced transplant coordinators, serving as sanctuaries of shared experience. In these groups, nurses can find camaraderie, exchange stories, and gain insights from those who have navigated similar challenges. Such circles will provide moral support and foster healing through shared experiences.
Counseling courses: Bridging professional and personal realities	Consider specialized counseling courses designed to address the complex family dynamics in organ donation scenarios. By incorporating this training into professional development, nurses will enhance their ability to support families and deepen their empathy and understanding of the emotional landscapes they encounter.
Illuminating the path: Community outreach programs	Figure an outreach initiative that engages the community in understanding organ donation. Educational programs demystifying brain death and organ donation through workshops and seminars can foster greater public understanding and support, bridging the gap between medical realities and public perception.

Table 2.
Recommendations in relation to each of theme 1 [30].

Theme 2	Recommendations
The evolution of donor care	It's a routine driven by protocol and urgency, with a focus on preserving organ function. Yet, beyond the clinical precision lies a realm of profound human connection—a realm where the true essence of care transcends the mechanical and embraces the holistic.
Reimagining donor care: A paradigm shift	To elevate the quality of donor care, we must embark on a transformative journey. Shift the paradigm from a mechanical approach to a more holistic, compassionate model.
Crafting the ultimate tutorial: A guide to holistic donor care	Imagine a tutorial or in-service training program designed not just to teach but to inspire. This program would be an immersive experience for health-care professionals, combining cutting-edge knowledge with empathetic practice. Through simulated scenarios and role-playing, nurses and physicians would learn to balance the technical aspects of donor management with the emotional needs of families. The goal: to optimize organ function while respecting the dignity and emotions of the donor and their loved ones.

Theme 2	Recommendations
The compulsory in-service training: A new standard	Figure a new era where every ICU nurse undergoes compulsory in-service training focused on donor management. This training is more than a requirement; it's an opportunity for growth and compassion. By integrating advanced simulation techniques and real-world case studies, nurses gain not only technical expertise but also the skills to offer emotional support to families, ensuring that care is both effective and empathetic.
Policy innovation: The holistic care framework	Envision a comprehensive policy or standard operating procedure dedicated to the care of brain-dead or potential organ donors. This framework would guide health-care professionals through a continuum of care that addresses both medical needs and family support. It emphasizes a holistic approach, ensuring that the care provided respects the donor's dignity and supports their loved ones through this challenging time.
Observational learning: Bridging the gap	Allowing professional nurses to observe the transplant process offers a profound opportunity for learning. By witnessing the intricate and compassionate aspects of transplantation, nurses can gain insights that enhance their daily care of brain-dead patients. This observational learning fosters a deeper understanding of the impact of their care, bridging the gap between clinical procedures and the human experience.
Community engagement: Voices of families	Engaging with families and communities through organ donation questionnaires and evaluations provides invaluable feedback. By actively seeking input, health-care providers can gain a better understanding of the needs and experiences of families. This engagement not only informs improvements in care but also strengthens the relationship between medical professionals and the communities they serve.
A new dawn for donor care	The journey from mechanical to meaningful donor care is a collective endeavor that requires dedication, empathy, and innovation. By implementing these recommendations, we can transform the experience of donor care into one that honors both the clinical and emotional dimensions of this crucial work. As we move forward, let us embrace a model of care that reflects the profound respect and compassion that every donor and his or her family deserve.

Table 3.
Recommendations in relation to each of theme 2 [30].

Theme 3	Recommendations
Cultural sensitivity in organ donation: A new frontier	*Educational initiatives*: Organize workshops titled "*The Art of Compassionate Care: Navigating Cultural Dimensions in Organ Donation*." Focus on evidence-based practices for caring for brain-dead patients and handling organ donation requests sensitively. *Professional development*: Encourage attendance at seminars, symposiums, and conferences focused on advancements in transplant care and cultural sensitivity. *Dissemination of knowledge*: Distribute relevant articles and research papers on organ donation practices and cultural considerations to health-care professionals. *Cultural sensitivity integration*: Collaborate with traditional healers to understand and integrate cultural beliefs into the organ donation process. *Cultural competency training*: Implement training programs focusing on cultural sensitivity and respect for diverse practices related to organ donation and care of brain-dead patients. *Community engagement*: Host open forums and discussions in community centers and online platforms to address cultural concerns and foster understanding about organ donation.

Table 4.
Recommendations in relation to each of theme 3 [30].

3.1 Close the gap: Recommendations in relation to nursing

Recommendations	
Recommendations for nursing practice: Nursing	Practice should establish institutional policies for caring for brain-dead patients and promoting awareness about the organ donation process. This transplant center can provide orientation, in-service, and continuing professional development programs for professional nurses who will care for brain-dead patients who are potential organ donors. The transplant team can form buddy systems or mentorship relationships with professional nurses in an intensive care unit to help them become more comfortable nursing brain-dead patients for potential organ donation. Transplant coordinators can do academic rounds in intensive care units to raise awareness and support among professional nurses who are caring for potential organ donors.
Recommendations for nursing management	Nursing managers have to demonstrate their support for professional nurses and transplant centers by informing them of counseling resources available at any time and allowing them to express their anxieties. If there are any uncertainties, unit managers or operational managers must support transplant centers and professional nurses who are caring for potential organ donors in selecting which procedures to implement. Attending in-service training, orientation, and continuing professional development programs about organ donation and transplantation should be encouraged. Another option is to create a mandatory referral policy to facilitate and support the referral of potential organ donors.
Recommendations for further research	The study's findings established an important understanding of nursing competency and added to the body of knowledge in studies on professional nurses' experiences caring for a potential organ donor. The study could be replicated at other hospitals in other locations to determine whether the results are associated. Additional research in nursing education, nursing practice, and transplantation would be beneficial on closing the gap in organ donation.

Table 5.
Recommendations in relation to nursing [30].

4. Conclusion

The research emphasized the significance of education, assistance, and knowledge for professional nurses who provide care for potential organ donors. When providing care for potential organ donors, professional nurses will always encounter challenges in the absence of formal, established training programs or support networks. The results showed that while professional nurses have difficulties when providing care for a potential organ donor, they also show joy when they understand that by ensuring a transplant would be successful, they are improving the life of another individual.

Acknowledgements

Thank you to all donor families for the gift of life.
Dr. Priya Walabh, thank you for your ongoing support and mentoring.
Unity in Transplant – together we are stronger.

Notes/thanks/other declarations

To my son, Miguel Menino, I am because of you.

Author details

Anja Meyer[1,2,3*] and Priya Walabh[2,4,5]

1 MCur, Department of Nursing, Faculty of Health Sciences, University of Johannesburg, South Africa

2 Gauteng Provincial Solid Organ Transplant Division, Johannesburg, South Africa

3 Department of Surgery, Charlotte Maxeke Johannesburg Academic Hospital, Johannesburg, South Africa

4 Department of Paediatrics and Child Health, Faculty of Health Sciences, School of Clinical Medicine, University of the Witwatersrand, Johannesburg, South Africa

5 Paediatric Gastroenterology, Hepatology and Nutrition Unit, Charlotte Maxeke Johannesburg Hospital, University of Witwatersrand, Johannesburg, South Africa

*Address all correspondence to: anjameyer85@yahoo.com

References

[1] Kunle A J. Organ donation in an African culture. Bangladesh Journal of Bioethics. 2018;**10**(1):21-25

[2] O'Leary GM. Deceased Donor Organ Donation: The Critical Care Nurse's Role. University in Philadelphia, Wolters Kluwer Health; 2018

[3] Dimo PM. Participating in organ donation: Issues among black South Africans. Global Journal of Health Science. 2019;**11**(1). ISSN 1916-9736, E-ISSN 1916-9744. DOI: 10.5539/gjhs.v11n1p71

[4] Lewis A, Koukoura A, Tsianos G, Gargavanis AA, Nielsen AA, Vassiliadis E. Organ donation in the US and Europe: The supply vs demand imbalance. Transplant Rev (Orlando). Apr 2021;**35**(2):100585. DOI: 10.1016/j.trre.2020.100585. Epub 2020 Oct 11

[5] Crymble K, Etheredge HR, Fabian J, Gaylard P. Nurses' knowledge about and attitudes toward organ donation in state and private hospitals in Johannesburg, South Africa. South African Journal Critical Care. 2017;**33**(2):52-57. DOI: 10.7196/SAJCC.2017.v33i2.322

[6] Valiee S, Shoaib D, Shiva M, Sahar D, Farzaneh K. Paper: Study of knowledge and attitude of nurses in Sanandaj city toward organ donation. Journal: Nursing Practice Today. 2019;**6**(2):74-82

[7] Payne K. Brain Death: 50 Years Later and Still Controversial. Southern Adventist University; 2018. Available from: https://discover.e.southern.edu/graduate-programs

[8] Fernandez-Alonso V, Moro-Tejedor MN, Palacio-Cena D, Paredes-Garza F, Gil-Carrasco MD, De La Matta Cant M, et al. Attitudes towards multi-organ donation among intensive care unit nurses in transplant hospitals. International Nursing Review. 2021;**68**:308-317

[9] Fernández-Alonso V, Palacios-Ceña D, Silva-Martin C, García-Pozo A. Facilitators and barriers in the organ donation process: A qualitative study among nurse transplant coordinators. International Journal of Environmental Research and Public Health. 2020;**17**:7996. DOI: 10.3390/ijerph17217996

[10] Thomson D. Organ donation in South Africa – A call to action. South Africa Journal Critical Care. 2017;**33**(2):36-37. DOI: 10.7196/SAJCC.2017.v33i2.352

[11] da Silva A, Aline F, Cunha SP, Débora Lira AC, Ribeiro J, Francisco J, et al. Brain death and organ maintenance: Knowledge of intensive care professionals. Journal of Nursing UFPE. 2018;**12**(1):51-58

[12] Akbulut S, Demyati K, Tamer M, Unsal S, Beyoglu S, Saritas H. Knowledge levels, attitudes, and awareness of nurses toward organ donation. Northern Clinics of Istanbul. 2022;**9**(4):367-375

[13] Koali SJ. Organ transplant trade: A moral examination. Open Journal of Philosophy. 2015;**5**:261-267. DOI: 10.4236/ojpp.2015.55033

[14] Slabbert M, Venter B. Routine referrals: A possible solution for transplantation shortages. South African Journal of Bioethics Law. 2017;**10**(1):15-19. DOI: 10.7196/SAJBL.2017.v10i1.498

[15] Li AH, Lo M, Crawshaw JE, Dunnett AJ, Naylor KL, Garg AX, et al. Interventions for increasing solid organ

donor registration. In: Cochrane Database of Systematic. Vol. 4. Canada: John Wiley & Sons; 2021. DOI: 10.1002/14651858. CD010829.pub2

[16] Whittingham. How you can support a patient to become an organ donor. British Journal of Community Nursing. 2018;**23**(9):460-461

[17] Jacob BD, Atluri S, Alexis Graham-Stephenson A, Ott M, Markham L, Sander S, et al. What Is the Effect of Organ Donation Authorization Rates When Utilizing a Standardized Effective Request Process?. Wolters Kluwer Health done at University of Missouri-Kansas City; 2022. DOI: 10.1097/ CCE.0000000000000615

[18] Svensson L. The Role of Relatives in Decision Making on Organ Donation – An Ethical Analysis. Sweden: School of Medical Sciences Örebro, University Örebro; 2020

[19] Tauetsile J. Employee engagement in non-western contexts: The link between social resources Ubuntu and employee engagement. International Journal of Cross Cultural Management. 2021;**21**(2):245-259. DOI: 10.1177/14705958211007874

[20] Ramollo DS. Ubuntu as a Self-Guiding Principle. University of Johannesburg, Department of Educational Psychology; 2022. Available from: https://www.ucatolica.edu.co/ portal/

[21] Drexler S, Kugler C, Farin E. Care of (potentially) brain-dead patients: A qualitative study protocol. Leading Global Nursing Research. 2019;**75**(11):3105-3110. DOI: 10.1111/ jan.14139

[22] Prins L, Human L. Early identification and referral of organ donors in five private hospitals: A survey to determine the knowledge and views of critical care professional nurses pre and post a powerpoint training intervention. South Africa Journal Critical Care. 2019;**35**(2):48-55. DOI: 10.7196/ SAJCC.2019.v35i2.370

[23] da Costa IF, Netto JJM, da Conceição M, Brito CC, Goyanna NF, dos Santos TC, et al. Weaknesses in the care for potential organ donors: The perception of nurses. Revista Bioética. 2017;**25**(1):130-137. DOI: 10.1590/1983-80422017251174

[24] Moghaddam HY, Manzari ZS, Heydari A, Mohammadi E. Mashhad. University of Medical Sciences. 2018;**10**(8):7205-7216. DOI: 10.19082/7205

[25] Simonsson J, Keijzer K, Södereld T, Forsberg A. Intensive critical care nurses' with limited experience: Experiences of caring for an organ donor during the donation process. Journal of Clinical Nursing. May 2020;**29**(9-10):1614-1622. DOI: 10.1111/jocn.15195. Epub 2020 Feb 7

[26] Wood VA. Honor guard: A ritual honoring patients and families who choose organ donation. Nursing in Critical Care. 2020;**15**(6):45-46

[27] Pediatric death and family organ donation: Bereavement support services in one pediatric health system. Journal of Patient Experience. 2024;**11**:1-7. © The Author(s) 2024 Article reuse guidelines: sagepub.com/journals-permissions DOI: 10.1177/23743735241226987

[28] r/nextfuckinglevel - Honor walk of Parker Vasquez, a true hero, whose organs will save or improve the lives of as many as 80 people

[29] Kentish-Barnes N, Siminoff LA, Walker W, Urbanski M, Charpentier J, Thuong M, et al. A narrative review of

family member's experience of organ donation request after brain death in the critical care setting. Intensive Care Medicine. 2019;**45**:331-342. DOI: 10.1007/s00134-019-05575-4

[30] Meyer A. Experiences of Professional Nurses Providing Care to Potential Organ Donors at a Public Institution in Gauteng. University of Johannesburg; 2022. Available from: https://hdl.handle.net/10210/501986

[31] Haor B, Wróblewska S, Daszuta K, Daszuta D. Confirming the Brain Death and the Nurse's Tasks in the Care of Potential Organ Donors and Their Families. The Journal of Neurological and Neurosurgical Nursing Poland. 2019. DOI: 10.15225/PNN.2019.8.3.5

[32] Magalhães ALP, Erdmann AL, de Sousa FGM, Lanzoni GM, da Silva EL, de Mello ALSF. Meaning of nursing care to brain dead potential organ donors. Revista Gaúcha de Enfermagem. 2018;**39**:e2017-e0274. DOI: 10.1590/1983-1447.2018.2017-0274

[33] Roberta A, Trapani S, Manzia TA, Lombardini L, Tisone G, Cardillo M. The COVID-19 Outbreak in Italy: Initial Implications for Organ Transplantation Programs. Rome, Italy: Italian National Transplant Center. Italian National Institute of Health; 2020. DOI: 10.1111/ajt.15904

[34] Sorensen SJ, Sofronas M, Hudson H, Wright DK. Supporting ethical ICU nursing practice in organ donation: An analysis of personhood. The Canadian Journal of Critical Care Nursing. 2021;**32**(1):18-26. DOI: 10.5737/23688653-3211826

[35] Contieroa PP, Wilson DN. Understanding ambivalence towards organ donation and transplantation: An exploratory study of nursing students. Nurse Education Today. 2019;**76**:191-195. DOI: 10.1016/j.nedt.2019.02.008

[36] Kerstis B, Widarsson M. When life ceases—Relatives' experiences when a family member is confirmed brain dead and becomes a potential organ donor—A literature review. Sage Open Nursing. 2020;**6**:1-15. DOI: 10.1177/2377960820922031

[37] Albaqawi HM, Butcon VE, Albagawi BS, Dayrit RD, Pangket P. Holistic nursing care among operating room nurses: Strengthening the standard of practice in Saudi Arabia. Belitung Nursing Journal. 2021;**7**(1):8-14. DOI: 10.33546/bnj.1279

[38] Cotrau P, Hodosan V, Bladu A, Daina C, Daina LG, Pantis C. Ethical socio-cultural and religious issues in organ donation. Maedica – A Journal of Clinical Medicine. 2019;**14**(1):12-14. DOI: 10.26574/maedica.2019.14.1.12

[39] Raewf MB, Mahmood YN. The cultural diversity in the workplace. Cihan University-Erbil Journal of Humanities and Social Sciences. 2021;**1**:1-6. DOI: 10.24086/cuejhss.vol5n1y2021.1-6

[40] De Gama BZ, Jones DG, Bhengu TT, Satyapal KS. Cultural practices of the Zulu ethnic group on the body and their influence on body donation. Anatomical Sciences Education. 2020;**0**:1-11. DOI: 10.1002/ase.1950

Chapter 7

Crossmatch and Histocompatibility

Antonio Paul, Rajamony Chellammal Arun Dileep and Noble Gracious

Abstract

Chronic kidney disease is a worldwide public health problem for which kidney transplantation results in an improved quality of life and social rehabilitation, and savings in overall healthcare costs. The human leukocyte antigen (HLA) system, also known as the major histocompatibility complex (MHC) in humans, plays a crucial role in the immune system. It is responsible for producing cell surface molecules that are specifically designed to convey antigenic peptides to the T-cell receptor (TCR) found on T cells. HLA determines whether a patient has already developed antibodies against the donor's antigens. Various platforms for crossmatching include CDC Crossmatch (CDC CXM), Flow cytometric crossmatch (FCXM), Luminex-based DSA Lysate crossmatch, and Virtual Crossmatch (VXM). VXM is a procedure used to determine the compatibility between a potential organ donor and recipient without physically mixing their blood samples. VXM does not function as a standalone laboratory test; instead, it depends on the analysis and interpretation of prior data obtained from the recipient's anti-HLA analysis using Single Antigen Bead (SAB) assays and donor HLA molecular type. Epitope-based matching is a novel method of histocompatibility matching that involves estimation of the eplet against the antibody in the recipient's serum based on the positive reaction pattern observed in the SAB assay.

Keywords: CDC crossmatch (CDCCXM), flow cytometric crossmatch (FCXM), virtual crossmatch (VXM), single antigen bead (SAB), HLA typing, eplet, donor-specific antibody (DSA), non-HLA antibody, K-SOTTO (Kerala state organ and tissue organization) for deceased donor organ transplantation

1. Introduction

Chronic kidney disease (CKD) poses a global public health challenge. Renal replacement therapy in this context can be achieved through either dialysis or organ transplantation. Nevertheless, dialysis is a lifelong treatment linked to diminished quality of life and heightened mortality risk. In contrast, kidney transplantation provides superior survival rates and improved quality of life for individuals suffering from end-stage kidney disease compared to dialysis. When comparing RRT to kidney transplantation, the latter leads to enhanced quality of life, increased social reintegration, and cost savings in healthcare. Pretransplant histocompatibility tests include a wide range of tests. Crossmatch is a technique used to ensure the donor's kidney is matched with the patient's and thus to avoid any immunological reactions resulting in rejection of the graft. There are different types of crossmatch techniques available to assess histocompatibility, which include CDC crossmatch, flow cytometry crossmatch, bead-based or solid-phase crossmatch, and virtual crossmatch. Each method has its own strengths and limitations; when used judiciously by the clinician, the best histocompatibility match is obtained, thereby improving the rejection-free survival of solid organ transplant recipients.

1.1 What is HLA

In 1952 Jean Dausset observed agglutination of leukocytes in the serum from the patients who had received multiple blood transfusions, which he attributed to an antibody in the serum directed against white blood cells. Further research led to the discovery of the Human leukocyte antigen (HLA) tissue system in 1958 [1].

Human leukocyte antigen (HLA) genes (genetic complex) are located on the short arm of the 6th chromosome. HLA genes encode proteins which are polymorphic molecules present or expressed on the surface of various cells, which play a crucial role in graft rejection. This genetic complex comprises the major histocompatibility complex (MHC) of humans.

The main function of the Human Leukocyte Antigen molecule is to present peptides produced from pathogens to T cells, which in turn triggers a T-cell-driven adaptive immune response.

The T cells can distinguish between foreign peptides and self-derived peptides. It is the recognition of HLA by the immune system that helps to distinguish self-cells from foreign cells. This phenomenon is known as MHC restriction. It is this discovery that established the role of histocompatibility in organ transplantation.

Major histocompatibility complex (MHC) is the most polymorphic genetic system known. More than 30,000 class I and 10,000 class II alleles have been detected and new alleles still are discovered. The IPD-IMGT/HLA database now holds more than 40,000 alleles (as of July 2024) of the human Major Histocompatibility Complex (MHC), which have been designated by the WHO Nomenclature Committee for Factors of the HLA System (**Figures 1** and **2**) [2].

The HLA class I molecule is composed of a heavy alpha-chain composed of three domains (alpha1, alpha2, and alpha3) and a beta2-microglobulin light chain. The HLA class II molecule is composed of two polypeptide chains, namely alpha- and beta-chains. Each chain is structured into two domains, specifically $\alpha 1$- and $\alpha 2$-domains for the alpha-chain, and $\beta 1$- and $\beta 2$-domains for the beta-chain. Every human leukocyte antigen possesses a peptide that originates from a protein antigen and is located on the surface of its grooves.

Human leukocyte antigen (HLA) Class I molecules (A, B, and C) are expressed by all nucleated cells in the body. However, the expression of HLA Class II molecules (DR, DP, and DQ) is limited to B cells, antigen-presenting cells, and activated microvascular endothelial cells. Nonclassical class I genes (HLA-E, -F, -G), and class I–like genes (MICA, MICB) (**Figure 3**) [4].

1.2 Nomenclature

Years ago, HLA typing was being performed using a serologic techniques like microlymphocytotoxicity using terasaki trays. Typing was found by analyzing the

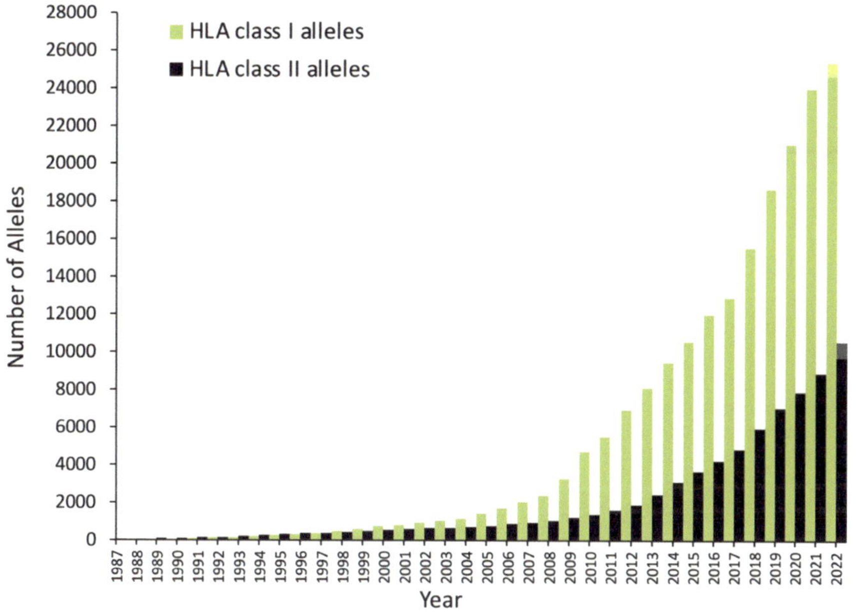

Figure 1.
The database's expansion in the quantity of alleles annually. The process of growth can be divided into two categories: HLA class I (shown by the color green) and HLA class II (represented by the color black). The year 2022 is projected to end with lighter tones. Figure adapted from IPD - IMGT/HLA website.

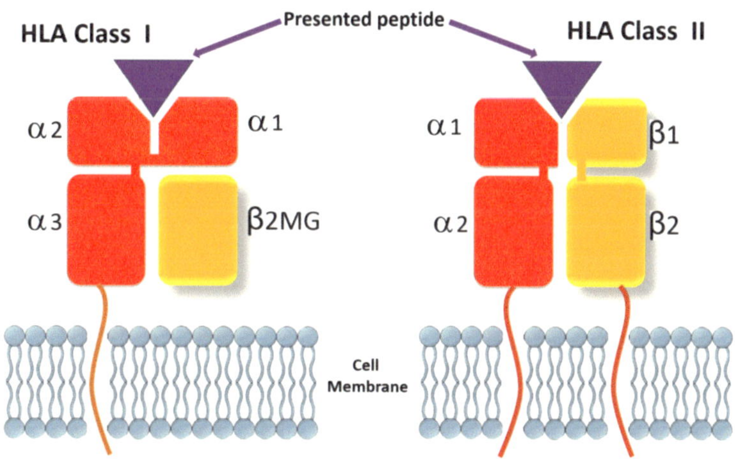

Figure 2.
Structure of human leukocyte antigen (HLA).

reactivity pattern in various wells. Since the introduction of modern molecular techniques like polymerase chain reaction PCR and more specific techniques like bead-based assays, typing has evolved to higher resolution, where specific HLA proteins can also be identified. The nomenclature includes the gene or locus (e.g., A, B, DRB1) followed by an asterisk (*). The first, second, third, and fourth 2-digit fields indicate allele group, specific HLA protein, silent mutation, and noncoding substitution, respectively. Each field is separated by colons. The first 2-digit field, which is the allele group, is equivalent to the serologically determined antigen (**Figure 4**) [5].

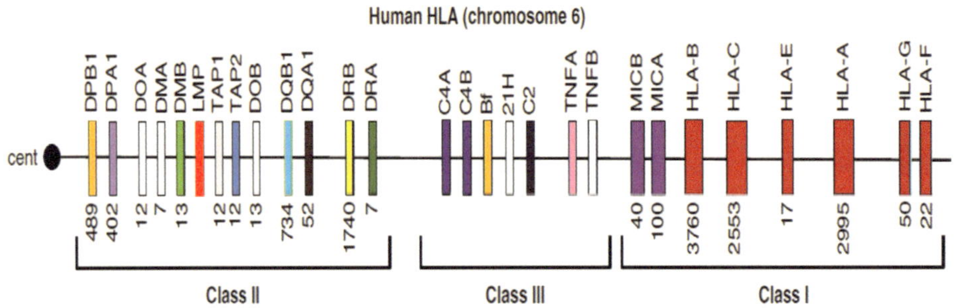

Figure 3.
Human major histocompatibility complex (MHC) genetic map. Diagram illustrating the arrangement of the major histocompatibility complex (MHC) on chromosome 6 in humans. The illustrations are not accurately proportioned. The centromere and major histocompatibility complex (HLA) are indicated in sequence. The number of unique proteins (alleles) produced by each human MHC gene is specified for each locus [3].

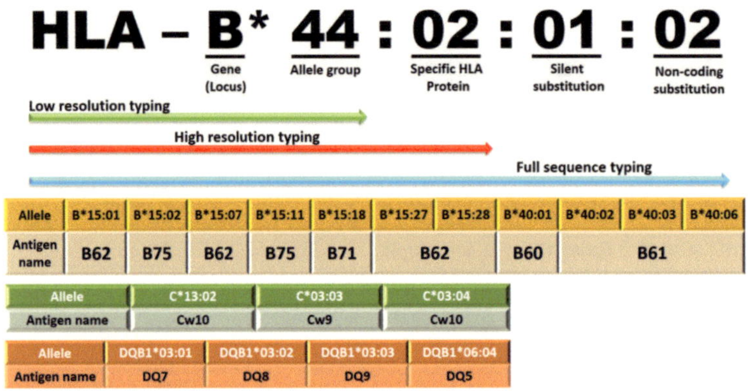

Figure 4.
The nomenclature of human leukocyte antigens (HLA) and the list of HLAs, in which the names of the antigens differ from the allele group, as determined by the molecular approach.

1.3 Anti-HLA antibodies

Anti-HLA antibodies can be developed in response to various sensitization events like blood transfusion, pregnancy, or even transplantation. Anti-HLA antibodies can be either IgG or IgM type. Those produced in response to pregnancy or transplantation are more likely to be of IgG type, whereas the sensitization due to blood transfusion can result in the development of either IgG or IgM antibodies.

2. Histocompatibility assessment in solid organ transplantation

Histocompatibility testing is primarily done in pretransplant testing. It relies on ensuring the match between the HLA of the donor and the recipient so that there will not be any immunological reactions leading to reduced graft survival or graft rejection. HLA typing, cell-based assays like complement-dependent cytotoxicity crossmatch and Flow cytometry crossmatch, and solid or bead-based assays like lysate crossmatch, panel-reactive antibodies (PRA), and virtual crossmatch (HLA typing and single antigen bead assay) are the key components related to histocompatibility assessment in solid organ transplantation evaluation.

2.1 Complement dependent cytotoxicity (CDC) crossmatch

The complement-dependent cytotoxicity crossmatch is a technique to detect preformed donor-specific antibodies through activation of the classical pathway of complement. It was introduced in 1960 by Patel and Terasaki. In their seminal paper published in 1969 they demonstrated that 24 out of 30 patients who suffered immediate graft failure had a positive crossmatch whereas only eight out of 195 patients with negative crossmatch suffered immediate graft rejection [6]. As a result of this study, prospective CDC crossmatching became the standard of care in histocompatibility assessment for kidney transplantation.

Presently, complement-dependent cytotoxicity crossmatch (CDCXM) remains the most frequently utilized pretransplant crossmatch technique across the globe. Either total lymphocytes or T & B lymphocytes can be used for this crossmatch technique. The recipient's serum is made to incubate with donor cells (lymphocytes) in a 72-well tersasaki plate, along with complement (often obtained from rabbit serum). If a donor-specific antibody is detected and attaches to donor lymphocytes, it triggers complement cascade activation and causes the creation of the membrane attack complex (MAC). MAC forms pores in the cell membrane itself, causing cell death and the release of inflammatory mediators that trigger the immune response. If donor-specific antibodies are not present, no lysis occurs and the result is deemed negative (**Figure 5**).

The crossmatch is interpreted by measuring the percentage of dead cells (proportion of lysed cells) in relation to living cells, as assessed using inverted phase contrast microscopy. The outcome can be evaluated based on the proportion of lysed cells, where a score of 0 indicates the absence of cell death. Scores of 2, 4, and 6 indicate progressively higher degrees of cell lysis. A score of eight signifies complete lysis of all cells, indicating the most intense reaction imaginable (**Table 1**) [7].

A negative complement-dependent cytotoxicity crossmatch (CDCXM) prior to transplantation is known to greatly decrease the likelihood of hyperacute graft rejection. Conversely, a positive crossmatch indicates the presence of human leukocyte antigen (HLA) antibodies, which can cause rejection or reduced graft survival (**Figures 6** and 7).

2.1.1 Modification for increasing the sensitivity of CDC-XM

Since the inception of CDC crossmatch in 1969, the test has undergone various technical modifications. The modifications include extended incubation time, different incubation temperatures, more robust techniques for lymphocyte isolation, and the use of different reagents like dithiothreitol (DTT) and antihuman globulin (AHG). All these modifications are aimed at enhancing the sensitivity and specificity of the test by making more favorable conditions for antigen-antibody interaction like more time, correct temperature, and better-quality viable lymphocytes. DTT is used to avoid the reactivity caused by IgM antibodies by breaking IgM pentamers into monomers, as IgM antibodies are not considered to be clinically significant in solid organ transplantation. Antihuman globulin (AHG) is aimed to enhance the reactivity when the antibody level is too low, by increasing the total number of Fc receptors available for the interaction resulting in a visible reaction even if the antibody levels are low [8, 9].

2.1.2 Limitations

Even though the CDC-XM has significantly decreased the incidence of acute graft rejection in solid organ transplantation, the risk still exists [10].

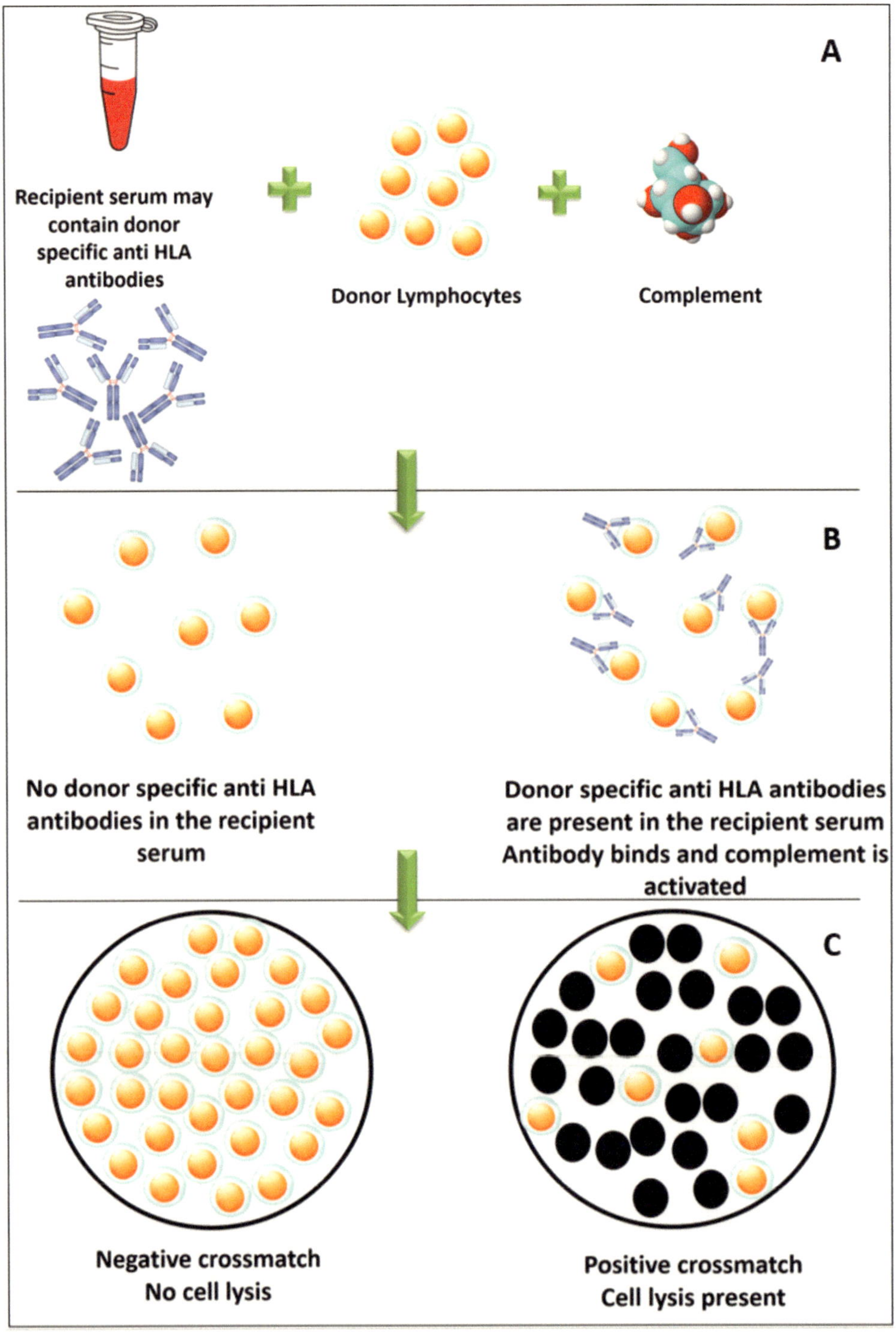

Figure 5.
The CDC crossmatch.

Score	Dead cells (%)	Intensity of the reaction
1	≤10	Negative
2 = +	11–20	Doubtful negative
4 = ++	21–50	Weak positive
6 = +++	51–80	Positive
8 = ++++	81–100	Strong positive

Table 1.
Complement dependent cytotoxicity-crossmatch (CDCXM) interpretation [7].

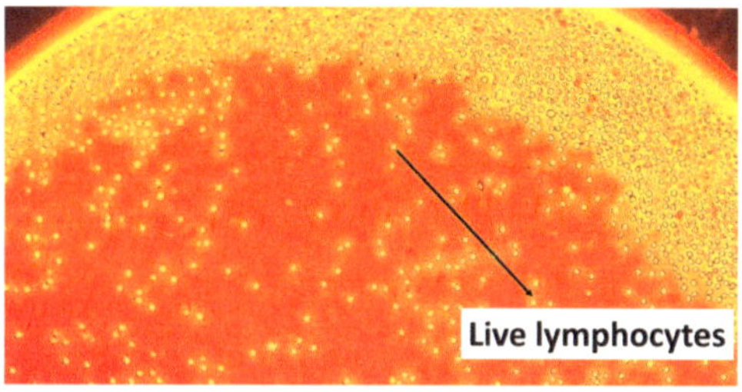

Figure 6.
A negative CDC crossmatch.

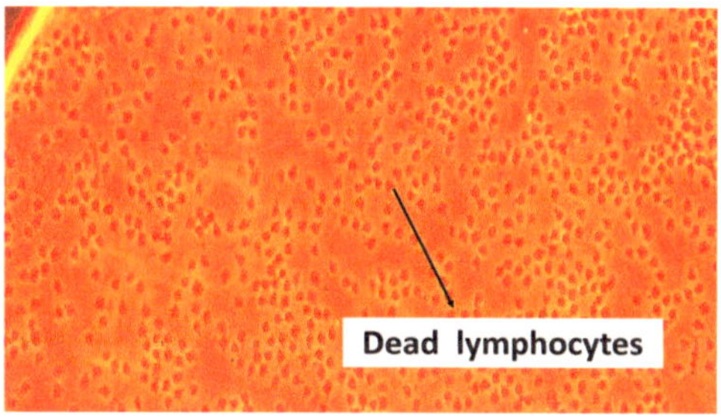

Figure 7.
A positive CDC crossmatch.

Positive fallacy IgM antibodies, which are frequently present in autoimmune illness patients, can also result in positive CDC-XMs. Furthermore, treatments like rituximab may cause a B-cell crossmatch to be falsely positive [11].

Other limitation of this technique is the viability of cells and low cell count in the sample which may interfere with the interpretation of the crossmatch. The challenge of having a low cell count in the case of cadaver patients has been addressed with new advancements in the techniques for cell separation. Commercially available lymphocyte isolation kits can be used to selectively remove or isolate lymphocytes based on the presence of specific cell surface antigens. This can be achieved through negative selection and depletion, or positive selection employing antibody complexes. The antibody complexes connect specific cells to magnetic particles that are commercially available. Labeled cells are pulled to the sides of the tube when the sample is placed in a magnet, while untouched cells can be simply poured or pipetted off into a new tube. The low cell viability can be addressed by rapid and appropriate transportation of the sample collected. The blood should be collected in an Acid Citrate Dextrose (ACD - Yellow Top) tube and the lymphocytes should be separated as early as possible as the number of viable lymphocytes may decline over a period of storage. If the sample collected must be transported, the storage conditions must be ensured with an appropriate temperature (2–6 degrees Celsius).

False-negative results may occur if there are low levels of DSA (antibody titer is too low to cause complement activation) or if the antibody isotype does not activate complement like HLA antibodies of the IgG2 and IgG4 subclasses.

The sensitivity of the CDCXM test in detecting anti-HLA class II antibodies is low, and the modification of CDCXM with AHG does not enhance this sensitivity since it binds nonspecifically to fragment crystallizable receptors (FcR) on B cells.

High levels of antibodies can also lead to false-negative crossmatch due to the phenomenon of Prozone. This can be addressed by performing the crossmatch in extended dilutions.

If a patient's serum contains an Anti-idiotypic antibody (antibody with specificity for that part of another antibody where it binds antigen) crossmatch reaction pattern will be like less reaction (fewer dead cells or negative reaction) in DTT untreated serum and more reaction (more dead cells or positive reaction) in the DTT treated serum. This challenge is usually seen in patients with rheumatoid arthritis and other autoimmune conditions.

The historical importance of CDCXM in solid organ transplantation is unquestionable; however, with the enormous evolution in histocompatibility testing methods over the years, it is believed that the CDCXM has outlived its usefulness. It is time to embrace a new gold standard in pretransplant histocompatibility testing [12].

2.1.3 Peak serum

Patients on the transplant waiting list should have sera collected at frequent intervals and perform CDCXM, so that there will be a clear picture of historic positivity, variations can be monitored and newly appearing anti-HLA antibodies can be detected. The serum with the highest titer, which exhibits the greatest reactivity, is commonly referred to as the 'peak serum.' This might have been collected some years ago, with the 'present serum' displaying much different reactivity. The antibodies detected in the sera at the highest level may still be significant, as they can raise the likelihood of early rejection due to previous sensitization and the resulting immunological memory.

2.2 Flow cytometry crossmatch

According to the pioneer study conducted by Patel and Terasaki, around 15% of kidney transplants that had negative CDCXM results suffered from early graft failure, despite the enhancements made to the assay. These observations prompted the development of more sensitive techniques, such as flow crossmatch by Garovoy in 1983, for detecting even low levels of anti-HLA antibodies [13].

In flow crossmatch fluorescein-labeled antibodies against human IgG (antihuman IgG F(ab)/FITC) are added to the incubated patient serum and donor lymphocytes (**Figure 8A**), whereas in CDC crossmatch, complement is added in this step. This fluorescein-labeled antibody will bind to all the IgG antibodies (thereby increasing the sensitivity of the assay) in the recipient serum. If a DSAb is present in the serum (**Figure 8B**), it gets bound to the donor lymphocytes. The complex that is formed (**Figure 8C**) between the DSA and antihuman IgG F(ab)/FITC is excited by lasers and the corresponding light emission measured as mean fluorescence intensity (MFI)

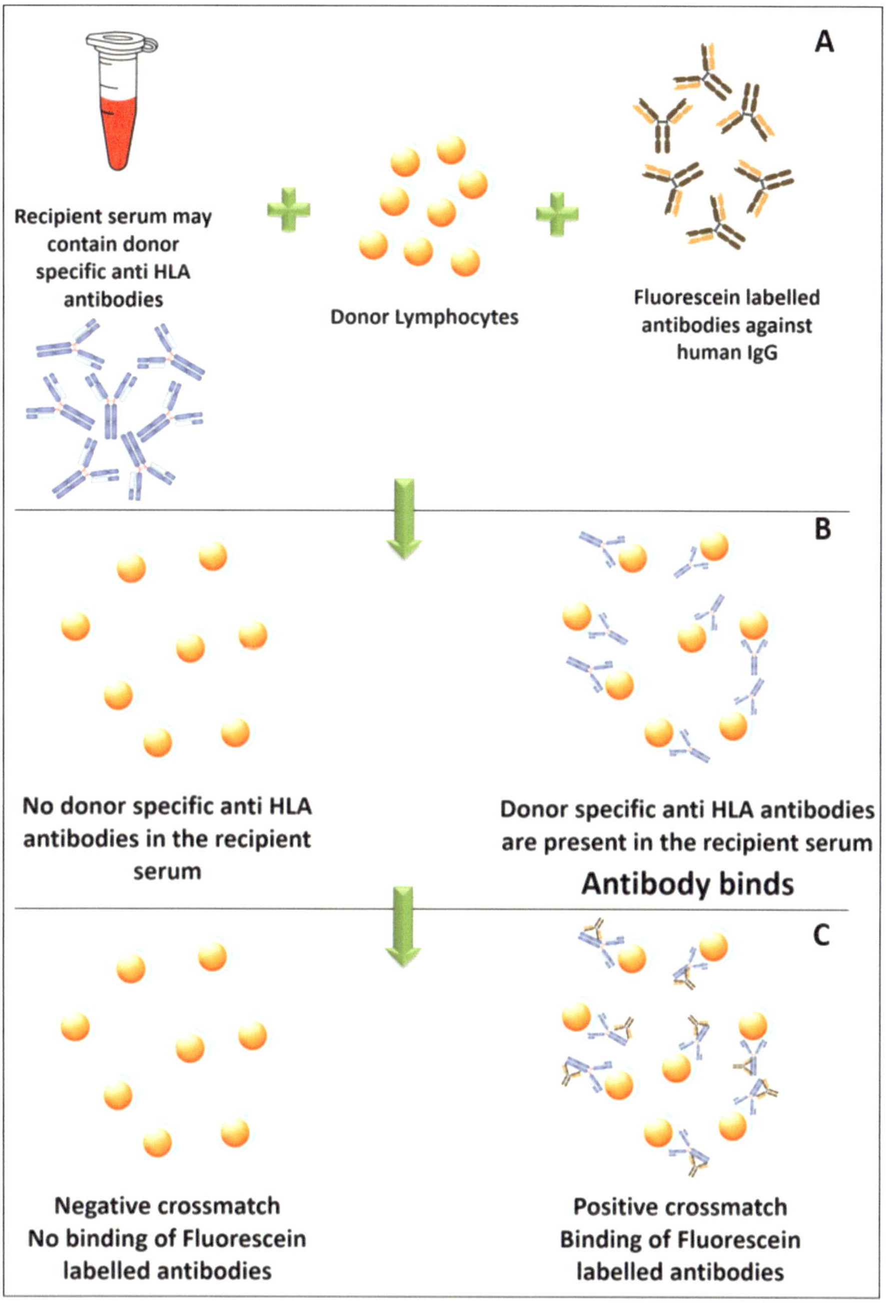

Figure 8.
The flow crossmatch.

is detected by a combination of filters and detectors. The difference in the MFI of the patient's serum and the negative control is called as median channel fluorescence (MCF) shift. It is typically quantified as a ratio or delta of the MCF, enabling a more objective interpretation of the results.

The utilization of anti-CD3 and anti-CD19 or CD20 monoclonal antibodies enables the differentiation of T and B lymphocyte subpopulations, facilitating the identification of antibodies against HLA class I (which is expressed by both T and B lymphocytes) and HLA class II (which is solely expressed by B lymphocytes).

2.2.1 Modifications

The FCXM has been enhanced with the implementation of three-color analysis and, more recently, a rapidly optimized technique that utilizes a 96-well plate format and other time-saving measures (referred to as the Halifax and Halifaster protocols). The purpose of these protocols is to decrease the amount of time required and streamline the setup process while maintaining the quality and sensitivity of the system. The implementation of the Halifax protocol improvements led to a reduction of over 60% in processing time compared to the standard protocol. The main modifications implemented included the adoption of a 96-well U-bottom tray, a modification in the ratio of cells to serum, decreased durations for incubation and washing steps, and an elevated incubation temperature. The Halifaster technique enhances the purity of lymphocytes to more than 90%, resulting in an increase in the sensitivity of the assay. A significant number of transplants centers throughout the world have implemented the Halifax protocol as a standard procedure in their clinical practice. The results obtained from different laboratories have shown a high level of agreement [14].

2.2.2 Advantages and limitations

Compared to the CDCXM, FCXM offers superior sensitivity since it can detect a wider spectrum of immunoglobulins of clinical value, such as complement-fixing and non-complement-fixing IgG antibodies [15].

Flow cytometric crossmatch (FCXM) is not perfect, and it occasionally produces false-positive or false-negative results, just like any other diagnostic test.

IgG binding to FcR in B cells, low background in the negative control, inadequate washing following antibody incubations, autoantibodies, surface antigens linked to lymphocytes other than HLA molecules and the use of therapeutic antibodies like anti-thymocyte globulin, rituximab (anti-CD20), alemtuzumab (anti-CD52), basiliximab (anti-CD25), and daclizumab (anti-CD25) are some of the possible causes of false-positive results [16, 17].

Many reasons for false-negative results in FCXM have been reported, including (a) low donor cell HLA expression levels; (b) an excess of lymphocytes resulting in prozone phenomenon; (c) low serum volume (inappropriate cell-to-serum ratio); (d) low levels of anti-HLA antibodies; (e) low lymphocyte purity (i.e., contaminants like platelets and dead lymphocytes); and (f) negative control serum with high background.

2.2.3 Interpretation

The result of the flow crossmatch can either be quantified or given simply as positive or negative. Fluorescence intensity above control is known as channel shifts.

Quantification can be done by performing serial dilution of the recipient serum samples to demonstrate the change in the levels of antibodies on diluting the serum. Positive flow cross matches in the presence of negative CDCXM are most likely to be the result of low-level, non-HLA, or non-complement-fixing antibodies.

Interpretation of the FXCM report is given in the **Table 2**.

2.3 Solid-phase DSA lysate crossmatch

2.3.1 Bead-based technology

In the 1990s, fluorescently tagged beads were introduced, which completely changed the HLA antibody testing process. Beads impregnated with varying ratios of two fluorochromes (10 distinct concentrations of red and infrared dyes are used to generate 100 distinct bead regions) are available as commercial kits. Each bead produces a unique signal and may have one or more types of HLA molecules attached. A distinct target analyte is coupled to every bead, of which the information is provided clearly in the lot sheet (**Figures 9** and **10A**).

The patient's serum is initially incubated with the beads. The serum will react with the bead expressing the relevant HLA molecule if the patient has HLA antibodies. Following washing, the beads are treated with a secondary antibody, often an antihuman IgG tagged with phycoerythrin (PE).

The two lasers used by the fluorocytometer stimulate the PE attached to the detection antibody and the fluorochrome in the bead, respectively (**Figure 10B**). As a result, the first output determines the bead's distinct signal and, in turn, the associated HLA molecule's specificity, while the second output tells whether the antibody is linked to the particular HLA molecule. Depending on the degree of testing being done, each bead has one or more distinct kinds of human leukocyte antigen (HLA) molecules attached. An HLA antibody present in the test serum will attach itself to the appropriate complementary HLA molecule (**Figure 10A**).

2.3.2 MFI

The change in a cell population's fluorescence intensity is called Mean Fluorescence Intensity (MFI). It is an indicator of the amount of antigen or

T-cell CXM	B-cell CXM	Interpretation
Negative	Negative	No DSAb to HLA class I or II or DSAb titer too low to cause a positive reaction or Non-complement-fixing DSAb
Positive	Positive	DSAb to HLA class I or Multiple DSAb to HLA class I +/− II
Negative	Positive	DSAb to HLA class II or Low levels of DSAb to HLA class I
Positive	Negative	Technical error (possibly related to B-cell viability) The test should be repeated

Table 2.
FCXM interpretation.

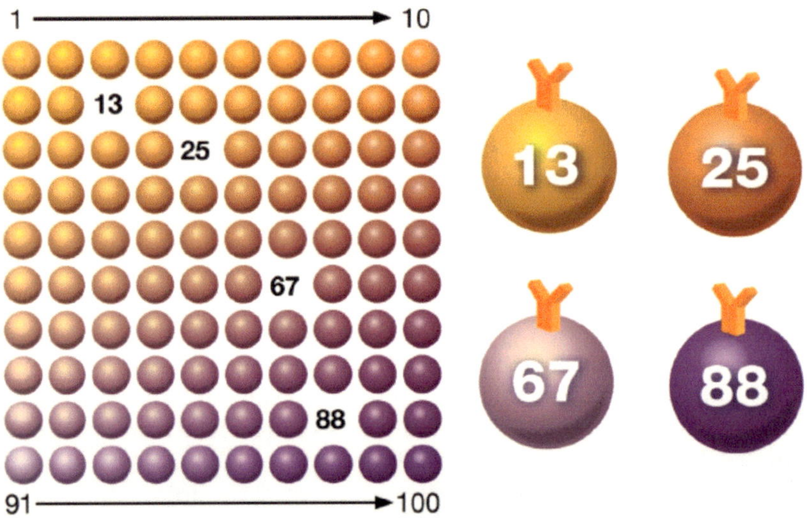

Figure 9.
Multiplex immunoassay technology refers to a method of simultaneously detecting and measuring multiple analytes in a sample using immunoassay techniques. The figure is sourced from Bio-Rad's Bio-Plex® suspension array system, specifically the xMAP technology overview. Link to the license - https://creativecommons.org/licenses/by/4.0/.

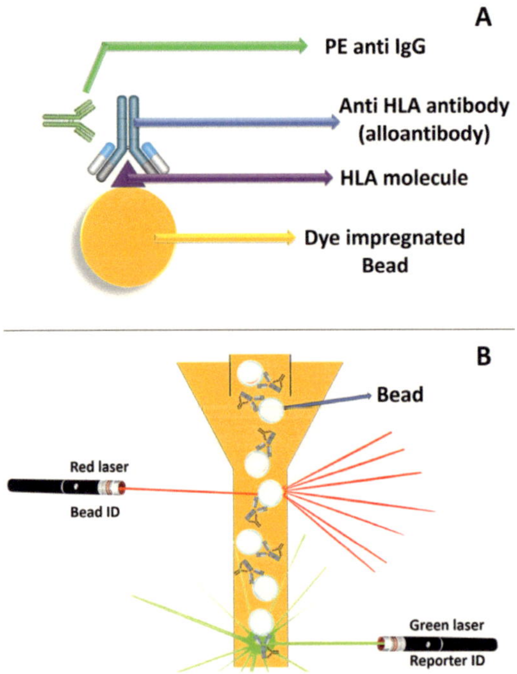

Figure 10.
Principle underlying the bead & fluorocytometer.

antibody that is present in the sample, depending upon the test that is being performed. A suggested "cut off" value for MFI positive does not exist. Most laboratories fix their "cut off" level to declare as positive based on levels measured with appropriate controls and on knowledge obtained from clinical outcomes. An effective strategy is to treat each patient as an individual, especially in the case of multiparous women or patients who have had previous grafting. For example, a patient who has had previous transplants, and whose MFI level for a particular HLA specificity was above the negative cut-off values but below the laboratory-established cut-off threshold (to label as positive), should be handled with caution. It might be a sign of pre-sensitization with extremely low antibody levels, which can be triggered upon exposure to the same antigen again with a different graft. When a patient has no prior history of possible HLA preimmunization, this result can be interpreted differently. Each testing facility must determine its own MFI "cut off" levels in cooperation with its clinical colleagues if there is no established standard for the execution of the bead-based assay [18].

2.3.3 Principle of lysate crossmatch

With donor lysates—which are made by lysing the donor's lymphocytes with a reagent—rather than living cells, which are more difficult to preserve for posttransplantation research, DSAXM enables us to carry out a true crossmatch.

Class I or Class II HLA-specific monoclonal antibodies have been coupled to two of the blend's beads. These two beads will collect the solubilized HLA when combined with a lysate, creating a donor-specific HLA target for antibodies in a serum sample. To ensure that the right conjugate has been used in the assay and to track the quantity of background in the experiment, control beads are also included in the bead blend. The beads are incubated with diluted patient serum. Antihuman IgG-phycoerythrin (PE) conjugate is added after another wash. After an incubation period, the fluorocytometer is used to examine the results. Software that yields a mean fluorescence index (MFI) value is utilized for result interpretation and analysis. Depending on the cut-off value, the MFI value is utilized to determine the positive and negative findings. The threshold value differs throughout laboratories. Generally speaking, the threshold for both Class I and Class II is 1000 (750–1500).

2.3.4 Advantages and limitations

It is possible to store the donor lysate, which is utilized in the crossmatch, for later examination. In fact, it has been demonstrated that this assay is more sensitive than cell-based assays for determining an organ's histocompatibility after solid organ transplantation.

Its downside is that the target cell is a lymphocyte with a wide variety of target molecules (non-HLA) on its surface, despite its high sensitivity. Solid-phase techniques that use isolated HLA molecules as targets (single antigen bead assay) for antibody detection have been developed as a workaround for this issue.

Luminex tests for DSA have the potential to be utilized for posttransplant surveillance to identify the emergence of *de novo* DSA in recipients of solid organ transplants, in addition to predicting the risk of rejection prior to transplantation.

2.4 Virtual crossmatch

The integration of solid-phase HLA antibody testing technologies, including single antigen beads (SAB), with the donor HLA type has greatly enhanced the sensitivity of antibody detection and facilitated a virtual assessment. The Virtual crossmatch (VXM) test, as established by the American Society for Histocompatibility and Immunogenetics (ASHI), is an assessment of immunological compatibility that compares a patient's alloantibody profile with a donor's histocompatibility antigens.

The VXM is not a direct laboratory test but rather relies on the analysis of previous results obtained from donor HLA molecular typing and Single Antigen Bead (SAB) assays conducted during the recipient's anti-HLA study.

2.4.1 Components of virtual crossmatch

2.4.1.1 Donor HLA typing

The first methods to identify HLA antigens were serological microlymphocytotoxicity techniques, which recognized different HLAs on the surface of lymphocytes using a battery of carefully chosen antisera. In clinical applications, increasingly accurate DNA-based typing approaches have supplanted serological methods over the last 20 years.

Sequencing-based typing (SBT), sequence-specific primer (SSP) directed amplification (**Figure 11**), and reverse sequence-specific oligonucleotide (rSSO) probe hybridization (**Figure 12**) are the three fundamental DNA-based HLA typing methods that are employed in conjunction with polymerase chain reaction (PCR). The main idea behind these techniques is that sequence-specific oligonucleotide probes (rSSO) hybridization, gel electrophoretic mobility (SSP), or direct DNA sequencing (SBT) are used to detect the specific polymorphisms after the HLA genes have been specifically amplified by PCR.

Using a special set of primers that are intended to have perfect matches with a single allele or collection of alleles and generate a product with a specific known size, we can type HLA using the SSP method. An image of an agarose gel electrophoresis

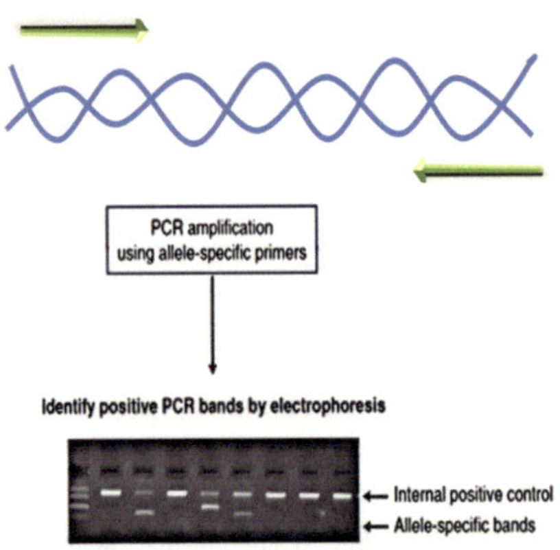

Figure 11.
HLA typing by SSP.

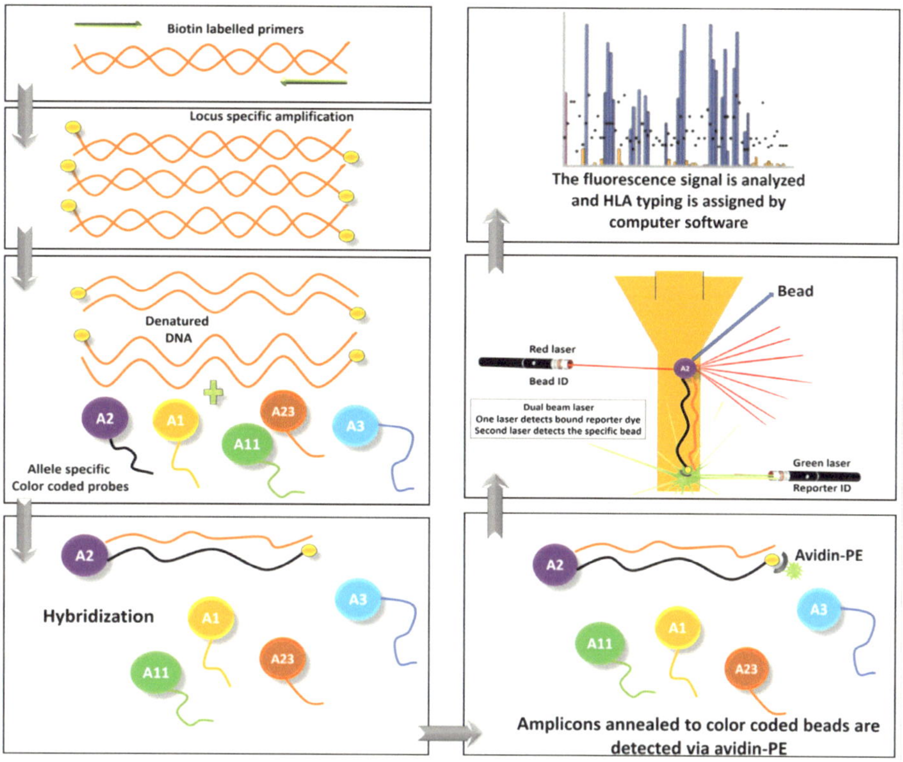

Figure 12.
HLA typing by reverse single-nucleotide probe hybridization (SSOP) method using bead-based assay.

displays the pattern of PCR products that are specific to the alleles or groups involved in the amplification of the HLA class I or class II genes (**Figure 11**).

Using locus-specific primers conjugated with biotin, DNA samples are amplified by PCR in the HLA typing by SSO approach. Streptavidin phycoerythrin (PE) is used to identify the hybridized polystyrene beads created from the denatured PCR products. A fluorocytometer is an equipment used to detect fluorescence signals. A software application analyzes the combined data and assigns an HLA type (**Figure 12**).

2.4.1.2 Single antigen bead assay on patient serum

Latex (polystyrene) microbeads coated with a single Human leukocyte antigen (single antigen assay for specific identification of antibodies) or multiple Human leukocyte antigens (for screening) extracted from gene-modified cells are used in solid-phase assays that use multiplex technology (developed by Luminex Corporation). The most sensitive solid-phase technique is the single antigen bead assay (SAB). Recipient serum is combined with these beads (**Figure 13A**). Any anti-HLA antibodies that are present, bind to the synthetic beads (**Figure 13B**) and are found using fluorocytometer with an isotype-specific detection antibody (**Figure 13C** and **D**). The HLA antigen specificity of each bead is indicated by distinct fluorochromes within the beads.

As to the criteria set by the European Federation for Immunogenetics, the patients who are suitable for VXM transplantation are those who meet the following conditions [19]:

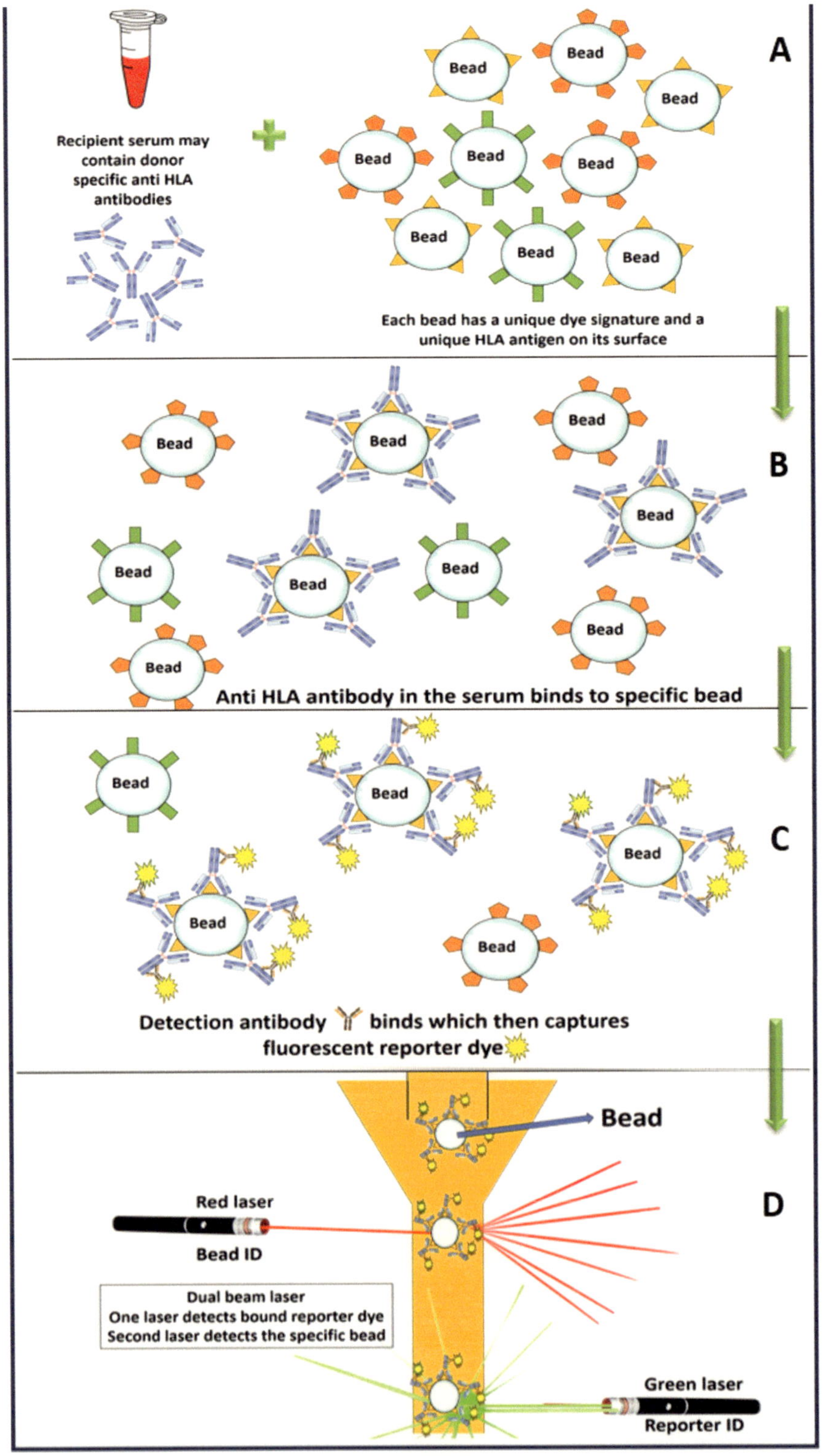

Figure 13.
The single antigen bead assay.

1. No events that could potentially cause sensitization have occurred since the last serum sample was tested.

2. A minimum of two distinct samples must have undergone testing, and at least one serum testing result received within the past 3 months must be included.

3. Clear and recorded definitions of acceptable and unacceptable mismatches have been established.

4. If a crossmatch is not performed on a recipient who has developed an immune response to foreign antigens, the identification of antibodies must be done using SAB technology.

Compared to other crossmatching methods, virtual crossmatching has the advantage of eliminating false positives caused by non-HLA antibodies, as seen in CDCXM and FXCM. Furthermore, since the antigens on beads are controllable, it is also clear which class of HLA they are binding to—keep in mind that class I and II antigens are present in B-cell crossmatching. In the event of a negative CDC crossmatch, the presence of a DSAb found by bead-based assays seems to be predictive of acute rejection risk and reduced graft survival.

Using an example (**Figure 14**), let us examine how virtual crossmatch functions. Only strong antibodies to the indicated specificities are shown by the patient. Given that the patient does not exhibit any DSA toward Donor 1, a virtual crossmatch between the two suggests that the pair might be compatible. Due to three strong DSAs that the patient exhibits toward Donor 2 (A2, B58, and DP401—highlighted in red), the patient and Donor 2 are incompatible. Donor 3 does not have sufficient HLA typing at the DP locus to support a virtual crossmatch.

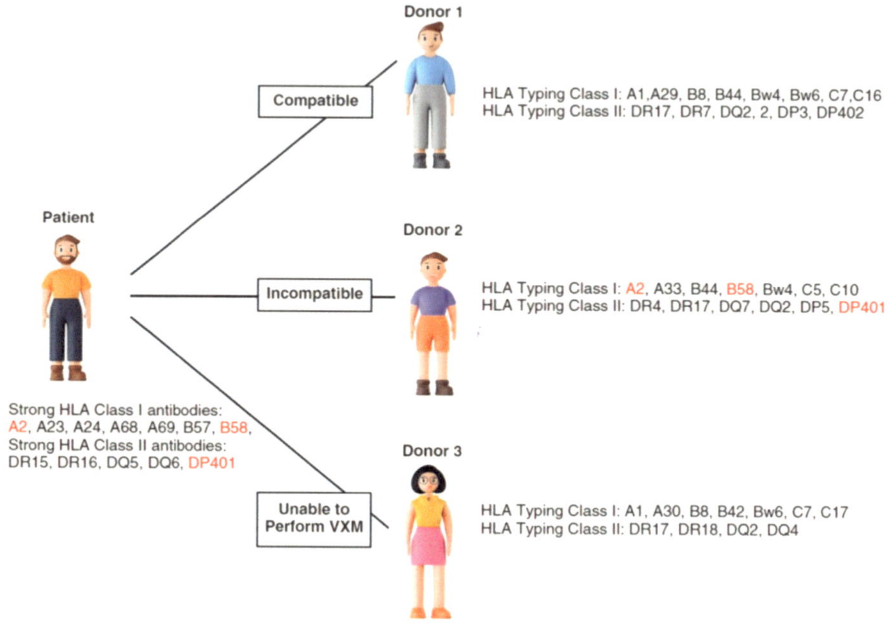

Figure 14.
The virtual crossmatch prediction.

2.4.2 Limitations and challenges

2.4.2.1 Lack of antigenic representation

LABScreen® Single Antigen (One Lambda) and LIFECODES ® Single Antigen (Werfen) are two popular SAB kits that have different antigen profiles, antigen densities, and detection sensitivity. The complement activation capabilities of antibodies cannot be assessed by the original SAB assay; some manufacturers offer C1q/C3d assays, which are modifications of the SAB assay that can assess the complement-binding capabilities of antibodies.

Currently, there are several commercial kits, known as extended or supplemental panels, that offer a greater number of alleles compared to the standard SAB panels. This decreases the probability of not detecting various antibodies that the patient might have developed against less common HLA (present in the donor). Furthermore, there is a higher level of presence of genetically varied genes from different ethnic backgrounds. This also enhances the extent of antigen coverage while simultaneously expanding the range and comprehensiveness of epitope coverage. Consequently, they more effectively complement molecular typing outcomes. Individuals who are most likely to derive advantages from these extended panels include transplant recipients who are highly sensitive, such as multiparous females, patients undergoing second or third transplants, and patients who received transplants from donors with incomplete typing. This is mainly accomplished by enhanced antibody profiling to obtain more accurate virtual crossmatches, higher precision in monitoring donor-specific antibodies (DSA), identification of acceptable alleles, and the utilization of epitope-based investigations to clarify the reactivity between antibodies and epitopes.

2.4.2.2 False positivity due to antigen configuration: antibodies to denatured HLA

Typically, regular HLA antigens are shown on the outer layer of cells as a complex made up of several molecules. Using class I as an illustration, there are substantial amounts of alpha-chain, beta2-microglobulin, and a peptide present within the grooves of the heavy alpha-chain. Nevertheless, the SAB reagent's beads can include HLA class I antigens in many forms, including native antigens, heavy alpha-chain alone, and peptide-free heavy alpha-chain with b2-microglobulin. Furthermore, these variations frequently exist as misfolded molecules, referred to as denatured HLA molecules. The existence of structural variations in the bead sets may hinder the precise evaluation of anti-HLA antibodies. In addition, patients may produce an antibody that does not bind to a specific region on the normal HLA antigen but instead binds to a region on the denatured HLA antigen. This might lead to a false-positive result in the SAB assay. If there is suspicion of false-positive reactivity, it maybe beneficial to reevaluate using alternative SAB kits or a new platform, such as a phenotypic beads assay or surrogate FCXM [20, 21].

2.4.2.3 Shared epitope phenomenon

An epitope refers to the specific region of an antigen that is recognized by an antibody (**Figure 14**). An antigen can exhibit many epitopes, which can either be exclusive to the antigen itself (private epitope) or shared by multiple antigens (public epitope). A cross-reactive group (CREG) is a collection of HLA antigens that have a shared public epitope and consistently show the same reactivity pattern. To obtain significant insights as DSAs, it is crucial to analyze the recipient's antibody profile with respect to the pre-identified CREGs (**Figure 15**).

The antibody's ability to recognize the epitope shared by numerous Human leukocyte antigens coated on the beads in the reagent maybe overestimated. This sharing of epitope by multiple antigens can result in a decreased MFI value for all impacted beads (as illustrated in **Figure 16b**), which is caused by the antibody attaching to competing targets (multiple, different antigen beads having the same epitope). When the concentration of the specific antibody is low, there is a higher chance of false-negative reactions occurring, leading to positive reactions being mistakenly identified as negative [5]. Antibodies when selectively attached to beads that possess the targeted eplet of the human leukocyte antigen (HLA), a greater mean fluorescence intensity (MFI) of 2500 can be obtained, as depicted in **Figure 16a**.

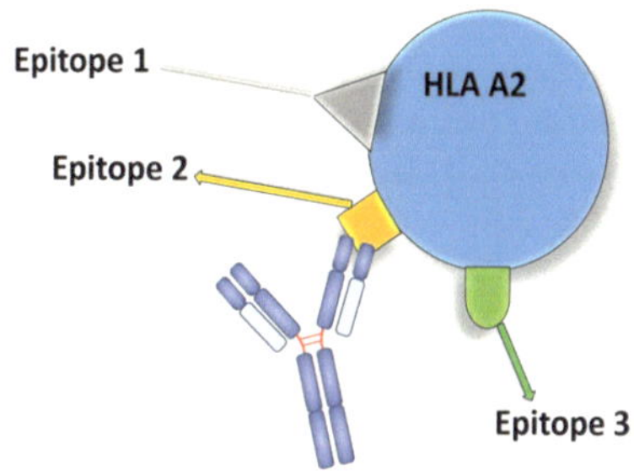

Figure 15.
Human leukocyte antigen with three different epitopes.

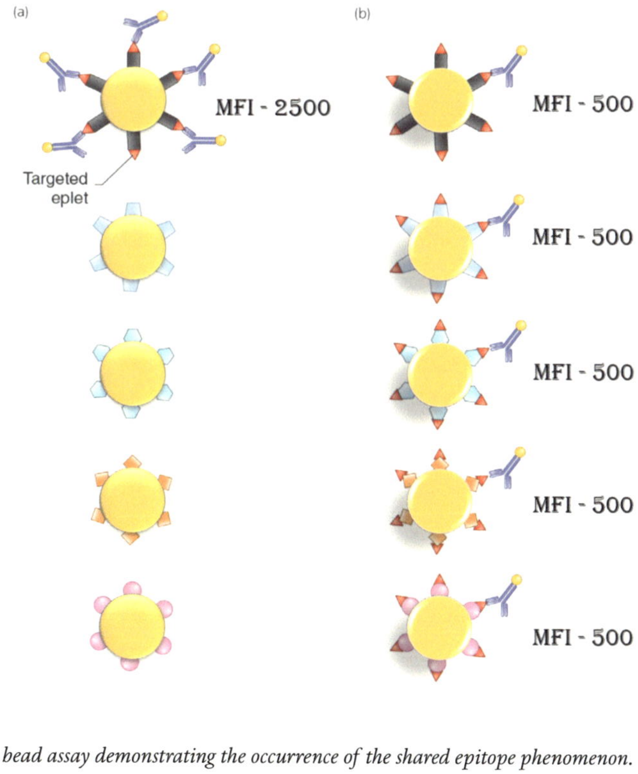

Figure 16.
The single antigen bead assay demonstrating the occurrence of the shared epitope phenomenon.

2.4.2.4 The prozone effect

Mean fluorescence intensity (MFI) can only rise to a certain point when the serum is overabundant with antibodies, saturating the antigens on the beads. We refer to this circumstance as the "prozone effect." Doing the assay with serum dilution (reducing the antibody titer so as to have an equal proportion of antigens and antibodies to react) maybe helpful in determining this impact [22, 23].

3. Comparison between various crossmatch methods

The highly sensitive solid-phase assays complement cell-based assays like CDC-XM and FCXM by almost eliminating immunological incompatibility in solid organ transplants. Comparison between various crossmatch methods is given in the **Table 3** [10].

The comparative investigations conducted on FCXM versus CDCXM reveal that around 15% of patients receiving primary grafts exhibit a negative CDCCXM but a positive FCXM, while this percentage increases to 34% for regrafts. Similarly, within the first 3 months, around 20% of primary grafts and 60% of regrafts have early graft loss when FCXM is positive. In contrast, the rates drop to 5% for primary grafts and 15% for regrafts when FCXM is negative [24].

The SAB test is currently the most sensitive approach for detecting anti-HLA antibodies, by which we can identify anti-HLA antibodies with a median fluorescence intensity (MFI) of 1000 or below (subject to variation based on the supplier of the bead-based assay). The FCXM would yield a positive result when the specific antibody (SAB) begins at a minimum fluorescence intensity (MFI) of 2500; however, this

Crossmatch	CDC CXM	Flow cytometry CXM	Virtual CXM
Target	Donor's lymphocytes	Donor's lymphocytes	Antigen coated beads
Type of antigens	Native Human leukocyte antigens on cell membrane	Native Human leukocyte antigens on cell membrane	Human leukocyte antigens extracted from gene-modified cells coated on latex microbeads
Type of antibodies detected	Cytotoxic IgG/IgM antibodies	IgG antibodies bound on the lymphocyte membrane	IgG antibodies bound to the HLA on beads
Specific for anti-HLA antibodies	No	No	Yes
Interpretation	Subjective: operator-dependent technique	Objective: Based on the difference in the intensity of fluorescence between test serum and negative control, referred to as channel shifts	Objective: Based on the MFI of specific antigens
Sensitivity	Low	High	High
Approximate processing time	4–5 hours	3 hours	<1 hour
Predicting the clinical outcome of the transplant	Hyperacute rejection	Acute rejection	Acute/chronic rejection

Table 3.
Comparison of different methods of crossmatches [10].

may vary depending on the locus, with a greater MFI required for HLA-C, DQB1, or DPB1. On the other hand, the CDCXM would produce a positive result when the MFI reaches a range of 8000–10,000. This information is valuable for establishing a connection between the outcomes acquired from the crossmatch tests and interpreting them within a therapeutic framework [25].

The VXM results have demonstrated a strong capacity to accurately forecast the outcomes of the physical crossmatch test, exhibiting a high degree of agreement. Furthermore, studies have shown that patients who have a negative FCXM result but a positive VXM result are at a heightened risk of antibody-mediated rejection (AMR) and have a shorter duration of graft life [26–29].

To provide an overall view of the various aspects that impact the decision-making process for transplants, a simple yet comprehensive review of these evaluations is systematically presented in a tabular format. This tabular representation is a valuable instrument that offers a structured and comprehensible overview of the several elements that must be considered when evaluating the feasibility of a kidney transplant (**Table 4**) [30].

CDCXM	FlowXM	SAB/Virtual XM	Interpretation
Positive	**Positive**	**Positive**	• Significant amount of DSA • Significant likelihood of experiencing hyperacute rejection
Negative	**Positive**	**Positive**	• Intermediate level of DSA • Non-complement-fixing DSA
Negative	*Negative*	**Positive**	• Little amount of DSA • False-positive SAB test and the possible causes include o High background due to serum factors binding to latex beads o Binding to denatured antigen o Setting a low threshold for designating an antibody as positive (overcalling)
Positive	**Positive**	*Negative*	• Binding of non-HLA antibodies • Drug interference (e.g., Rituximab, ATG, alemtuzumab, IVIG). • False-negative SAB test and the reason could be: o The bead panel lacks representation of the donor antigen/allele o The presence of inhibitors in serum, causes a “prozone” effect. o IgM/IVIG binding to the beads, masking the detection of IgG alloantibody o Low-level anti-HLA antibody against a shared epitope, which is “diluted out” across multiple beads, leading to an under-representation of the true antibody burden (**Figure 16**)
Positive	*Negative*	*Negative*	• IgM antibody (either anti-HLA or non-HLA) o Can be confirmed by treating the serum with DTT
Negative	**Positive**	*Negative*	• Low-level IgG non-HLA antibody • False-negative SAB test

Bold indicates a positive crossmatch result and italic indicate a negative crossmatch result

Table 4.
Illustration of different scenarios following pretransplant histocompatibility tests [30].

4. Algorithmic approach to pretransplant histocompatibility testing

Having an algorithm for pretransplant histocompatibility testing is very beneficial. It will help the healthcare professionals to have a uniform systematic approach and better utilization of the resources. We suggest an algorithm (**Figures 17** and **18**) based

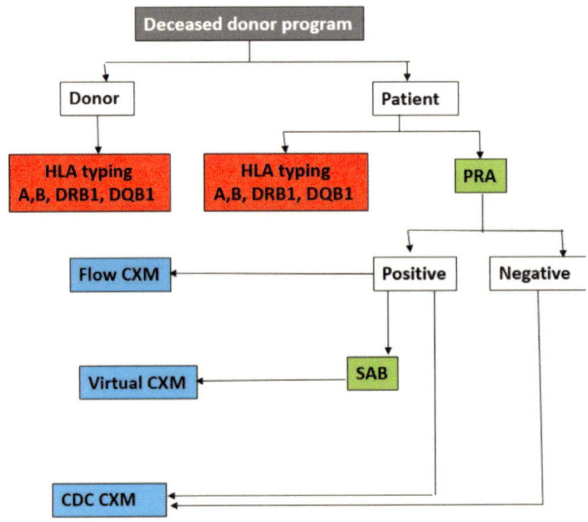

Figure 17.
Transplant immunology testing algorithm for deceased donor organ transplantation.

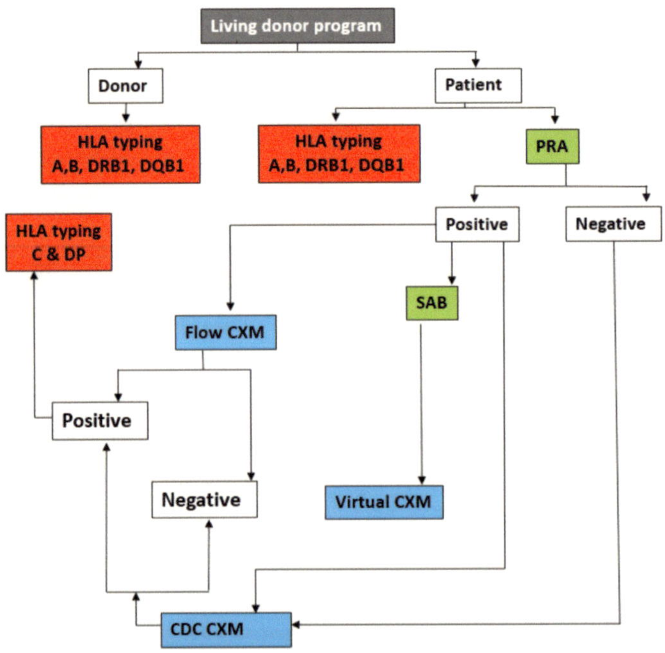

Figure 18.
Transplant immunology testing algorithm for living donor organ transplantation.

on recommendations suggested in **Tables 5** and **6**, for the deceased as well as the living donor transplantation program. This recommendation has been developed considering the cost, feasibility, and accessibility of diagnostic resources.

Deceased donor program					
Deceased donor			**Patient/recipient**		
1	HLA typing - A, B, DR B1, DQ B1		1	HLA typing - A, B, DR B1, DQ B1	
	Recommendation	Desirable		Recommendation	Mandatory
	Method	SSO/SSP/NGS		Method	SSO/SSP/NGS
			2	Screen for anti-HLA antibodies	
				PRA	Mandatory
				SAB	Desirable (if PRA is negative)
					Mandatory (if PRA is positive for class I or II)
Crossmatch					
Nonsensitized recipient (Negative PRA)			Sensitized recipient (Positive PRA)		
	CDC CXM	Mandatory		CDC CXM	Mandatory
	Flow CXM	Desirable		Flow CXM	Mandatory
	Virtual CXM	Desirable		Virtual CXM	Mandatory

Table 5.
Transplant immunology testing recommendations for deceased donor organ transplantation.

Living donor program					
Living donor			Patient/recipient		
1	HLA typing - A, B, DR B1, DQ B1		1	HLA typing - A, B, DR B1, DQ B1	
	Recommendation	Mandatory		Recommendation	Mandatory
	Method	SSO/SSP/NGS		Method	SSO/SSP/NGS
	HLA typing – C, DP		2	Screen for Anti-HLA antibodies	
	Recommendation	Desirable		PRA	Mandatory
		Mandatory (if the recipient has Anti HLA-C or Anti HLA-DP antibodies along with a positive crossmatch by flow/CDC)		SAB	Desirable (if PRA is negative)
					Mandatory (if PRA is positive for class I or II)
	Method	SSO or SSP			
Crossmatch					
Nonsensitized recipient (Negative PRA)			Sensitized recipient (Positive PRA)		
•	CDC CXM	Mandatory	•	CDC CXM	Mandatory
•	Flow CXM	Desirable	•	Flow CXM	Mandatory
•	Virtual CXM	Desirable	•	Virtual CXM	Mandatory

Table 6.
Transplant immunology testing recommendation for living donor organ transplantation.

5. Epitope-based HLA matching: a new histocompatibility paradigm

An antibody's antigenic determinant or recognition point is called an epitope. Every HLA comprises of several epitopes, many of which are shared by various antigens and have polymorphic sequences. Epitope analysis is a method used to determine the recipient's serum antibody reactivity against the eplet expressed on donor HLA.

To prolong long-term graft survival and prevent the production of donor-specific HLA antibodies, donors and recipients should be matched for epitopes. A single amino acid can define an epitope, even if the constellation of epitopes is what separates one antigen from another. Epitopes can be classified as structural or functional; functional epitopes are called eplets (**Figure 19**). The most common definition of an eplet that stimulates the synthesis of antibodies (a functional feature) is a linear or conformational sequence of three amino acids (previously called triplets), at least one of which differs from the antibody producer.

Functional epitopes, or eplets, are distinguished from structural epitopes by the following analogy. We are using the example of a suspension bridge intended to link two islands divided by a body of water to explain the distinction between structural epitopes and functional epitopes. The functional part of the bridge, which connects the islands horizontally, is equivalent to an eplet or functional epitope. But until structural elements—the suspension cables—support that portion of the bridge over the water, it is unable to perform that role. An operational bridge, or structural epitope, is the end product of the collective [31].

The epitope-centered HLA matching principle has been included in the algorithms of two computational methods, HLA Matchmaker and PIRCHE-II, in order to determine the best donor for a recipient. These programs use state-of-the-art artificial intelligence algorithms to determine which eplets are targets of antibodies found on platforms with a single antigen bead. HLA Matchmaker matches these structures precisely using Microsoft Excel and looks for antibody responses to particular regions of these structures. Any other antigen that expresses the same eplet that an antibody is produced against will attach to it. Currently, a lot of centers are employing these platforms to find mismatched eplets [32, 33].

The degree of match between donor and recipient can be investigated on a more detailed and physiologically appropriate categorization system by dissecting each HLA molecule into a collection of epitopes. *De novo* donor-specific antibodies are likely to be developed by the recipient of the donor with zero HLA allele mismatches but a few eplet-level mismatches. Studies have shown that kidney transplants with

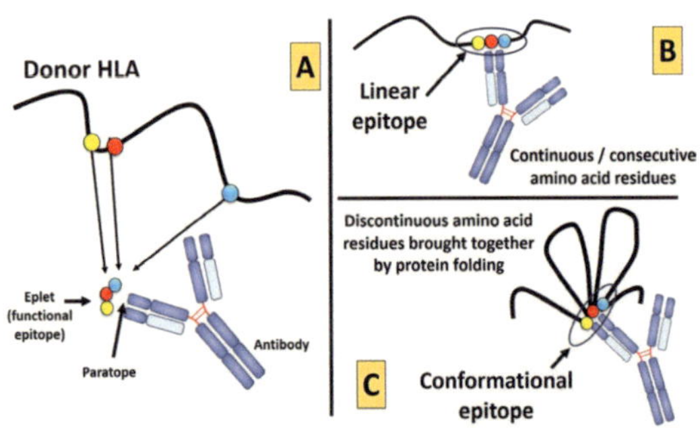

Figure 19.
Eplets and epitope.

eplet mismatches have reduced survival, even though donor-recipient pair had zero HLA allele mismatches [34–36].

6. Non-HLA antibodies

Numerous non-HLA antibodies have been linked to poor kidney transplant outcomes when they target endothelial, epithelial, or different proteins. Some of the reported non-HLA antibodies are those against the following: vimentin (AVA), tubulin (anti-Kα1 tubulin), collagens (anti-Col), angiotensin II type 1 receptor (AT1R-Ab), endothelin-1 type A receptor (ETAR), Major Histocompatibility complex class I chain-related antigen A & B (MICA-Ab), and anti-endothelial cell antibodies (AECA). Other collagen type IV, fibronectin, perlecan, vimentin, agrin, peroxisomal trans-2-enoyl-CoA reductase (PECR), protein kinase C zeta type (PRKCZ), Rho guanine nucleotide exchange factor 2 (Ant-ARHGDIB-Ab), and H-Y antigen [37].

The generation of non-HLA antibodies is influenced by both autoimmunity and alloimmunity in a complementary and integrated manner. Advances in transcriptomics and genomewide evaluation tools have made significant strides in our understanding of the mechanisms behind antibody creation.

Before transplantation, when some endothelial injury happens neoantigens or cryptic antigens are exposed, which is the first step in the development of non-HLA antibody formation. This injury can be caused by acute kidney injury, chronic kidney disease, lupus nephritis, focal segmental glomerulosclerosis, diabetes, or preeclampsia. Acute graft pyelonephritis, BKV nephropathy, anti-HLA antibodies, rejection, and specific transplant-associated factors are some of the complex factors that contribute to the formation of non-HLA antibodies in the posttransplant setting. Other factors include the interaction between autoimmunity and alloimmunity. The formation of non-HLA alloantibodies does not always need endothelial damage (**Table 7**) [38–41].

These antibodies identify non-HLA antigens found in a variety of tissues and cells, including immune cells, podocytes, mesangial cells, tubular epithelial cells,

Antibody type	Auto/alloantibody	Mechanism of injury
Ant-AT1R-Ab	Autoantibody	Complement independent
Ant-ETAR-Ab	Autoantibody	Complement independent
Ant-MICA-Ab	Auto and alloantibody	Complement dependent
Ant-perlecan-Ab	Autoantibody	Complement dependent
Ant-agrin-Ab	Autoantibody	Complement dependent
Ant-collagen type IV, III & I -Ab	Autoantibody	—
Ant-fibronectin-Ab	Autoantibody	—
Ant-vimentin-Ab	Autoantibody	Complement dependent
Ant-H-Y-Ab	Alloantibody	Complement dependent
Ant-ARHGDIB-Ab	Autoantibody	Complement dependent
Ant-PECR-Ab	Autoantibody	Complement dependent
Ant-PRKCZ-Ab	Autoantibody	—

Table 7.
Non-HLA antibodies.

endothelium vascular cells, and smooth muscle vascular cells. The majority of antigens that cause the development of non-HLA autoantibodies are endothelial autoantigens because the vascular endothelium serves as the primary barrier between the recipient's immune system and the transplanted kidney [38, 42].

In the past 15 years, AT1R-Ab has been the most extensively studied and well-known form of non HLA antibody. Reduced graft function, steroid-refractory vascular rejection, and malignant hypertension were all linked to the presence of AT1R-Ab [43].

6.1 Endothelial cell crossmatching

It is a technique for identifying antibodies against non-HLA endothelial cells. Anti-endothelial cell antibodies (AECA) are not detected by standard lymphocyte crossmatching methods. Endothelial cells are made to incubate with the patient's serum (with the assumption that serum contains anti-endothelial cell antibodies). During the incubation the anti-endothelial cell antibodies, if present will attach to its corresponding antigen. A fluorescent-tagged antibody directed against this anti-endothelial cell antibody is added following which a flow cytometer is used to measure the fluorescence intensity, which is correlated with the quantity of AECAs bound to the cell (**Figure 20**).

Another cutting-edge endothelial cell flow cytometry crossmatch method is the XM-One assay, which selects precursor endothelial cells directly from donor blood using magnetic beads coated with a Tie-2 antibody. Patient serum is then reacted with these cells to identify AECAs. It is an endothelial FCXM technology that has been approved by the FDA. This test has the advantage of detecting DSA and being able to screen for antibodies to endothelial cells, T lymphocytes, and B lymphocytes all in one assay [44].

7. Financial aspect of transplant immunology tests

The cost that a patent incurs for doing various transplant immunology tests varies widely across the globe. Multiplex-bead assays are costly and yield variable measurements that limit the comparison of results between laboratories. Laboratories modify the manufacturers' methods to reduce reagent costs or enhance assay sensitivity. Despite the excellent sensitivity of the SAB assay for antibody detection, the CDC-XM test is still the most widely utilized in middle-income and low-income countries nations (LMIC) owing to its easy availability and financial constraints [45, 46].

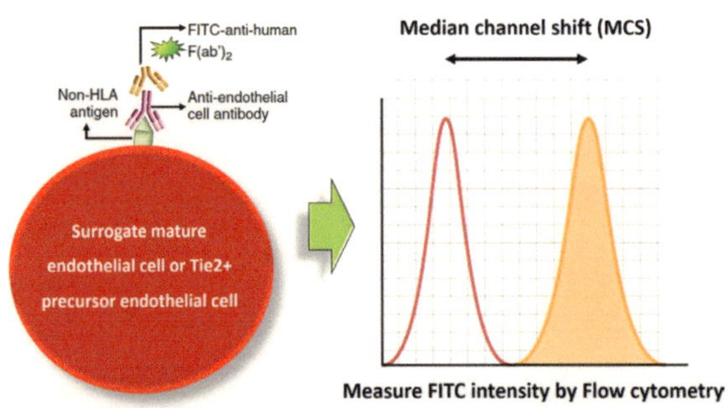

Figure 20.
Endothelial cell crossmatching.

8. Summary

With improved sensitivity of crossmatching has come an improvement in clinical outcomes. Every one of the aforementioned approaches has advantages and disadvantages of its own; no test is meant to serve as the exclusive indicator of transplant immunologic risk.

While there is no perfect test, it can be rather helpful to be able to evaluate DSA using different testing methods in these kinds of intricate scenarios.

In resource-limited settings transplant clinicians rely only on CDC crossmatch, but the preferred method would be identifying the DSAbs in the recipient serum by Flow crossmatch bead-based assays, and single antigen bead assay (virtual crossmatching).

When it comes to donor selection, the computational-based method—that is, epitope matching algorithms—is still relatively new in the field of organ transplantation. Still, there is a good chance that this novel approach will become a crucial instrument for risk evaluation and improved donor choice. This is a promising area for additional research in the field of transplantation, with great prospects for their wider application in the future as physicians progressively harness the power of artificial intelligence and machine learning algorithms.

Conflict of interest

The authors declare no conflict of interest.

Author details

Antonio Paul[1,2], Rajamony Chellammal Arun Dileep[1] and Noble Gracious[3,4]*

1 ACTIMoS (Advanced Centre for Transplant Immunology and Molecular Science), Kochi, Kerala, India

2 Medical Trust Hospital, Kochi, Kerala, India

3 Nephrology, Govt Medical College, Alappuzha, Kerala, India

4 K-SOTTO (Kerala State Organ and Tissue Transplantation Organization), Kerala, India

*Address all correspondence to: noblegracious@hotmail.com

References

[1] Dausset J. Leuco-agglutinins. IV. Leuco-agglutinins and blood transfusion. Vox Sanguinis. 1954;**4**:190-198

[2] IPD-IMGT/HLA Database|Nucleic Acids Research|Oxford Academic. [Internet]. Available from: https://academic.oup.com/nar/article/51/D1/D1053/6814448?login=false [Accessed: May 1, 2024]

[3] Zhang Q, Locke AF, Alvarez AC, Cabarong ML, Liv LC, Alfaro BGP, et al. Advancing precision in histocompatibility and immunogenetics: a comprehensive review of the UCLA exchange program. Frontiers in Genetics. 1 Feb 2024;**15**:1352764

[4] Robinson J, Malik A, Parham P, Bodmer JG, Marsh SG. IMGT/HLA database--A sequence database for the human major histocompatibility complex. Tissue Antigens. 2000;**55**(3):280-287

[5] Nishikawa K, Masui S, Ishida H. Virtual crossmatching and epitope analysis in kidney transplantation: What the physician involved in kidney transplantation should know? International Journal of Urology: Official Journal of the Japanese Urological Association. 2023;**30**(1):7-19

[6] Terasaki PI, Patel R. Significance of the positive crossmatch test in kidney transplantation. The New England Journal of Medicine. 1969;**280**(14):735-739

[7] Altermann W, Seliger B, Sel S, Wendt D, Schlaf G. Comparison of the established standard complement-dependent cytotoxicity and flow cytometric crossmatch assays with a novel ELISA-based HLA crossmatch procedure. Histology and Histopathology. 2006;**21**:1115-1124

[8] Jaramillo A, Ramon DS, Stoll ST. Technical aspects of crossmatching in transplantation. Clinics in Laboratory Medicine. 2018;**38**:579-593

[9] Jayant K, Reccia I, Julie BM. Role of crossmatch testing when Luminex-SAB is negative in renal transplantation. Polski Przeglad Chirurgiczny. 2018;**90**:41-46

[10] Mahowald GK. The CDC crossmatch in the era of flow cytometric cross-match and single antigen beads. Jornal Brasileiro de Nefrologia. 2021;**43**(3):299-300

[11] Okuno T, Kondelis N. Evaluation of dithiothreitol (DTT) for inactivation of IgM antibodies. Journal of Clinical Pathology. 1978;**31**(12):1152-1155

[12] Tafulo S, Osório E, Mendes C, Liwski R. Complement-dependent cytotoxicity crossmatch in solid organ transplantation: The gold standard or golden history? Human Immunology. 2024;**85**(1):110734

[13] Garovoy MR, Rheinschmidt MA, Bigos M, Colombe B, Feduska N. Flow cytometry analysis: A high technology crossmatch technique facilitating transplantation. Transplantation Proceedings. 1983;**15**(3):1939-1944

[14] Liwski RS. Rapid optimized flow cytometric crossmatch (FCXM) assays: The Halifax and Halifaster protocols. Human Immunology. 2017;**79**(1):28-38

[15] Jaramillo A, Ramon D. Chapter 11 - The crossmatch assay in solid organ transplantation. In: Introduction to Flow Cytometry. 1st ed. Nova Science Publishers, Inc.; 2019. pp. 237-273

[16] Maguire O, Tario JD, Shanahan TC. Flow cytometry and solid organ transplantation: A perfect match. Immunological Investigations. 2014;**43**:756-774

[17] Guillaume N. Improved flow cytometry crossmatching in kidney transplantation. HLA. 2018;**92**:375-383

[18] Tait BD. Detection of HLA antibodies in organ transplant recipients - Triumphs and challenges of the solid phase bead assay. Frontiers in Immunology. 2016;7:570

[19] EFI. Standards for Histocompatibility & Immunogenetics Testing. European Federation for Immunogenetics (EFI); 2019. Available from: https://efi-web.org/ [Accessed: August 4, 2022]

[20] Ravindranath MH, Jucaud V, Ferrone S. Monitoring native HLA-I trimer specific antibodies in Luminex multiplex single antigen bead assay: Evaluation of beadsets from different manufacturers. Journal of Immunological Methods. 2017;**450**:73-80

[21] Pandey S, Harville TO. Epitope analysis aids in transplant decision making by determining the clinical relevance of apparent pre-transplant donor specific antibodies (DSA). Annals of Clinical and Laboratory Science. 2019;**49**(1):50-56

[22] Phanish MK. Immunological risk assessment and human leukocyte antigen antibody testing in kidney transplantation. Indian Journal of Nephrology. 2016;**26**(2):80-85

[23] Tambur AR, Wiebe C. HLA diagnostics: Evaluating DSA strength by titration. Transplantation. 2018;**102**(1S Suppl. 1):S23-S30

[24] Gebel HM, Bray RA, Nickerson P. Pre-transplant assessment of donor-reactive, HLA-specific antibodies in renal transplantation: Contraindication vs. risk. American Journal of Transplantation: Official Journal of the American Society of Transplantation and the American Society of Transplant Surgeons. 2003;**3**(12):1488-1500

[25] Rocha Y, Jaramillo A, Neumann J, Hacke K, Palou E, Torres J. Crossmatch assays in transplantation: Physical or virtual?: A review. Medicine (Baltimore). 2023;**102**(50):e36527

[26] Johnson CP, Schiller JJ, Zhu YR, Hariharan S, Roza AM, Cronin DC, et al. Renal transplantation with final allocation based on the virtual crossmatch. American Journal of Transplantation: Official Journal of the American Society of Transplantation and the American Society of Transplant Surgeons. 2016;**16**(5):1503-1515

[27] Amico P, Hirt-Minkowski P, Hönger G, Gürke L, Mihatsch MJ, Steiger J, et al. Risk stratification by the virtual crossmatch: A prospective study in 233 renal transplantations. Transplant International: Official Journal of the European Society for Organ Transplantation. 2011;**24**(6):560-569

[28] Morris AB, Sullivan HC, Krummey SM, Gebel HM, Bray RA. Out with the old, in with the new: Virtual versus physical crossmatching in the modern era. HLA. 2019;**94**(6):471-481

[29] Peräsaari JP, Jaatinen T, Merenmies J. Donor-specific HLA antibodies in predicting crossmatch outcome: Comparison of three different laboratory techniques. Transplant Immunology. 2018;**46**:23-28

[30] Schinstock CA, Gandhi MJ, Stegall MD. Interpreting anti-HLA antibody testing data: A practical

guide for physicians. Transplantation. 2016;**100**(8):1619

[31] Bezstarosti S, Kramer CSM, Claas FHJ, de Fijter JW, Reinders MEJ, Heidt S. Implementation of molecular matching in transplantation requires further characterization of both immunogenicity and antigenicity of individual HLA epitopes. Human Immunology. 2022;**83**(3):256-263

[32] Duquesnoy RJ, Marrari M. Correlations between Terasaki's HLA class I epitopes and HLAMatchmaker-defined eplets on HLA-A, -B and -C antigens. Tissue Antigens. 2009;**74**(2):117-133

[33] Duquesnoy RJ, Marrari M, Mulder A, da Mata Sousa LCD, da Silva AS, do Monte SJH. First report on the antibody verification of HLA-ABC epitopes recorded in the website-based HLA epitope registry. Tissue Antigens. 2014;**83**(6):391-400

[34] Kramer CSM, Israeli M, Mulder A, Doxiadis IIN, Haasnoot GW, Heidt S, et al. The long and winding road towards epitope matching in clinical transplantation. Transplant International: Official Journal of the European Society for Organ Transplantation. 2019;**32**(1):16-24

[35] Tafulo S, Malheiro J, Santos S, Dias L, Almeida M, Martins LS, et al. HLA class II eplet mismatch load improves prediction of dnDSA development after living donor kidney transplantation. International Journal of Immunogenetics. 2021;**48**(1):1-7

[36] Bryan CF, Chadha V, Warady BA. Donor selection in pediatric kidney transplantation using DR and DQ eplet mismatching: A new histocompatibility paradigm. Pediatric Transplantation. 2016;**20**(7):926-930

[37] Sorohan BM, Baston C, Tacu D, Bucșa C, Țincu C, Vizireanu P, et al. Non-HLA antibodies in kidney transplantation: Immunity and genetic insights. Biomedicine. 2022;**10**(7):1506

[38] Zhang Q, Reed EF. The importance of non-HLA antibodies in transplantation. Nature Reviews Nephrology. 2016;**12**(8):484-495

[39] Kim D, Gimferrer I, Warner P, Nelson K, Sibulesky L, Bakthavatsalam R, et al. Preformed angiotensin II type-1 receptor antibodies are associated with rejection after kidney transplantation: A single-center, cohort study. Transplantation Proceedings. 2018;**50**(10):3467-3472

[40] Philogene MC, Zhou S, Lonze BE, Bagnasco S, Alasfar S, Montgomery RA, et al. Pre-transplant screening for non-HLA antibodies: Who should be tested? Human Immunology. 2018;**79**(4):195-202

[41] Kimball PM, Gupta G, McDougan F. Circulating angiotensin type II receptor: Possible marker for antibody mediated rejection after renal transplantation? Human Immunology. 2017;**78**(10):629-633

[42] Sorohan BM, Ismail G, Leca N, Tacu D, Obrișcă B, Constantinescu I, et al. Angiotensin II type 1 receptor antibodies in kidney transplantation: An evidence-based comprehensive review. Transplantation Reviews. 2020;**34**(4):100573

[43] Dragun D, Müller DN, Bräsen JH, Fritsche L, Nieminen-Kelhä M, Dechend R, et al. Angiotensin II type 1-receptor activating antibodies in renal-allograft rejection. The New England Journal of Medicine. 2005;**352**(6):558-569

[44] Alheim M, Johansson SM, Hauzenberger D, Grufman P,

Holgersson J. A flow cytometric crossmatch test for simultaneous detection of antibodies against donor lymphocytes and endothelial precursor cells. Tissue Antigens. 2010;**75**(3):269-277

[45] Mulley WR, Kanellis J. Understanding crossmatch testing in organ transplantation: A case-based guide for the general nephrologist. Nephrology (Carlton, Vic.). 2011;**16**(2):125-133

[46] Kamburova EG, Wisse BW, Joosten I, Allebes WA, van der Meer A, Hilbrands LB, et al. How can we reduce costs of solid-phase multiplex-bead assays used to determine anti-HLA antibodies? HLA. 2016;**88**(3):110-119

Chapter 8

Evaluating Hypothermic Machine Perfusion in Liver Transplantation

Hetal Lad, Tiffany Hsiung, Aditya Kasina and Arpit Amin

Abstract

Static cold storage (SCS) has been the standard-of-care preservation technique for liver grafts utilized for liver transplantation (LT). However, there remains a significant mismatch in the number of SCS liver grafts utilized for LT compared to the number of potential liver recipients on the waitlist. This has led to renewed interest in evaluating application of machine perfusion preservation techniques like hypothermic machine perfusion (HMP) to expand the overall pool of available liver grafts. The initial focus of this chapter is to describe the mechanistic benefits of HMP in preservation of liver grafts. Thereafter, we highlight the clinical benefits of HMP in decreasing early allograft dysfunction (EAD) rates and decreased biliary complications in LT recipients. Lastly, we discuss future potential use of HMP in pediatric LT via ex-vivo liver graft splitting and potential for combining HMP with normothermic regional perfusion (NRP) in liver grafts obtained from donors after circulatory death (DCD).

Keywords: donation after brain death (DBD) liver grafts, donation after circulatory death (DCD) liver grafts, hypothermic machine perfusion (HMP), static cold storage (SCS), ischemia-reperfusion injury (IRI), liver transplantation (LT)

1. Introduction

Liver transplantation (LT) emerged as a viable treatment option for patients suffering from end-stage liver disease in the 1980s. The discovery of the University of Wisconsin solution coupled with static cold storage (SCS) for liver graft preservation paved the way for rapid adoption of LT across the world. With the advent of additional transplant oncology related indications for LT for select patients suffering from hepatocellular carcinoma, cholangiocarcinoma, colorectal liver metastases, and neuroendocrine liver metastases, there continues to be a demand for donor liver grafts as reflected by an ever-increasing liver transplant waitlist [1].

This supply-demand mismatch for liver grafts can be attributed to limitations of SCS preservation technique, which result in high discard rates of donation after circulatory death (DCD) liver grafts [2, 3]. Additionally, there is a high discard rate after SCS preservation of donation after brain death (DBD) liver grafts if the donor liver is classified as an extended criteria donor (ECD) by criteria such as advanced donor age

(age > 65 years) or macrosteatosis >30% [2, 3]. DCD liver grafts and ECD-DBD liver grafts that undergo SCS preservation suffer from severe ischemia-reperfusion injury (IRI) during LT [2, 3]. This leads to an increased risk of primary non-function (PNF), early allograft dysfunction (EAD), and biliary strictures after LT, which explains the rationale behind high discard rates of SCS DCD and SCS ECD-DBD liver grafts.

Hence, there has been a significant interest within the liver transplant community to evaluate machine perfusion technologies like hypothermic machine perfusion (HMP), normothermic machine perfusion (NMP), and normothermic regional perfusion (NRP) to mitigate the IRI associated with SCS DCD liver grafts and ECD-DBD liver grafts, so that we can increase the supply of available donor liver grafts for LT. The main objective of this chapter is to summarize the clinical evidence supporting the application of HMP in clinical LT. We will explore the mechanistic benefits of HMP in liver graft preservation and different HMP modalities currently utilized in clinical LT. We will present clinical evidence demonstrating decreased EAD rates and deceased biliary complication rates with HMP, resulting in improved LT graft and recipient survival. Discussion on basics of NMP and/or NRP in LT are beyond the scope of this chapter and will be discussed in a separate chapter. Lastly, we will discuss potential future evolution of HMP in LT focusing on application of ex vivo liver splitting with HMP, and potential hybrid application of HMP with NRP or NMP technologies.

2. Hypothermic machine perfusion of liver grafts—Mechanistic benefits and modalities

Under physiologic conditions, there is forward electron transport between mitochondrial complex I and mitochondrial complex II, resulting in adenosine triphosphate (ATP) production essential for cellular metabolism (**Figure 1A**) [4–6]. During SCS, liver grafts are preserved at temperatures between 0 and 4°C under hypoxic conditions [4–6]. As cold ischemia time increases, lack of oxygen leads to hepatocyte and cholangiocyte injury through disruption of the forward electron transport between mitochondrial complex I and complex II. This results in diminished ATP production as well as accumulation of flavin mononucleotide (FMN) and succinate (**Figure 1B**) [4–8]. Subsequently, after liver graft reperfusion with normothermic oxygenated blood in a succinate rich microcellular environment, there is a pathologic initial reverse flow of electrons from mitochondria complex II to mitochondrial complex I. This leads to the production of reactive oxygen species (ROS) in hepatocytes and cholangiocytes, termed reperfusion injury (**Figure 1C**) [4–8]. Mitochondrial ROS leads to hepatocyte and cholangiocyte damage/death and release of danger-associated molecular patterns, which activates the host immune system through complex interplay between neutrophils, lymphocytes, and Kupffer cells [4–8]. Depending on the severity of IRI to hepatocytes/cholangiocytes at LT, liver grafts may develop EAD/PNF as well as biliary strictures/ischemic cholangiopathy (IC) (**Figure 2**) [4–8].

During HMP, liver grafts are preserved at temperatures between 4 and 10°C (**Figure 3**). There are various HMP modalities, each with its own unique nomenclature, currently in clinical application. Understanding this unique nomenclature is important to analyzing mechanistic benefits of HMP. *Hypothermic oxygenated machine perfusion (HOPE)* refers to the hypothermic preservation of a liver graft using a continuous oxygenated preservation solution [Belzer KPS University of Wisconsin solution]

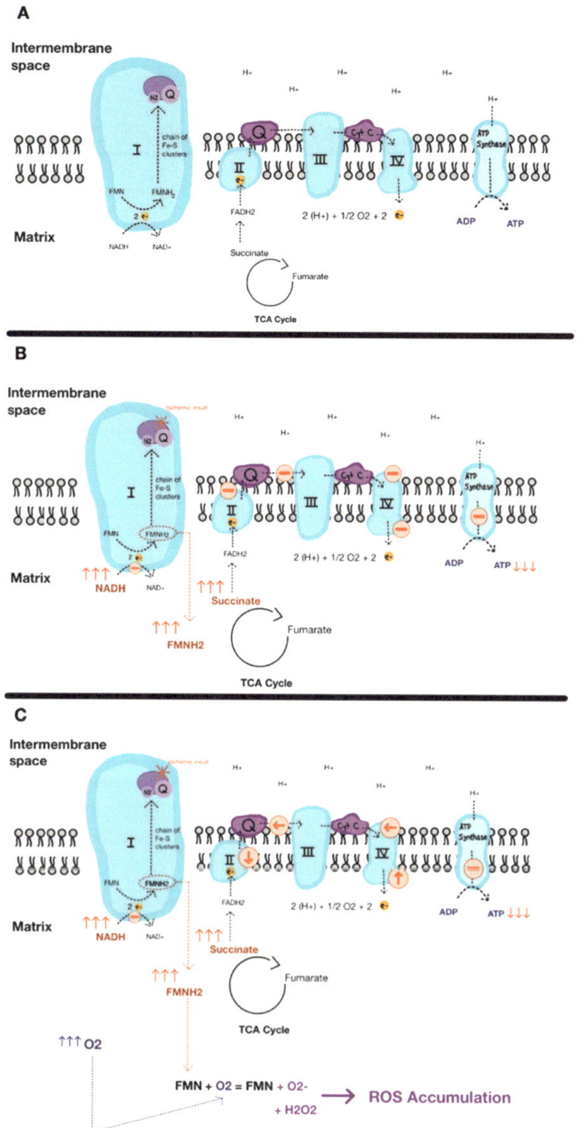

Figure 1.
Insult to liver graft mitochondrial electron transport chain during Ischemia and reperfusion. A. Physiologic state of mitochondrial electron transport chain in liver graft prior to cross-clamp. Under normal physiologic conditions, the electron transport chain (ETC) exhibits forward electron flow from complex I to IV. Reduced form of flavin mononucleotide (FMNH2), reduced form of nicotinamide adenine dinucleotide (NADH), and succinate from the Citric Acid Cycle contribute to the electrons in complex I and II, and are subsequently oxidized to their respective counterparts FMN, NAD, and fumarate. This culminates in the production of ATP. B. Ischemic injury to mitochondrial electron transport chain of liver graft during static cold storage. Under ischemic conditions, the mitochondrial ETC chain is compromised by injury to complex I. Insult to the ubiquinone-site (Q-site) within complex I inhibits forward flow of electrons. This inhibits downstream ATP formation. Additionally, FMNH2 dissociates from complex I, building up in the mitochondrial matrix. The lack of FMN in complex I consequently inhibits oxidation of NADH, causing a buildup of NADH. There is also a buildup of succinate due to lack of forward electron flow. C. Reperfusion injury to mitochondrial electron transport chain of liver graft after static cold storage. During reperfusion there is a rush of oxygen (O_2) into the mitochondria with already accumulated succinate, FMNH2, and NADH. Electrons overwhelm the transport chain, causing retrograde electron flow and decreased ATP production. Combination of reversed electron transfer and increased O2 results in a reaction with FMN to create reactive oxygenated species (ROS) like superoxide anions and hydrogen peroxide, that cause further insult to the mitochondria and ultimately cell.

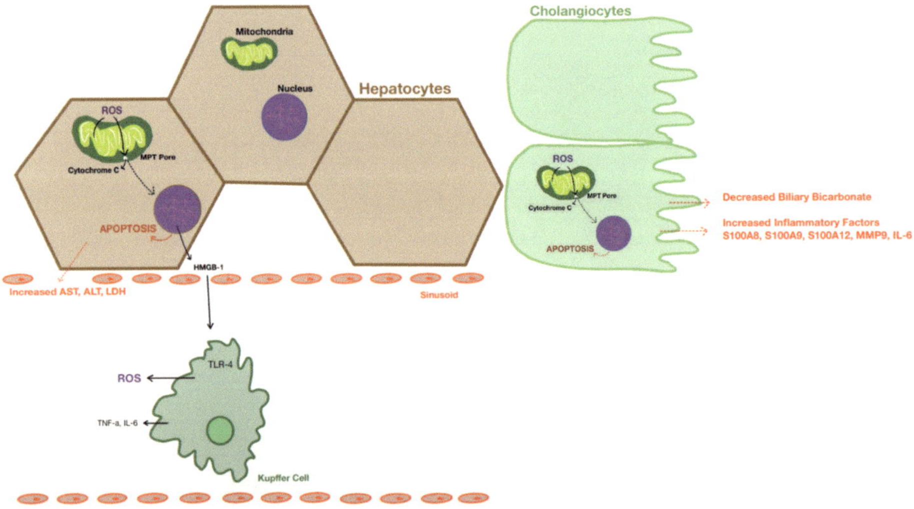

Figure 2.
Ischemia reperfusion injury in liver graft during liver transplant. During ischemia reperfusion injury (IRI), reactive oxygen species (ROS) accumulate in the mitochondria and trigger apoptosis by opening of the mitochondrial permeability transition pore (MPT pore) and release of Cytochrome C. ROS causes release of hepatocyte danger associated molecular patterns such as high mobility group box-1 (HMGB-1). HMGB-1 then activates the toll-like receptor-4 (TLR-4) pathway in Kupffer cells, promoting production of proinflammatory cytokines such as tumor necrosis factor-alpha (TNF-a) and interleukin-6 (IL-6). Apoptosis of hepatocytes leads to increased aspartate aminotransferase (AST), alanine aminotransferase (ALT), and lactate dehydrogenase (LDH), ultimately increasing the risk for early allograft dysfunction. On the other hand, cholangiocyte apoptosis leads to decreased biliary bicarbonate and acidic biliary pH, increased inflammatory factors such as S100 calcium binding protein A8 (S100A8), S100 calcium binding protein A9 (S100A9), matrix metalloproteinase 9 (MMP9), IL 6, which ultimately leads to persistent peribiliary inflammation resulting in biliary strictures.

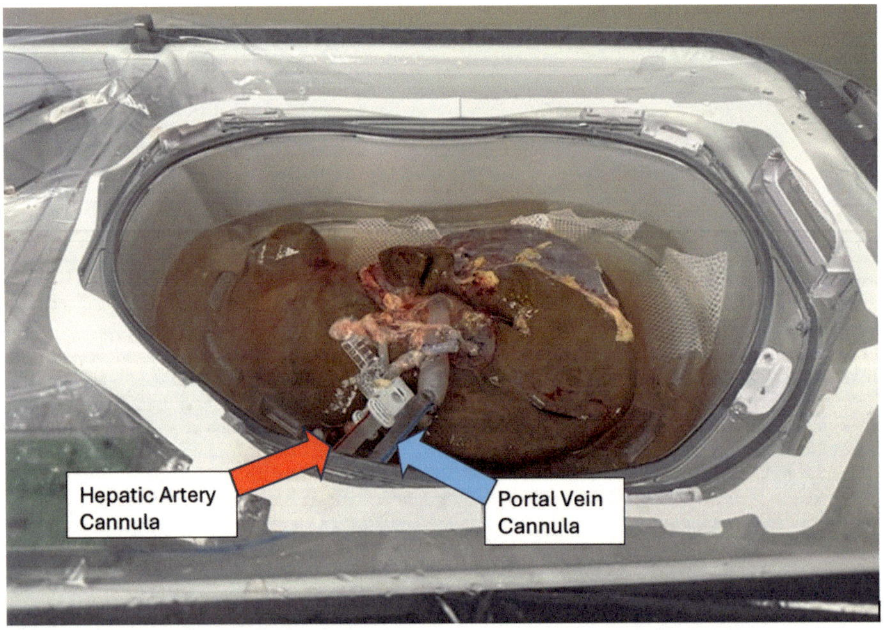

Figure 3.
Liver graft on oxygen "Pre-charged" portable hypothermic machine perfusion (HMP-O_2).

administered via portal vein cannulation, with flow rates of 150–200 ml/min and portal pressures of 3 mm Hg [9]. *Dual hypothermic oxygenated machine perfusion (dHOPE)* refers to the hypothermic preservation of a liver graft using continuous oxygenated preservation solution [Belzer MPS University of Wisconsin solution] administered via both arterial and portal vein cannulation, with hepatic arterial pressures at 25 mm Hg and portal vein pressures at 5 mm Hg [10]. Another modality, referred to as *portable HMP-*O_2, involves oxygen precharging of a portable closed chamber hypothermic machine circuit with 100% oxygen at 10 L/min for >20 minutes followed by liver graft preservation using this pre-oxygenated preservation solution [Vasosol solution], administered via both arterial and portal vein cannulation, with adjusted hepatic arterial and portal vein pressures based on flow rates of 0.667 ml/g liver tissue / minute (**Figure 3**) [11].

Due to the continuous perfusion of liver grafts during HMP, hypothermic conditions are maintained, resulting in decreased metabolic demand of hepatocytes and cholangiocytes, along with concomitant removal of metabolic waste products [7–8]. The availability of oxygen in HMP circuits, either through continuous oxygenation of preservation solution (HOPE/dHOPE) or through oxygen precharging of preservation solution (HMP-O_2), allows for the maintenance of low-flux forward electron transport between mitochondrial complex I and mitochondrial complex II [9–11]. This leads to continuous ATP production and reduced succinate accumulation within 1–2 hours of HMP (**Figure 4**) [7–8]. As a result, liver grafts preserved with HMP exhibit decreased production of ROS upon reperfusion, leading to a lower degree of IRI in LT recipients.

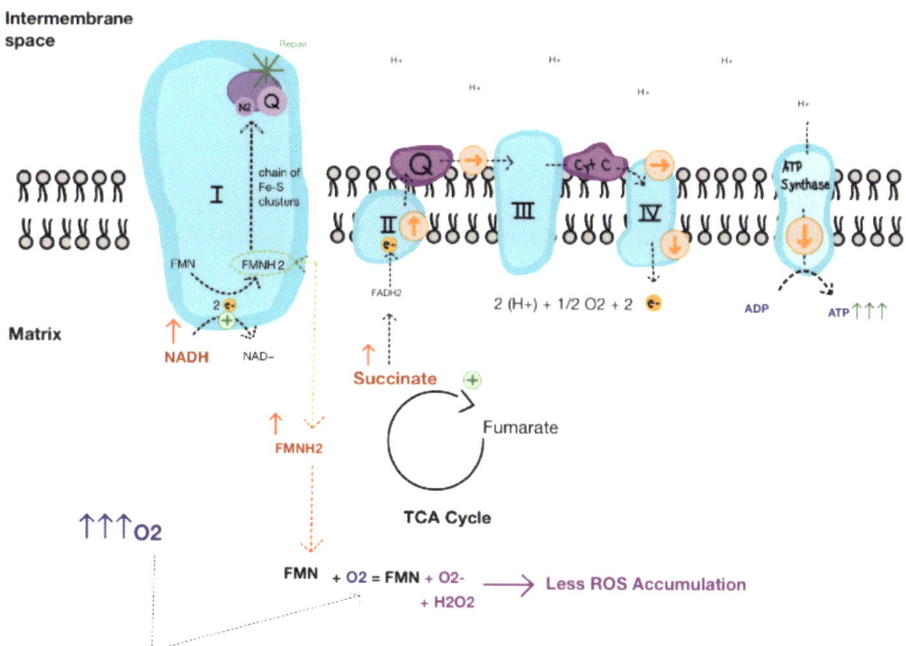

Figure 4.
Protective effect of oxygenated hypothermic machine perfusion on mitochondrial electron transport chain of liver graft. Hypothermic machine perfusion has been shown to protect mitochondria by allowing for repair of complex I's Q site. This results in low flux forward electron flow, allowing for ATP production. Additionally, there is decreased dissociation of FMNH2 from complex I, allowing for increased metabolism of NADH, FMN, and succinate. This ultimately reduces FMN associated production of ROS during reperfusion of liver grafts preserved by oxygenated hypothermic machine perfusion.

3. Clinical evidence for HMP in LT

3.1 Clinical studies evaluating HMP-O2

Guarrera and colleagues published the first clinical series on HMP in LT in the United States of America (USA) in 2010 [12]. In the HMP group (n = 20, DBD livers), livers were procured at the donor hospital, underwent SCS for transport, and were placed on HMP at the recipient hospital using both hepatic artery and portal vein cannulation, with a median perfusion duration of 4.3 hours [12]. Of note, no active oxygenation was utilized but there was ambient room air exchange with the HMP chamber, resulting in mean perfusate effluent partial pressure of oxygen of 137 mm Hg [12]. The study followed the HMP group and a control group of 20 matched LT recipients, who received SCS DBD liver grafts, for 12 months [12]. The EAD rate was noted to be 5% in the HMP group compared to 25% in the SCS group [12]. The biliary stricture rate was noted to be 5% in the HMP group compared to 15% in the SCS group [12]. While the EAD rate and biliary stricture rate in the HMP group did not show a statistically significant difference compared to the SCS group, there was a trend towards lower rates of EAD and biliary strictures in the HMP group [12]. 1-year graft and recipient survival was 90% in both groups [12]. These authors noted that the length of hospital stay was statistically significantly lower in the HMP group (10 days) compared to SCS group (15 days) [12]. This seminal study provided proof-of-concept that HMP can be safe and may have potential clinical benefits for LT recipients.

Building on their initial work, *Guarrera and colleagues* reported the application of HMP in preventing discard of extended criteria "orphan" DBD livers, which were declined by other transplant centers in their United Network for Organ Sharing region in USA in 2015 [13]. These ECD-DBD "orphan" livers met at least one of the following criteria: donor age > 65 years, donor liver with greater than 25% macrosteatosis, donor Hepatitis C positive liver with greater than 15% macrosteatosis, or donor liver with significant ischemic injury defined as aspartate aminotransferase (AST) level > 1000 IU/L or alanine aminotransferase (ALT) level > 1000 IU/L at time of organ offer [13]. In the HMP group (n = 31), donor livers were transported using SCS from the donor hospital to the recipient hospital and back-to-base HMP was utilized at the recipient hospital for a median perfusion duration of about 3.8 hours [13]. The mean perfusate oxygen pressure was noted to be 228 mm Hg due to ambient air exchange at the organ chamber [13]. The control group consisted of 30 SCS ECD-DBD liver recipients, which were matched to HMP liver recipients for donor/recipient age, model for end-stage liver disease (MELD) score, donor risk index (DRI), and cold ischemia time [13]. Follow-up duration for the study was 1 year [13]. EAD rate was equivalent in both groups (19% in HMP group vs. 30% in SCS group) [13]. Biliary stricture rate was noted to be statistically significantly lower in the HMP group (13%) compared to the SCS group (33%) [13]. 1-year graft survival was equivalent in both groups (81% in the HMP group vs. 80% in SCS group) [13]. 1-year recipient survival was equivalent in both groups (84% in HMP group vs. 80% in SCS group) [13]. This study demonstrated that HMP application can help decrease discard rate of ECD-DBD liver grafts [13]. Additionally, this study showed lower biliary stricture rate in LT recipients, who received HMP preserved ECD-DBD liver grafts [13].

Given the large travel distances in the USA between donor centers and recipient hospitals, which result in accumulation of IRI in liver grafts due to SCS transport, back-to-base application of HMP in the USA may have limited utility for livers procured at distant donor hospitals. Additionally, there are aviation regulatory restrictions on transport of compressed oxygen gas chambers in the USA, which limit the application of continuously oxygenated HMP circuits for air transport. To overcome this logistical hurdle, *Guarrera and colleagues* developed a novel technique termed HMP-O_2. This involves precharging the HMP circuit with 100% oxygen, delivered at 10 L/min at the donor hospital, with immediate placement of the donor liver on the HMP circuit at the donor hospital to initiate continuous HMP-O_2. This allows for extended HMP-O_2 perfusion time, minimizes SCS related IRI, and facilitates air transport of donor livers over longer distances [11]. Through dual hepatic artery and portal vein cannulation, they demonstrated that HMP-O_2 circuit had a perfusate oxygen tension of 700 mm Hg at onset of preservation and subsequent oxygen tension values up to 150 mmHg after 90 min of HMP-O_2 [11].

Subsequently, a prospective multicenter randomized control trial (RCT) involving nine transplant centers in the USA evaluated HMP-O_2 and SCS in LT, with the results published in 2023 [14]. Both the study group (HMP-0_2, n = 63) and control group (n = 73) included liver grafts from DBD (HMP-O_2, n = 48; SCS, n = 52), ECD-EBD (HMP-O_2, n = 10; SCS, n = 11), and DCD (HMP-O_2, n = 5; SCS, n = 10) [14]. The median perfusion duration across groups was 2.8 hours [14]. From a logistical perspective, the HMP-O_2 circuit was utilized in an end-ischemic fashion at the recipient hospital in 36 (57%) cases, and continuous fashion in 27 (43%) of cases, beginning at the donor hospital, depending on investigator preference [14]. Additionally, amongst the 27 continuous HMP-O_2 cases, HMP-O_2 circuit was transported via air in 22 (81%) of cases, demonstrating the safe portability of the circuit [14]. Risk of graft failure based on Liver Graft Assessment following transplant score at seven days (L-GRAFT$_7$) was found to be statistically significantly lower in HMP-O_2 group (3.4%) compared to SCS group (4.5%) [14]. While the EAD rate and biliary stricture rate in the HMP-O_2 group did not reach a statistically significant difference to SCS group, there was trend towards lower EAD rate and biliary stricture rate in HMP-O_2 group (EAD: 11%; biliary stricture: 11%) compared to SCS group (EAD: 16%; biliary stricture: 22%) [14].1-year graft survival was similar between HMP-O_2 group (94%) and SCS group (93%) [14]. 1-year recipient survival was similar between HMP-O_2 group (94%) and SCS group (97%) [14]. This pivotal multicenter RCT was able to demonstrate non-inferiority of HMP-O_2 and SCS in clinical LT as per Food and Drug Administration (FDA) guidelines in the USA. FDA has granted continued access use of HMP-O_2 at participating transplant centers in the USA currently and final FDA regulatory approval of HMP-O_2 use is pending at the time of writing of this manuscript. All the HMP-O_2 cohort and RCTs have been summarized in **Tables 1** and **2** respectively.

In summary, given the clinical benefits and portability of the HMP-O_2 circuit, there is a potential for broader adoption of HMP-O_2 in the USA for preservation of DBD, ECD-DBD, and DCD livers once regulatory FDA approval is obtained.

3.2 Clinical studies evaluating HOPE

End-ischemic HOPE application for liver graft preservation was pioneered by *Dutkowski and colleagues* in Switzerland in 2014 [9]. In this pilot study, 8 DCD livers [median functional warm ischemia time (fWIT) of 31 minutes] were initially stored with SCS for a median time of 2.4 hours followed by end-ischemic HOPE for a median duration of 2 hours prior to LT [9]. Control group consisted of 8 DBD LT recipients, who were matched to the study group based on total preservation time, donor/

Study	N	Donor type	Perfusion logistics and route	Perfusion duration, median (IQR), hours	Results
Horné et al. Germany 2022* [20]	50 HOPE; 50 SCS	DBD	Back-to-Base HOPE	2.73 (2.3–3.2)***	EAD: HOPE 14 (28.0%); SCS 25 (50.0%) (p = 0.04) 1-Month Graft Survival: HOPE 49 (98%); SCS 47 (94%) (p = 0.36) 1-Month Patient Survival: HOPE 49 (98%); SCS 47 (94%) (p = 0.36)
Patrono et al. Italy 2022* [26]	121 dHOPE; 723 SCS	ECD-DBD	Back-to-Base dHOPE	2.3 (2.0–3.0)***	EAD: Not Available 6-Month Graft Survival: dHOPE 118 (97.5%); SCS 648 (89.6%) (p = 0.002)
Rayar et al. France 2021** [19]	25 HOPE; 69 SCS	ECD-DBD	Back-to-Base HOPE	2.0 (1.3–4.2)	EAD: HOPE 7 (28%); SCS 29 (42%) (p = 0.22) 1-Year Biliary Complications: HOPE 2 (8%); SCS 8 (11.6%) (p = 1.0) 1-Year Graft Survival HOPE 22 (88%); SCS 62 (89.5%) (p = 1.0) 1-Year Patient Survival HOPE 23 (91%); SCS 63 (91.3%) (p = 1.0)
Mueller et al. Switzerland 2020* [17]	70 HOPE; 70 SCS	DCD/DBD	Back-to-Base HOPE	2.0 (1.7–2.5)	5-Year HCC Recurrence-Free Patient Survival: HOPE 46 (92%; SCS 37 (73%) (p = 0.027)
Ravaioli et al. Italy 2020** [18]	10 HOPE; 30 SCS	ECD-DBD	Back-to-Base HOPE	2.2 (1–3.5)***	EAD: HOPE 0 (0%); SCS 7 (23.3%) 1-Year Biliary Strictures: HOPE 1 (10%); SCS 3 (10%) 1-Year Graft Survival: HOPE 10 (100%); SCS 27 (90.0%)
Schlegel et al. Switzerland 2019* [16]	50 HOPE; 50 SCS	DCD	Back-to-Base HOPE	2 (1.6–2.4)	1-Year Biliary Non-anastomotic Strictures: HOPE 4 (8%); SCS 11 (22%) (p = 0.09) 1-Year Graft Survival: HOPE 43 (86%); SCS 32 (64%) (p = 0.005)
Patrono et al. Italy 2019* [25]	25 dHOPE; 50 SCS	DBD	Back-to-Base dHOPE	3.1 (2.3–3.9)	EAD: dHOPE 8 (32.0%); SCS 17 (34.0%) (p = 1.00) 6-Month Biliary Complications: dHOPE 6 (24.0%); SCS 9 (18.0%) (p = 0.76)

DOI: http://dx.doi.org/10.5772/intechopen.1007569

van Rijn et al. Netherlands 2017** [10]	10 dHOPE; 20 SCS	DCD	Back-to-Base dHOPE	2.1 (2.1–2.3)	EAD: dHOPE 0 (0%); SCS 2 (10%) (p = 1.0) 1-Year Graft Survival: dHOPE 10 (100%); SCS 13 (67%) 1-Year Patient Survival: dHOPE 10 (100%); SCS 17 (85%) (p = 0.209)
Guarrera et al. United States 2015** [13]	31 HMP-O_2; 30 SCS	ECD-DBD	Back-to-Base HMP-O_2	3.8 (2.9–4.7)	EAD: HMP 6 (19%); SCS 9 (30%) (p = 0.384) 1-Year Biliary Stricture: HMP 3 (10%); SCS 10 (33%) (p = 0.031) 1-Year Patient/Graft Survival: HMP 26 (83.8%); SCS 24 (80.0%) (p = 0.761)
Dutkowski et al. Switzerland 2015** [15]	25 HOPE; 50 SCS	DCD	Back-to-Base HOPE	2.0 (1.7–2.5)	EAD: HOPE 5 (20%); SCS 22 (44%) (p = 0.046) 1-Year Biliary Complications: HOPE 5 (20%); SCS 23 (46%) (p = 0.042) 1-Year Graft Survival: HOPE 23 (90%); SCS 35 (69%) (p = 0.035)
Dutkowski et al. Switzerland 2014** [9]	8 HOPE; 8 SCS	DCD / DBD	Back-to-Base HOPE	2.0 (1.7–2.7)	EAD: HOPE 0 (0%); SCS 0 (0%) (p = NS) 6-Month Biliary Complications: HOPE 2 (25%); SCS 2 (25%) 6-Month Graft Survival: HOPE 8 (100%); SCS 8 (100%)
Guarrera et al. United States 2010** [12]	20 HMP-O_2; 20 SCS	DBD	Back-to-Base HMP-O_2	4.3 (3.4–5.2)	EAD: HMP-O_2 1 (5%), SCS; 5 (25%) (p = 0.08) 1-Year Biliary Strictures: HMP-O_2 1 (5%), SCS 3 (15%) (p = NS) 1-Year Patient/Graft Survival: HMP-O_2 18 (90%), SCS 18 (90%) (p = NS)

*Retrospective.
**Prospective.
***Reported as Mean [95% CI].
Abbreviations: donation after brain death, DBD; donation after circulatory death, DCD; dual hypothermic oxygenated machine perfusion, dHOPE; early allograft dysfunction, EAD; hypothermic oxygenated machine perfusion, HCC, hepatocellular carcinoma; HOPE; hypothermic machine perfusion-02, HMP-0$_2$; interquartile range, IQR; not significant, NP; p-value, P; static cold storage, SCS.

Table 1.
Observational studies utilizing hypothermic machine perfusion of liver grafts for transplantation.

Study	N	Donor type***	Perfusion logistics and route	Perfusion duration, median (IQR) (Hours)	EAD within first week, N (%)			Biliary stricture development, N (%)			1-year graft survival, N (%)			1 year patient survival, N (%)		
					Study	Control	P	Study	Control	P	Study	Control	P	Study	Control	P
Panayotova et al. United States 2023 [14]	63 HMP-O_2; 73 SCS	DBD/ ECD-DBD/ DCD	Continuous HMP-O_2	2.8 (1.8–3.6)	7 (11.1)	12 (16.4)	0.37	7 (11.1)	16 (21.9)	0.18	59 (93.7)	68 (93.2)	0.92	59 (93.7)	71 (97.3)	0.99
Grat et al. Finland 2023 [28]	26 dHOPE; 78 SCS	DBD	Back-to-Base dHOPE	2.0 (NA)	7 (26.9)	26 (33.3)	0.63	0 (0.0)	4 (5.1)	NA	26 (100)	75 (96.2)	0.57	25 (96.2)	72 (92.4)	NA
van Rijn et al. Netherlands 2021 [27]	78 dHOPE; 78 SCS	DCD	Back-to-Base dHOPE	2.2 (2.0–2.6)	20 (25.6)	31 (39.7)	0.61 (0.39–0.96)****	5 (6.4)*******	14 (17.9)	0.03	66 (84.6)******	67 (85.9)	NA	72 (92.3)******	74 (94.9)	1.46 (0.41–5.21)****
Schlegal et al. Europe* 2023 [24]	85 HOPE; 85 SCS	DBD	Back-to-Base HOPE	1.6 (1.2–2.3)	14 (16.5)	39 (45.9)	NA	15 (17.6)*****	19 (22.4)	0.44	81 (95.3)	78 (91.8)	0.36	81 (95.2)	81 (95.3)	1
Ravaioli et al. Italy 2022 [23]	55 HOPE; 55 SCS	DBD	Back-to-Base HOPE	2.4 (2–3.1)	7 (12.7)	19 (34.5)	0.007	2 (3.6)	2 (3.6)	NA	54 (98.2)	48 (87.3)	0.058	54 (98.2)	52 (94.5)	NA

Czigany et al. Europe** 2021 [21]	23 HOPE; 23 SCS	ECD-DBD	Back-to-Base HOPE	2.4 (1.7–3.4)	4 (17.4)	8 (34.8)	0.314	4 (17.4)******	6 (26.1)	0.72	21 (91.0)	18 (78.0)	0.25	21 (91.3)	19 (82.6)	0.44

*Patients from England, Belgium, Netherlands, France, Austria, Switzerland.
**Patients from Germany, Czech Republic.
***All studies included extended criteria donors.
****Treatment effect (95% CI).
*****Incidence of all biliary complications.
******6-month outcome.
*******Non-anastomotic biliary stricture only [Anastomotic: 23 (29) dHOPE; 22 (28) SCS, $p = 1.07$].
Abbreviations: donation after brain death, DBD; donation after circulatory death, DCD; dual hypothermic oxygenated machine perfusion, dHOPE; early allograft dysfunction, EAD; hypothermic oxygenated machine perfusion, HOPE; hypothermic machine perfusion-02, HMP-0_2; interquartile range, IQR; not available, NA; P-value, P; static cold storage, SCS.

Table 2.
Randomized control trials utilizing HOPE liver grafts for transplantation.

recipient age, MELD score, and graft steatosis [9]. They reported equivalent EAD rates (0% in both groups), similar biliary complications (25% in both groups), and equivalent 6-month graft / patient survival (100% in both groups) [9].

Building on their pilot HOPE study, *Dutkowski and colleagues* published their outcomes in LT recipients, who received 25 HOPE-treated DCD liver grafts with a median fWIT of 31 minutes at their center [15]. Matched control group consisted of 50 SCS DBD LT recipients and 50 SCS DCD LT recipients at their center and two additional European centers in the Netherlands and United Kingdom [15]. Median duration of end-ischemic HOPE was 2 hours prior to LT [15]. They demonstrated that the EAD rate (20%) in the HOPE-treated DCD group was statistically significantly lower than EAD rate (44%) in SCS DCD group [15]. Additionally, they found that the EAD rate (20%) in the HOPE-treated DCD group was equivalent to the EAD rate (22%) in the SCS DBD group [15]. Biliary complication rate (20%) in HOPE-treated DCD group was found to be statistically significantly lower than biliary complication rate in SCS DCD group (46%) [15]. Also, the biliary complication rate (20%) in the HOPE-treated DCD group was equivalent to that in the SCS DBD group (22%) [15]. 1-year graft survival in HOPE-treated DCD group (90%) was found to be statistically significantly higher than SCS DCD group (69%) and equivalent to SCS DBD group (96%) [15].

Subsequently, *Dutkowski and colleagues* reported that 5-year graft survival [censored for hepatocellular carcinoma (HCC) tumor recurrence] of their first 50 HOPE-treated DCD liver grafts (94%) was statistically significantly higher than that of SCS DCD liver grafts (79%) [16]. In addition, they found that 14% of SCS DCD liver grafts were lost due to IC at 5-year follow-up while none of HOPE treated DCD liver grafts were lost due to ischemic cholangiopathy highlighting the protective effect of HOPE on DCD liver grafts with respect to biliary complications [16]. Additionally, *Dutkowski and colleagues* studied the effect of HOPE on HCC recurrence in LT recipients by comparing 70 HOPE-treated DCD liver grafts to 70 SCS DCD liver grafts [17]. They found that 5-year HCC recurrence-free survival in the HOPE treated DCD LT cohort was 92% compared to 73% in SCS DCD LT cohort [17]. These findings suggest that the lower IRI with HOPE may exert anti-tumor protective effects in potential LT recipients with HCC. In summary, initial single center trials by Dutkowski and colleagues demonstrated lower EAD rates, improved biliary complications, and improved graft survival in recipients of HOPE treated DCD liver grafts [17].

Encouraged by promising results of HOPE reported by *Dutkowski and colleagues*, adoption of HOPE in LT occurred in other European countries with several single center studies published on this topic. *Ravaioli and colleagues* evaluated the outcomes of end-ischemic HOPE in ECD-DBD liver grafts in Italy in 2020 [18]. Study group consisted of 10 ECD-DBD liver grafts preserved with end-ischemic HOPE and the control group consisted of 30 ECD-DBD liver grafts preserved with SCS [18]. Mean perfusion time was reported to be 2.2 hours [18]. While they did not detect statistically significant differences between the two groups, they reported that EAD rate tended to be lower in HOPE ECD-DBD group (0%) compared to SCS ECD-DBD group (23%) and 1-year graft survival tended to be higher in HOPE ECD-DBD group (100%) compared to SCS ECD-DBD group (90%) [18]. *Rayar and colleagues* reported their outcomes of end-ischemic HOPE in ECD-DBD liver grafts in France in 2021 [19]. Study group consisted of 25 ECD-DBD liver grafts preserved with end-ischemic HOPE and the control group consisted of 69 ECD-DBD liver grafts preserved with SCS [19]. They reported that the EAD rate was similar between the HOPE ECD-DBD group (28%) and SCS ECD-DBD group (42%) [19]. Similarly, the biliary complication rate was similar between the HOPE ECD-DBD group (8%) and SCS ECD-DBD group (12%) [19]. They found that the intensive care unit (ICU) length of stay and hospital stay was statistically significantly lower in the HOPE ECD-DBD group (ICU stay: 3 days; hospital stay: 15 days) compared to SCS ECD-DBD group. Group (ICU stay: 5 days; hospital stay 20 days) [19]. 1-year graft survival was similar between the HOPE ECD-DBD group (88%) and SCS ECD-DBD group (90%) [19]. *Horne and colleagues* reported their experience of end-ischemic HOPE on DBD liver grafts in Germany in 2022 [20]. Study group consisted of 50 HOPE DBD liver grafts and the control group consisted of matched 50 SCS DBD liver grafts [20]. They reported that intraoperative post-reperfusion syndrome (defined as drop in mean arterial pressure > 30% occurring within 5 minutes of graft unclamping and lasting greater than 1 minutes) occurred at a statistically significantly lower rate in HOPE DBD liver grafts (12%) compared to SCS DBD liver grafts (42%) [20]. Additionally, the EAD rate was statistically significantly lower in the HOPE DBD LT group (28%) compared to the SCS DBD LT group (50%) [20]. In short, single center studies at other European centers evaluating end-ischemic HOPE application in DBD and ECD-DBD grafts revealed potential benefit of HOPE in reducing post-reperfusion syndrome rate and EAD rate with subsequent reduction in ICU and hospital length of stay of LT recipients.

Clinical momentum built based on favorable outcomes of single-center studies evaluating end-ischemic HOPE in LT led to further interest in conducting RCTs in Europe. The first multicenter RCT based at 4 European centers in Germany and Czech Republic comparing outcomes of end-ischemic HOPE ECD-DBD LT recipients (n = 23) to SCS ECD-DBD LT (n = 23) was published by Czigany and colleagues in 2021 [21]. While not statistically significant, a trend towards lower EAD rate was noted in HOPE ECD-DBD LT group (17%) compared to SCS ECD-DBD group (35%) [21]. Clavien-Dindo grade 3–5 complication rates were noted to be lower in HOPE ECD-DBD LT group (44%) compared to SCS ECD-DBD group (74%) [21]. ICU length of stay was shorter in HOPE ECD-DBD LT group (5 days) compared to SCS ECD-DBD LT group (8 days) [21]. Similarly, hospital length of stay was shorter in ECD-DBD LT group (20 days) compared to SCS ECD-DBD LT group (36 days) [21]. 1-year graft survival was higher in HOPE ECD-DBD LT group (91%) compared to SCS ECD-DBD LT group (78%) [21]. Czigany and colleagues subsequently reported long-term outcomes and showed an improved 5-year graft survival trend (albeit not statistically significant) for HOPE ECD-DBD LT group (95%) compared to SCS ECD-DBD LT group (69%) (**Table 3**) [22].

Subsequently, a single-center RCT evaluating outcomes of end-ischemic HOPE ECD-DBD LT recipients (n = 55) compared to SCS ECD-DBD LT recipients (n = 55) was conducted by *Ravaioli and colleagues* in Italy in 2022 [23]. Median end-ischemic HOPE perfusion duration was 2.4 hours [23]. EAD rate was found to be statistically significantly lower in HOPE ECD-DBD LT recipients (13%) compared to SCS ECD-DBD LT recipients (35%) [23]. Biliary stricture rate was found to be equivalent in both groups at 4% [23]. 1-year graft survival was statistically significantly higher in HOPE ECD-DBD LT recipients at 98% compared to SCS ECD-DBD LT recipients at 87% [23]. Lastly, a European multicenter RCT led by Dr. Schlegel and Dr. Dutkowski reported outcomes of end-ischemic HOPE DBD LT recipients (n = 85) compared to SCS DBD LT recipients (n = 85) in 2023 [24]. Median end-ischemic HOPE perfusion duration was 1.5 hours [24]. Authors reported that liver-graft related Clavien-Dindo class 3B-5 complications (PNF, biliary complications, vascular complications) were significantly lower in HOPE DBD LT group (10%) compared to SCS DBD LT group

Study	N	Donor type	Median follow-up, months (95% CI)	Perfusion logistics and route	Perfusion duration, median (IQR) (Hours)	Late-onset biliary stricture development, N (%)			Late-onset graft failure, N (%)			Mortality, N (%)		
						Study**	Control***	P	Study**	Control***	P-Value	Study**	Control***	P
Eden et al. Europe 2024 [29]	1202 HOPE/ dHOPE/ NRP-HOPE	DBD/ DCD	34.8 (13.2–56.4)	Back-to-Base HOPE/ dHOPE/ NRP-HOPE	2.3 (1.8–3.4)	1-Year: 43 (10)	1-Year: 18 (2.3)	<0.01	1-Year: 35 (8)	1-Year: 38 (5)	<0.01	1-Year: 39 (9)	1-Year: 69 (9)	0.13
						2-Year: 50 (11.5)	2-Year: 19 (2.5)		3-Year: 56 (13)	3-Year: 54 (7)		3-Year: 69 (16)	3-Year: 100 (13)	
									5-Year: 82 (19)	5-Year: 77 (10)		5-Year: 95 (22)	5-Year: 115 (15)	
Czigany et al. Europe 2023 [22]	21 HOPE; 20 SCS	DBD	48 (41–55)	Back-to-Base HOPE	2.4 (1.7–3.4)	5-Year: 3 (14.3)	5-Year: 3 (15)	>0.99	5-Year: 1 (4.8)*	5-Year: 5 (25)	0.093	5-Year: 1 (4.8)*	5 Year: 5 (25)	NA

Occurring after 6 months.
**Study = DCD in Eden et al.*
***Control = DBD in Eden et al.*
Abbreviations: donation after brain death, DBD; donation after circulatory death, DCD; dual hypothermic oxygenated machine perfusion, dHOPE; hypothermic oxygenated machine perfusion, HOPE; interquartile range, IQR; not available, NA; normothermic regional perfusion-hypothermic oxygenated machine perfusion, NRP-HOPE; P-value, P; static cold storage, SCS.

Table 3.
Long term outcomes following utilization of HOPE liver grafts for transplantation.

(37%) [24]. There was no statistically significant difference in 1-year graft survival between HOPE DBD LT group (95%) and SCS DBD LT group (92%) [24]. All the HOPE cohort and RCT studies have been summarized in **Tables 1** and **2** respectively.

In summary, HOPE application in clinical LT has significant potential advantages in reducing liver-graft related complications in DBD LT recipients. In ECD-DBD LT recipients, HOPE has potential to lower the frequency of reperfusion syndrome, decrease EAD rates and reduce ICU/hospital length of stay in ECD-DBD LT recipients. In DCD LT recipients, HOPE has been shown to reduce EAD rate, decrease biliary stricture rate, and reduce HCC recurrence risk. Given these robust findings, rapid clinical adoption of HOPE in clinical LT is anticipated at multiple European centers once country-specific regulatory requirements are overcome. In the USA, a multicenter prospective randomized control trial evaluating HOPE vs. SCS in LT is currently in progress [NCT05045794] and results are anticipated over the next year.

3.3 Clinical studies evaluating dHOPE

Van Rijn and colleagues published the first clinical study evaluating end-ischemic dHOPE application in 10 DCD LT recipients in the Netherlands in 2017 [10]. Control group consisted of 20 matched DCD LT recipients [10]. Median warm ischemia time was similar in the dHOPE group (27 minutes) and SCS group (32 minutes) [10]. Median end-ischemic dHOPE perfusion duration was 2.1 hours [10]. EAD rates were equivalent in the dHOPE DCD LT group (0%) and SCS DCD LT group (10%) [10]. None of the dHOPE DCD LT recipients required re-LT while 25% of SCS DCD LT recipients required re-LT within 1 year due to IC [10]. Their study demonstrated a protective effect of dHOPE on biliary complications in LT recipients.

Patrono and colleagues published their clinical study comparing outcomes of end-ischemic dHOPE in 25 ECD-DBD LT recipients with 50 matched SCS ECD-DBD LT recipients in Italy in 2019 [25]. Median end-ischemic dHOPE perfusion duration was 3.1 hours [25]. EAD rates were equivalent in dHOPE ECD-DBD LT group (32%) and SCS ECD-DBD LT group (34%) [25]. No difference in biliary complications were detected between dHOPE ECD-DBD LT group (24%) and SCS ECD-DBD LT group (18%) at 6-month follow-up [25]. They noted that the postoperative rate of stage 2–3 acute kidney injury was statistically significantly lower in dHOPE ECD-DBT LT group (16%) compared to SCS ECD-DBD LT group (42%) [25]. Subsequently, *Patrono et al* published their updated experience with dHOPE in 121 ECD DBD LT recipients compared to 723 SCS ECD DBD LT recipients in 2022 [26]. After matching both groups on recipient age, recipient gender, MELD score, donor age, donor body mass index, donor liver macrosteatosis, and anastomoses time in recipient, d-HOPE ECD DBD LT recipients were found to have significantly reduced rate of in early allograft failure, reduced rate of Clavien-Dindo grade 3 or higher complications, reduced rate of comprehensive complication index and reduced severity of IC rates compared to SCS ECD DBT LT recipients [26]. 6-month graft survival in d-HOPE ECD DBD LT group (98%) was statistically significantly higher than 6-month graft survival in SCS group (90%) [26].

Building on the momentum of these single center studies showing favorable outcomes of dHOPE, Van Rijn and colleagues published a pivotal multicenter European RCT comparing outcomes of dHOPE DCD LT recipients (n = 78) to SCS DCD LT recipients [27]. Warm ischemia time was comparable in both dHOPE group (29 minutes) and SCS group (27 minutes) [27]. Median end-ischemic dHOPE perfusion duration was 2 hr. and 12 minutes [27]. They reported statistically significantly lower post-reperfusion syndrome in dHOPE DCD LT group (12%) compared to SCS DCD

LT group (27%) [27]. EAD rate was statistically significantly lower in dHOPE DCD LT group (26%) compared to SCS DCD LT group (40%) [27]. At 6-month follow-up, anastomotic biliary stricture rate was equivalent in both groups (dHOPE 29% vs. SCS 28%) [27]. At 6-month follow-up, they found that non-anastomotic biliary stricture rate was statistically significantly lower in dHOPE DCD LT group (6%) compared to SCS DCD LT group (18%) [27]. 1-year graft survival was equivalent between both dHOPE DCD LT group (85%) and SCS DCD LT group (86%) [27]. The findings of this RCT showing beneficial effect of dHOPE in decreasing non-anastomotic biliary strictures are significant since treatment of non-anastomotic biliary strictures is challenging after DCD LT and frequently requires re-LT.

Subsequently, Grat and colleagues focused on evaluating outcomes of dHOPE DBD LT recipients (n = 26) and SCS DBD LT recipients (n = 78) in a single-center RCT [28]. Median dHOPE perfusion duration was 2 hours. EAD rate was noted to be equivalent in dHOPE DBD LT group (27%) and SCS DBD LT group (33%) [28]. There was no statistically significant difference in reperfusion rate in the dHOPE DBD LT group (23%) compared to SCS DBD LT group (19%) [28]. Authors performed subgroup analysis involving high-risk DBD liver donors defined as having DRI > 1.7 and found that dHOPE was associated with improved early allograft function and lower rate of comprehensive complication index in this higher risk DBD subgroup compared to SCS [28]. All the dHOPE cohort studies and dHOPE RCTs have been summarized in **Tables 1** and **2** respectively.

In summary, end-ischemic dHOPE application in clinical LT has significant potential benefits in DCD LT in reducing severity of post-reperfusion syndrome and decreasing rate of non-anastomotic biliary stricture rates. Also, clinically relevant protective effects (decreased EAD rate, decreased IC rate, and decreased Clavien-Dindo grade 3 or higher complications) of dHOPE appear to be more pronounced in ECD-DBD LT recipients. Given these promising findings, there is potential for increased dHOPE utilization at European transplant centers once country-specific regulatory approvals are obtained and institutional expertise is attained. To our knowledge, no studies evaluating effectiveness of dHOPE liver preservation at transplant centers in the USA have been published.

4. Future directions of HMP

Excellent short-term (1-year) clinical outcomes have been reported in LT recipients, who received HMP preserved liver grafts. Long-term (5-year and 10-year) single and multicenter outcomes of LT recipients, who received HMP preserved liver grafts are eagerly anticipated over the next-decade. A recent observational multicenter international European cohort study focusing on long-term liver graft outcomes preserved with either HOPE alone, dHOPE alone, or NRP-HOPE reported excellent long-term outcomes in both DBD and DCD LT recipients [29]. For HOPE/dHOPE/NRP-HOPE preserved liver DBD grafts, LT recipients were found to have 1-year, 3-year, and 5-year death censored graft survival of 95%, 92%, and 91% respectively (**Table 3**) [29]. Similarly, for HOPE/dHOPE/NRP-HOPE preserved liver DCD grafts, LT recipients were found to have 1-year, 3-year, and 5-year death-censored graft survival of 92, 87, and 81% (**Table 3**) [29]. Additionally, authors found that the 1-year cumulative incidence of non-anastomotic strictures was statistically significantly lower in DCD liver grafts treated with NRP-HOPE / NRP-dHOPE combination (3.8%) compared to DCD liver grafts treated with HOPE alone/dHOPE alone (12.6%) [29].

These findings highlight cumulative benefit of sequential NRP-HOPE/NRP-dHOPE application in DCD liver grafts, however further prospective studies exploring this topic are required [29].

Viability assessment of liver grafts during HMP is challenging because liver grafts are maintained under hypothermic conditions and there is no bile production observed during HMP. Initial efforts of viability assessment by Patrono et al. focused on evaluating HMP perfusate AST, ALT, LDH, lactate; however they only found a weak correlation between these cytosolic injury markers and postoperative EAD [30]. Given our increased understanding of IRI mechanisms at cellular level, Muller et al. focused on evaluating FMN levels as a surrogate for mitochondrial injury through real-time fluorescence spectroscopy and mass spectrometry in 54 HOPE treated liver grafts [31]. They demonstrated that HOPE preserved liver grafts with FMN level exceeding 10,000 A.U on fluorescence spectroscopy or 100 ng FMN/ml perfusate on mass spectrometry after 30 minutes of HOPE was highly predictive of 90-day graft loss. Their study, also, confirmed findings of prior studies showing weak correlation between perfusate cytosolic markers (AST, ALT, LDH, and lactate) and EAD [31]. Findings of this study are a promising breakthrough since real-time FMN analysis during HMP may be utilized by LT surgeons in their decision making to accept or discard DCD liver grafts. However, validation of FMN as a predictive marker of EAD with additional studies using various modalities of HMP is required.

There has, also, been an increased interest in applying HMP to ex-vivo liver splitting in pediatric LT. Rossignol et al. reported their experience with utilization of HOPE for ex-vivo splitting of DBD liver grafts (n = 15) compared to SCS ex-vivo splitting of DBD liver grafts (n = 17) in pediatric LT [32]. They were able to demonstrate a lower rate of reperfusion syndrome in HOPE-split grafts (13%) compared to SCS split grafts (3%) and similar 1-year graft/recipient survival in both HOPE-split/SCS-split LT recipients [32].

Lastly, it must be stated that the HMP-O_2 circuit is completely portable since the preservation solution is pre-charged with oxygen at the beginning of machine preservation alleviating the need to further oxygenate the circuit during air transportation. On the other hand, HOPE and dHOPE circuits require continuous oxygenation and their application is limited to end-ischemic utilization at the recipient hospital. Since portability of compressed oxygen cylinders is prohibited due to current aviation regulations, additional clinical innovation is required for HOPE/dHOPE circuits to enhance their safe portability during air transport. Also, future clinical studies are required to determine the optimal level of oxygen tension and optimal duration of HMP required to safely preserve liver grafts under hypothermic conditions.

5. Conclusion

Significant progress has been made in the clinical application of HMP in LT over the last decade. Single-center studies and multicenter RCTs evaluating different HMP modalities have shown significant clinical benefit in reducing EAD, biliary complications, and reducing ICU/hospital length of stay in LT recipients compared to SCS. Different HMP modalities (HMP-O_2, HOPE, dHOPE) have been successfully integrated at pioneering LT centers in both Europe and the USA to help reduce waitlist times for potential LT recipients by increasing the use of ECD-DBD and DCD liver grafts. The next steps in the evolution of HMP in clinical LT include overcoming regulatory hurdles in various countries to broaden the availability and application of these HMP modalities.

Conflict of interest

The authors declare no conflict of interest.

Abbreviations

AST	aspartate aminotransferase
ATP	adenosine triphosphate
DBD	donation after brain death
DCD	donation after circulatory death
dHOPE	dual hypothermic oxygenated machine perfusion
DRI	donor risk index
EAD	early allograft dysfunction
ECD	extended criteria donor
FDA	food and drug administration
FMN	flavin mononucleotide
fWIT	functional warm ischemia time
HCC	hepatocellular carcinoma
HMP-O_2	oxygen “precharge” hypothermic machine perfusion
HMP	hypothermic machine perfusion
HOPE	hypothermic oxygenated machine perfusion
IC	ischemic cholangiopathy
IRI	ischemia-reperfusion injury
L-GRAFT$_7$	liver graft assessment following transplant score at seven days
LT	liver transplantation
MELD	model for end-stage liver disease
NMP	normothermic machine perfusion
NRP	normothermic regional perfusion
PNF	primary non-function
RCT	randomized control trial
ROS	reactive oxygen species
SCS	static cold storage
USA	United States of America

Author details

Hetal Lad, Tiffany Hsiung, Aditya Kasina and Arpit Amin*
Department of Surgery, Rutgers New Jersey Medical School, Newark, NJ, USA

*Address all correspondence to: arpit.amin@rutgers.edu

References

[1] Kwong AJ, Kim WR, Lake JR, Schladt DP, Schnellinger EM, Gauntt K, et al. OPTN/SRTR 2022 annual data report: Liver. American Journal of Transplantation. 2024;**24**(2s1):S176-s265

[2] Karangwa S, Panayotova G, Dutkowski P, Porte RJ, Guarrera JV, Schlegel A. Hypothermic machine perfusion in liver transplantation. International Journal of Surgery. 2020;**82s**:44-51

[3] Amin A, Panayotova G, Guarrera JV. Hypothermic machine perfusion for liver graft preservation. Current Opinion in Organ Transplantation. 2022;**27**(2):98-105

[4] Sousa Da Silva RX, Weber A, Dutkowski P, Clavien PA. Machine perfusion in liver transplantation. Hepatology. 2022;**76**(5):1531-1549

[5] Chouchani ET, Pell VR, Gaude E, Aksentijević D, Sundier SY, Robb EL, et al. Ischaemic accumulation of succinate controls reperfusion injury through mitochondrial ROS. Nature. 2014;**515**(7527):431-435

[6] Pell VR, Chouchani ET, Murphy MP, Brookes PS, Krieg T. Moving forwards by blocking back-flow: The Yin and Yang of MI therapy. Circulation Research. 2016;**118**(5):898-906

[7] Schlegel A, Muller X, Dutkowski P. Hypothermic liver perfusion. Current Opinion in Organ Transplantation. 2017;**22**(6):563-570

[8] Schlegel A, de Rougemont O, Graf R, Clavien PA, Dutkowski P. Protective mechanisms of end-ischemic cold machine perfusion in DCD liver grafts. Journal of Hepatology. 2013;**58**(2):278-286

[9] Dutkowski P, Schlegel A, de Oliveira M, Müllhaupt B, Neff F, Clavien PA. HOPE for human liver grafts obtained from donors after cardiac death. Journal of Hepatology. 2014;**60**(4):765-772

[10] van Rijn R, Karimian N, Matton APM, Burlage LC, Westerkamp AC, van den Berg AP, et al. Dual hypothermic oxygenated machine perfusion in liver transplants donated after circulatory death. The British Journal of Surgery. 2017;**104**(7):907-917

[11] Panayotova GG, Rosado J, Paterno F, Deo D, Dikdan G, McCarty MA, et al. Novel oxygenation technique for hypothermic machine perfusion of liver grafts: Validation in porcine donation after cardiac death (DCD) liver model. The American Journal of Surgery. 2020;**220**(5):1270-1277

[12] Guarrera JV, Henry SD, Samstein B, Odeh-Ramadan R, Kinkhabwala M, Goldstein MJ, et al. Hypothermic machine preservation in human liver transplantation: The first clinical series. American Journal of Transplantation. 2010;**10**(2):372-381

[13] Guarrera JV, Henry SD, Samstein B, Reznik E, Musat C, Lukose TI, et al. Hypothermic machine preservation facilitates successful transplantation of "orphan" extended criteria donor livers. American Journal of Transplantation. 2015;**15**(1):161-169

[14] Panayotova GG, Lunsford KE, Quillin RC 3rd, Rana A, Agopian VG, Lee-Riddle GS, et al. Portable hypothermic oxygenated machine

perfusion for organ preservation in liver transplantation: A randomized, open-label, clinical trial. Hepatology. 2024;**79**(5):1033-1047

[15] Dutkowski P, Polak WG, Muiesan P, Schlegel A, Verhoeven CJ, Scalera I, et al. First comparison of hypothermic oxygenated PErfusion versus static cold storage of human donation after cardiac death liver transplants: An international-matched case analysis. Annals of Surgery. 2015;**262**(5):764-770; discussion 70-1

[16] Schlegel A, Muller X, Kalisvaart M, Muellhaupt B, Perera M, Isaac JR, et al. Outcomes of DCD liver transplantation using organs treated by hypothermic oxygenated perfusion before implantation. Journal of Hepatology. 2019;**70**(1):50-57

[17] Mueller M, Kalisvaart M, O'Rourke J, Shetty S, Parente A, Muller X, et al. Hypothermic oxygenated liver perfusion (HOPE) prevents tumor recurrence in liver transplantation from donation after circulatory death. Annals of Surgery. 2020;**272**(5):759-765

[18] Ravaioli M, De Pace V, Angeletti A, Comai G, Vasuri F, Baldassarre M, et al. Hypothermic oxygenated new machine perfusion system in liver and kidney transplantation of extended criteria donors: First Italian clinical trial. Scientific Reports. 2020;**10**(1):6063

[19] Rayar M, Beaurepaire JM, Bajeux E, Hamonic S, Renard T, Locher C, et al. Hypothermic oxygenated perfusion improves extended criteria donor liver graft function and reduces duration of hospitalization without extra cost: The PERPHO study. Liver Transplantation. 2021;**27**(3):349-362

[20] Horné F, Drefs M, Schirren MJ, Koch DT, Cepele G, Jacobi SJ, et al. Hypothermic oxygenated machine perfusion (HOPE) prior to liver transplantation mitigates post-reperfusion syndrome and perioperative electrolyte shifts. Journal of Clinical Medicine. 2022;**11**(24):7381

[21] Czigany Z, Pratschke J, Froněk J, Guba M, Schöning W, Raptis DA, et al. Hypothermic oxygenated machine perfusion reduces early allograft injury and improves post-transplant outcomes in extended criteria donation liver transplantation from donation after brain death: Results from a multicenter randomized controlled trial (HOPE ECD-DBD). Annals of Surgery. 2021;**274**(5):705-712

[22] Czigany Z, Uluk D, Pavicevic S, Lurje I, Froněk J, Keller T, et al. Improved outcomes after hypothermic oxygenated machine perfusion in liver transplantation-long-term follow-up of a multicenter randomized controlled trial. Hepatology Communications. 2024;**8**(2):e0376

[23] Ravaioli M, Germinario G, Dajti G, Sessa M, Vasuri F, Siniscalchi A, et al. Hypothermic oxygenated perfusion in extended criteria donor liver transplantation-a randomized clinical trial. American Journal of Transplantation. 2022;**22**(10):2401-2408

[24] Schlegel A, Mueller M, Muller X, Eden J, Panconesi R, von Felten S, et al. A multicenter randomized-controlled trial of hypothermic oxygenated perfusion (HOPE) for human liver grafts before transplantation. Journal of Hepatology. 2023;**78**(4):783-793

[25] Patrono D, Surra A, Catalano G, Rizza G, Berchialla P, Martini S, et al. Hypothermic oxygenated machine perfusion of liver grafts from brain-dead donors. Scientific Reports. 2019;**9**(1):9337

[26] Patrono D, Cussa D, Sciannameo V, Montanari E, Panconesi R, Berchialla P, et al. Outcome of liver transplantation with grafts from brain-dead donors treated with dual hypothermic oxygenated machine perfusion, with particular reference to elderly donors. American Journal of Transplantation. 2022;**22**(5):1382-1395

[27] van Rijn R, Schurink IJ, de Vries Y, van den Berg AP, Cortes Cerisuelo M, Darwish Murad S, et al. Hypothermic machine perfusion in liver transplantation—A randomized trial. The New England Journal of Medicine. 2021;**384**(15):1391-1401

[28] Grąt M, Morawski M, Zhylko A, Rykowski P, Krasnodębski M, Wyporski A, et al. Routine end-ischemic hypothermic oxygenated machine perfusion in liver transplantation from donors after brain death: A randomized controlled trial. Annals of Surgery. 2023;**278**(5):662-668

[29] Eden J, Brüggenwirth IMA, Berlakovich G, Buchholz BM, Botea F, Camagni S, et al. Long-term outcomes after hypothermic oxygenated machine perfusion and transplantation of 1,202 donor livers in a real-world setting (HOPE-REAL study). Journal of Hepatology. 3 Jul 2024:S0168-8278(24)02341-9

[30] Patrono D, Catalano G, Rizza G, Lavorato N, Berchialla P, Gambella A, et al. Perfusate analysis during dual hypothermic oxygenated machine perfusion of liver grafts: Correlations with donor factors and early outcomes. Transplantation. 2020;**104**(9):1929-1942

[31] Muller X, Schlegel A, Kron P, Eshmuminov D, Würdinger M, Meierhofer D, et al. Novel real-time prediction of liver graft function during hypothermic oxygenated machine perfusion before liver transplantation. Annals of Surgery. 2019;**270**(5):783-790

[32] Rossignol G, Muller X, Hervieu V, Collardeau-Frachon S, Breton A, Boulanger N, et al. Liver transplantation of partial grafts after ex situ splitting during hypothermic oxygenated perfusion-the HOPE-Split pilot study. Liver Transplantation. 2022;**28**(10):1576-1587

Chapter 9

Current Status in Live Liver Donation: Donor Selection, Surgical Technique, Long-Term Outcome

Chan Woo Cho and Gyu-Seong Choi

Abstract

Living donor liver transplantation (LDLT) has been one of the most remarkable steps in the field of liver transplantation. Live liver donation significantly expands the scarce donor pool in countries with a shortage of available cadaveric grafts. Live liver donation has clinical benefits over deceased liver donation, such as shortening wait time, scheduling convenience, and increasing long-term success. In that healthy people undergo major surgery for their loved ones, the physical and psychological sacrifices of donors are immense. Thus, donor safety is one of the most important issues in performing LDLT. Recently, due to a better understanding of liver anatomy and technical innovations in donor surgery, live liver donor selection criteria have expanded, and good results are reported with securing donor safety. In this chapter, we introduce expanded selection criteria for live liver donation and innovative donor surgery, including minimally invasive approaches, and provide information regarding the current overview of donor postoperative quality of life and long-term outcomes.

Keywords: liver transplantation, living donors, donor selection, outcomes, minimal invasive surgery, hepatectomy

1. Introduction

Living donor liver transplantation (LDLT) represents a groundbreaking advancement in the field of liver transplant surgery, providing an effective alternative to deceased donor liver transplantation. One of the most significant advantages of LDLT is its ability to expand the donor organ pool, thereby offering new hope to patients with end-stage liver disease or hepatocellular carcinoma. Unlike the unpredictable nature of organs from deceased donors, live liver donors can be carefully assessed, ensuring a timely and effective transplantation process. Importantly, live liver donors undergo comprehensive preoperative evaluations that consider their medical history, and psychological well-being, ultimately contributing to improved graft quality and both donor and recipient outcomes.

The selection criteria for live liver donors are multifaceted and designed to prioritize donor safety and optimize outcomes. Factors like donor age, body mass index (BMI), blood type, graft volume, and graft quality play pivotal roles in determining eligibility and ensuring good results for both donor and recipient. While traditionally, younger and healthier individuals were favored as donors, recent research is reshaping these parameters, allowing for older donors and those with varying BMI ranges to contribute effectively. Understanding these updated criteria is key to broadening the donor base and meeting the rising demand for liver transplantation.

Moreover, innovative surgical techniques have emerged, such as minimal invasive donor hepatectomy (MIDH), which minimizes donor morbidity and enhances recovery experiences. As these surgical methods evolve, they promise better outcomes for donors, making the idea of living donation more appealing and accessible.

As we delve into the details of donor selection criteria, the evolution of donor surgery, and the long-term outcomes for living liver donors, we invite readers to explore the possibilities and implications of living liver donation. The focus of this chapter is to foster a deeper understanding of how these advancements in live liver donation can improve the lives of sick people with liver disease and why they matter to anyone impacted by liver disease or organ donation.

2. Selection of the live liver donor

LDLT requires careful selection of donors to ensure safety and optimal outcomes. The selection criteria for live liver donors include age, BMI, blood type, minimum graft volume, and graft quality.

2.1 Donor age

LDLT has expanded to include older donors, with many centers accepting donors up to 60 years old or even older [1, 2]. Studies have shown that carefully selected elderly donors (≥55–60 years) can safely undergo right lobe donation without compromising donor safety or recipient outcomes [3, 4]. However, some research indicates that advanced donor age may be associated with lower graft and recipient survival [5]. The use of left lobe grafts from older donors may require extra caution due to a higher incidence of small-for-size syndrome [6]. Proper donor selection criteria, including preservation of the middle hepatic vein, adequate remnant liver volume, and absence of fatty liver, are crucial for ensuring good outcomes with older donors [1, 4]. Collectively, age itself is not a contraindication for a living donor hepatectomy, but the careful use of elderly donors can help expand the donor pool without compromising safety [7–9].

2.2 Donor body mass index

The impact of BMI on liver transplantation outcomes remains controversial. Several studies suggest that grafts from obese donors (BMI >30) can be safely transplanted without negatively affecting long-term patient outcomes [10–12]. However, higher donor BMI is associated with an increased risk of hepatic steatosis [13, 14] and wound complications [15]. BMI alone may not be a reliable predictor of complications, as age and socioeconomic factors do not significantly influence serious complications in living donors. While donor BMI does not appear to affect graft and patient survival in adult recipients, it may impact outcomes in pediatric liver transplantation when adult donors have severe obesity (BMI ≥35) [16]. Overall, careful evaluation of potential donors with higher BMI, including assessment of hepatic steatosis, can help expand the donor pool without compromising transplant outcomes.

2.3 ABO-compatibility

Recent studies have shown that ABO-incompatible (ABOi) LDLT can be performed safely with outcomes comparable to ABO-compatible (ABOc) LDLT. Improved desensitization protocols, including rituximab, plasma exchange, and intravenous immunoglobulin, have significantly enhanced the success of ABOi LDLT [17, 18]. While some studies reported lower graft volumes and increased cytomegalovirus infection rates in ABOi LDLT [19, 20], others found no significant differences in overall patient and graft survival between ABOi and ABOc LDLT [18, 21]. Exchange donor programs have been implemented to overcome ABO incompatibility [22]. Although ABOi LDLT may have a higher risk of biliary and vascular complications, it remains a viable option when ABO-compatible donors are unavailable, especially with the development of simplified and effective desensitization protocols [17, 23].

2.4 Graft volume

Graft volume selection is crucial in LDLT to ensure donor safety and recipient outcomes. Most centers consider a graft-to-recipient weight ratio (GRWR) of 0.7 or less and a remnant liver volume of 30% as acceptable minimums [2]. At our center, LDLT is performed when the GRWR is 0.8 or more and the remnant liver is 30% or higher. The left lobe is preferred for donor safety, but right lobe grafts maybe necessary for recipients with higher Model for End-Stage Liver Disease (MELD) scores or older donors [24]. Preoperative CT volumetry is essential for accurate graft size estimation [25]. Some centers use algorithms considering graft-to-recipient body weight ratio, remnant liver volume, and estimated congestion ratio to guide graft selection [26]. Despite differences in early postoperative liver function, long-term outcomes are comparable between left and right lobe grafts when both meet volumetric criteria [27]. The right posterior sector graft is a viable option when the left lobe volume is inadequate [28].

2.5 Graft quality

Graft quality, particularly hepatic steatosis, is a critical factor in live liver donation for LDLT. While moderate to severe steatosis can increase the risk of primary graft nonfunction [29, 30], mild steatosis appears to have minimal impact on outcomes [31]. Noninvasive evaluation methods, such as CT liver-to-spleen attenuation ratio (CTL-S) and Magnetic Resonance Imaging Proton Density Fat Fraction (MRI-PDFF), can accurately estimate graft steatosis [32, 33]. In our center, a preoperative biopsy is recommended when the CTL-S is –7 or less and the MRI-PDFF is 15% or higher. Short-term intensive treatments combining diet, exercise, and medication can effectively reduce steatosis in potential donors [34]. While using steatotic grafts expands the donor pool, careful selection and management are crucial. On the whole, the use of mildly steatotic grafts (macrovesicular fatty change <30%) in LDLT appears justified, but moderate to severe steatosis requires careful consideration of risks and benefits [29, 31].

3. Innovation of donor surgery

The evolution of donor hepatectomy for LDLT has focused on minimizing donor risk while preserving graft viability. With innovative surgical techniques such as selective vascular occlusion, and hanging maneuver proposed [35], donor morbidity has decreased significantly with experience, from 53.8 to 9.2% in one study [36]. Early techniques involved large incisions, but have progressed to minimally invasive approaches [37]. Laparoscopic and robotic techniques have emerged, offering better cosmesis, less pain, and improved quality of life [38].

3.1 Implementation and various approaches of minimal invasive donor hepatectomy

MIDH has emerged as a promising approach to reduce donor morbidity in LDLT. Various techniques have been developed, including hand-assisted, laparoscopic-assisted, pure laparoscopic, and robotic approaches [39, 40]. While left lateral sectionectomy has become standard in experienced centers, major left, and right liver donations remain challenging to perform with minimally invasive approaches [39]. The right posterior sector graft is a viable option when left lobe volume is inadequate. Our center reported the results of pure laparoscopic donor right posterior sectionectomy (PLDRPS) in living donors with insufficient remnant left lobe volume and PV anomaly. Studies have shown that PLDRPS is technically feasible and safe when performed by experienced surgeons, with no open conversions or perioperative blood transfusions reported. Comparative studies between PLDRPS and pure laparoscopic donor right hemihepatectomy (PLDRH) have found similar donor outcomes, although recipient outcomes may require further evaluation [41, 42]. Expert consensus guidelines emphasize donor safety and recommend careful donor selection and standardized techniques [43]. MIDH requires significant expertise in liver transplantation, hepatobiliary surgery, and minimally invasive techniques [40].

3.2 Development of surgical equipment in MIDH

MIDH for LDLT has gained attention in recent years as laparoscopic and robotic approaches using three-dimensional (3D) cameras have emerged as the dominant modality. Flexible 3D laparoscopy provides improved depth perception and hand-eye coordination compared to conventional 2D techniques, allowing more realistic and detailed visualization of the surgical field (**Figure 1**) [44, 45]. In addition, the small space was easily manipulated by a flexible scope that provided a variety of surgical views, including bird's-eye, low-angle, and lateral views [46]. Several expertized centers have reported successful cases of pure laparoscopic donor hepatectomies, including left hemihepatectomy, right hemihepatectomy, extended right hepatectomy, and right posterior sectionectomy with complex biliary and vascular anatomy [41, 46–48]. Indocyanine green fluorescence cholangiography has been utilized to enhance biliary visualization and transection line refinement during MIDH [45]. Robotic donor hepatectomy has also shown promise, offering advantages such as tremor elimination and increased freedom of movement [49].

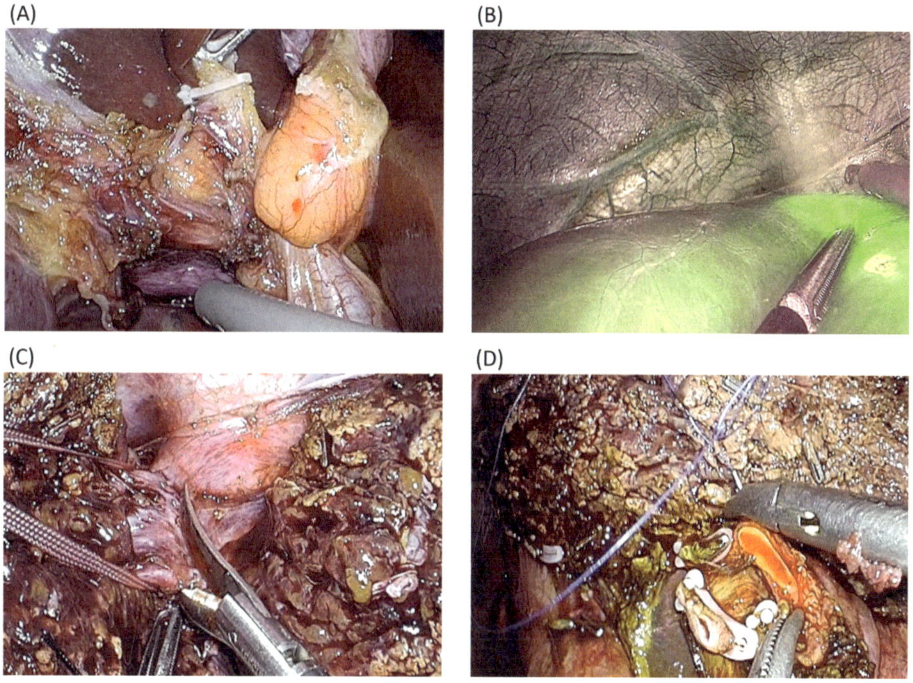

Figure 1.
Surgical fields of flexible 3D laparoscopy in PLDRH. (A) Identification of the right hepatic artery and right portal vein; (B) Indocyanine green fluorescence image for the demarcation line; (C) Division of the right hepatic vein; and (D) Closure of the right hepatic duct.

3.3 Expanding selection criteria for MIDH

While minimally invasive approaches offer benefits like improved cosmesis and faster recovery, careful donor selection remains crucial. The selection of the donors must also be done in a stepwise fashion just like with the surgical procedure. Factors such as donor age, remnant liver volume, graft volume, and anatomical complexity should be considered when choosing between laparoscopic or robotic and open techniques. In order to start a safe program of MIDH, the suggested recommendations are as follows: GRWR of more than 1.0, modest donor BMI score of less than 30 a remnant liver volume of more than 35%, graft weight of less than 700 g, normal vascular and biliary anatomy, and a nonemergent setting [43, 50]. As experience accumulates, selection criteria for PLDH have expanded to include donors with anatomical variations, higher BMI, and larger graft weights [41, 44, 51, 52]. Despite these advancements, careful consideration is still needed for donors with advanced age, limited remnant liver volume, or multiple anticipated vessel openings, as these factors may impact recipient outcomes [53].

4. Outcomes of live liver donors

Since living donor liver transplantation carries small but significant risks for donors, donor safety is a primary concern after donation. Many studies report improved outcomes with increased experience, developed surgical techniques, and strict donor selection over time.

4.1 Postoperative morbidity and mortality

Donor hepatectomy for LDLT is generally safe, with no reported donor mortality across multiple studies [54–57]. The overall complication rates range from 9.3 to 39.6% across studies, with most being minor and manageable [54, 58]. Biliary complications are the most frequent, occurring in 3.4–8.6% of donors [59–62]. Other common complications include ileus, atelectasis, and hernias [63, 64]. Right lobe donation carries a higher risk of complications compared to left lobe or left lateral segment donation [55, 65]. Strict donor selection criteria and improved surgical techniques have reduced complication rates over time [66].

4.2 Liver regeneration

Liver regeneration is crucial for the safety and outcomes of live liver donors. Studies show that donor livers regenerate rapidly, reaching 65–80% of the original volume within 2 weeks and 88–90% by 6 months [67, 68]. Factors affecting regeneration include remnant liver volume, graft type, age, gender, initial graft size, and intraoperative blood loss [69–71]. Right lobe donors may experience more complications but achieve similar regeneration as left lobe donors [68, 72]. While complete regeneration may not occur within the first year, donors maintain normal liver function and can safely resume daily activities [67, 72, 73].

4.3 Quality of life restoration and the impact of MIDH

Live liver donors generally maintain a good quality of life (QOL) post-donation, with most returning to baseline levels within 6 months [74]. Physical QOL typically decreases initially but recovers within 3–6 months [75, 76]. Mental QOL often remains stable or improves post-donation [75]. However, some donors experience poor QOL outcomes, particularly those with postoperative complications or whose recipients expire [77, 78].

MIDH has shown promising results in terms of quality of life and postoperative outcomes. Studies have demonstrated that MIDH, including laparoscopic and robotic approaches, leads to faster mobility recovery, better body image satisfaction, and improved quality of life compared to open donor hepatectomy [79, 80]. Donors undergoing MIDH experienced less pain, reduced incision-related complications, and a faster return to work [81, 82]. Both laparoscopic and robotic techniques have been successfully applied to right hepatectomy, demonstrating feasibility and safety [81, 83]. Overall, MIDH appears to offer improved donor satisfaction and quality of life without compromising safety or recipient outcomes [80, 84].

4.4 Long-term outcomes of live liver donation

Live liver donors generally report positive long-term outcomes and satisfaction with their decision to donate [85]. A large-scale study of 10,116 live liver donors found increased mortality risk compared to healthy controls without contraindications to donation [86]. Similarly, a U.S. study of 4111 donors found comparable long-term mortality in healthy individuals [87]. Mental health outcomes are generally stable or improved post-donation, with some donors reporting increased anxiety or alcohol use disorders [88]. Despite these risks, donor survival rates remain high, with one study reporting 98.8% 15-year survival. Long-term follow-up, including psychosocial support, is recommended for live liver donors [86].

5. Conclusion

LDLT is a transformative solution for bridging the gap between the growing demand for liver transplants and the limited availability of deceased donor organs. This prospective and timely alternative not only addresses the urgent needs of patients with end-stage liver disease but also offers hope and life-saving opportunities.

LDLT constitutes a significant advancement in the field of organ transplantation, offering an effective alternative to deceased donor liver transplantation. The expanded selection criteria for live liver donors have broadened the donor pool, thereby contributing to alleviating the critical shortage of donor organs for individuals suffering from end-stage liver disease or hepatocellular carcinoma.

The introduction of innovative surgical techniques, particularly MIDH, has further improved the safety and feasibility of the donation procedure. These techniques not only reduce postoperative complications but also promote faster recovery and better overall QOL for donors. The positive long-term outcomes for live liver donors and their high satisfaction rates regarding the decision to donate reinforce the attractiveness of living liver donation as a treatment option. By fostering greater awareness and understanding of the benefits of living organ donation, we can inspire more individuals to participate in this noble cause, ultimately saving lives and bridging the gap in organ availability.

As we continue to advance donor selection and surgical techniques, the role of LDLT will only become more critical in enhancing organ donation efforts. In doing so, we can ensure that more patients receive the life-saving transplants they need, thereby fulfilling the promise of bridging the gap and saving lives through organ donation.

Acronyms and abbreviations

ABOc	ABO-compatible
ABOi	ABO-incompatible
BMI	body mass index
CTL-S	CT liver-to-spleen attenuation ratio
GRWR	graft-to-recipient weight ratio
LDLT	living donor liver transplantation
MIDH	minimal invasive donor hepatectomy
MELD	model for end-stage liver disease
MRI-PDFF	magnetic resonance imaging proton density fat fraction
PLDRH	pure laparoscopic donor right hemihepatectomy
PLDRPS	pure laparoscopic ronor right posterior sectionectomy
3D	three-dimensional
QOL	quality of life

Author details

Chan Woo Cho[1] and Gyu-Seong Choi[2]*

1 Department of Surgery, Yeungnam University College of Medicine, Daegu, Korea

2 Department of Surgery, Samsung Medical Center, Sungkyunkwan University School of Medicine, Seoul, Korea

*Address all correspondence to: gyuseong.choi@samsung.com

References

[1] Hoon Kim S, Duke Lee S, Kyu-Kim Y, Park SJ. Living donors ages 60 or older in right lobe living donor liver transplantation. Transplantation. 2015;**99**(3):e16-e17

[2] Soin AS, Chaudhary RJ, Pahari H, Pomfret EA. A worldwide survey of live liver donor selection policies at 24 Centers with a combined experience of 19 009 adult living donor liver transplants. Transplantation. 2019;**103**(2):e39-e47

[3] Kadohisa M, Inomata Y, Uto K, Hayashida S, Ohya Y, Yamamoto H, et al. Impact of donor age on the outcome of living-donor liver transplantation: Special consideration to the feasibility of using elderly donors. Transplantation. 2021;**105**(2):328-337

[4] Kim SH, Lee EC, Shim JR, Park SJ. Right lobe living donors ages 55 years old and older in liver transplantation. Liver Transplantation. 2017;**23**(10):1305-1311

[5] Busquets J, Xiol X, Figueras J, Jaurrieta E, Torras J, Ramos E, et al. The impact of donor age on liver transplantation: Influence of donor age on early liver function and on subsequent patient and graft survival. Transplantation. 2001;**71**(12):1765-1771

[6] Ikegami T, Taketomi A, Ohta R, Soejima Y, Yoshizumi T, Shimada M, et al. Donor age in living donor liver transplantation. Transplantation Proceedings. 2008;**40**(5):1471-1475

[7] Grande L, Matus D, Rimola A, Manyalic M, Cabrer C, Garcia-Valdecasas JC, et al. Expanded liver donor age over 60 years for hepatic transplantation. Clinical Transplants. 1998:297-301

[8] Kuramitsu K, Egawa H, Keeffe EB, Kasahara M, Ito T, Sakamoto S, et al. Impact of age older than 60 years in living donor liver transplantation. Transplantation. 2007;**84**(2):166-172

[9] Kim JM, Joo DJ, Hong SK, You YK, Hwang S, Ryu JH, et al. Outcomes of sexagenarian living liver donors in Korea: A multicenter study. Liver Transplantation. 2023;**29**(7):698-710

[10] Moss J, Lapointe-Rudow D, Renz JF, Kinkhabwala M, Dove LM, Gaglio PJ, et al. Select utilization of obese donors in living donor liver transplantation: Implications for the donor pool. American Journal of Transplantation. 2005;**5**(12):2974-2981

[11] Andert A, Becker N, Ulmer F, Schoning W, Hein M, Rimek A, et al. Liver transplantation and donor body mass index >30: Use or refuse? Annals of Transplantation. 2016;**21**:185-193

[12] Knaak M, Goldaracena N, Doyle A, Cattral MS, Greig PD, Lilly L, et al. Donor BMI >30 is not a contraindication for live liver donation. American Journal of Transplantation. 2017;**17**(3):754-760

[13] Rinella ME, Alonso E, Rao S, Whitington P, Fryer J, Abecassis M, et al. Body mass index as a predictor of hepatic steatosis in living liver donors. Liver Transplantation. 2001;**7**(5):409-414

[14] Peng CJ, Yuan D, Li B, Wei YG, Yan LN, Wen TF, et al. Body mass index evaluating donor hepatic steatosis in living donor liver transplantation. Transplantation Proceedings. 2009;**41**(9):3556-3559

[15] Lin JS, Muhammad H, Lin T, Kamel I, Baghdadi A, Rizkalla N, et al.

Donor BMI and post-living donor liver transplantation outcomes: A preliminary report. Transplantation direct. 2023;**9**(2):e1431

[16] Takagi K, de Wilde RF, Polak WG, JNM IJ. The effect of donor body mass index on graft function in liver transplantation: A systematic review. Transplantation Reviews (Orlando, Fla.). 2020;**34**(4):100571

[17] Lee TB, Ko HJ, Shim JR, Choi BH, Ryu JH, Yang K. ABO-incompatible living donor liver transplantation with a simplified desensitization and immunosuppression protocol: A single-Center retrospective study. Experimental and Clinical Transplantation. 2021;**19**(7):676-685

[18] Kim JD, Choi DL, Kim SG, Lee AJ. Single-Center experience of ABO-incompatible living-donor liver transplantation with a new simplified intravenous immunoglobulin protocol: A propensity score-matching analysis. Transplantation Proceedings. 2016;**48**(4):1134-1138

[19] Ikegami T, Yoshizumi T, Soejima Y, Uchiyama H, Shirabe K, Maehara Y. Feasible usage of ABO incompatible grafts in living donor liver transplantation. HepatoBiliary Surgery and Nutrition. 2016;**5**(2):91-97

[20] Chae MS, Lee N, Choi HJ, Chung HS, Park CS, Lee J, et al. Comparison of liver graft regeneration between ABO-compatible and ABO-incompatible living donor liver transplantation: A propensity score matching analysis. Annals of Transplantation. 2018;**23**:507-519

[21] Testa G, Vidanovic V, Chejfec G, Gangemi A, Iqpal R, Porubsky M, et al. Adult living-donor liver transplantation with ABO-incompatible grafts. Transplantation. 2008;**85**(5):681-686

[22] Hwang S, Lee SG, Moon DB, Song GW, Ahn CS, Kim KH, et al. Exchange living donor liver transplantation to overcome ABO incompatibility in adult patients. Liver Transplantation. 2010;**16**(4):482-490

[23] Kim JM, Kwon CH, Joh JW, Han SB, Sinn DH, Choi GS, et al. Case-matched comparison of ABO-incompatible and ABO-compatible living donor liver transplantation. The British Journal of Surgery. 2016;**103**(3):276-283

[24] Manatsathit W, Samant H. Graft selection strategy in adult-to-adult living donor liver transplantation: When both hemiliver grafts meet volumetric criteria. Liver Transplantation. 2016;**22**(12):1741-1742

[25] Kawasaki S, Makuuchi M, Matsunami H, Hashikura Y, Ikegami T, Chisuwa H, et al. Preoperative measurement of segmental liver volume of donors for living related liver transplantation. Hepatology. 1993;**18**(5):1115-1120

[26] Asakuma M, Fujimoto Y, Bourquain H, Uryuhara K, Hayashi M, Tanigawa N, et al. Graft selection algorithm based on congestion volume for adult living donor liver transplantation. American Journal of Transplantation. 2007;**7**(7):1788-1796

[27] Kurihara T, Yoshizumi T, Yoshida Y, Ikegami T, Itoh S, Harimoto N, et al. Graft selection strategy in adult-to-adult living donor liver transplantation: When both hemiliver grafts meet volumetric criteria. Liver Transplantation. 2016;**22**(7):914-922

[28] Kim BW, Xu W, Wang HJ, Park YK, Lee K, Kim MW. Volumetry-based selection of right posterior sector grafts for adult living donor liver transplantation. Liver Transplantation. 2011;**17**(9):1046-1058

[29] Soejima Y, Shimada M, Suehiro T, Kishikawa K, Yoshizumi T, Hashimoto K, et al. Use of steatotic graft in living-donor liver transplantation. Transplantation. 2003;**76**(2):344-348

[30] Noujaim HM, de Ville de Goyet J, Montero EF, Ribeiro CM, Capellozzi VL, Crescentini F, et al. Expanding postmortem donor pool using steatotic liver grafts: A new look. Transplantation 2009;87(6):919-925

[31] Zhang QY, Zhang QF, Zhang DZ. The impact of steatosis on the outcome of liver transplantation: A meta-analysis. BioMed Research International. 2019;**2019**:3962785

[32] Iwasaki M, Takada Y, Hayashi M, Minamiguchi S, Haga H, Maetani Y, et al. Noninvasive evaluation of graft steatosis in living donor liver transplantation. Transplantation. 2004;**78**(10):1501-1505

[33] Ahn J, Choi HJ, Park SE, Seo CH, Hong TH, You YK. Noninvasive evaluations to estimate graft steatosis in living donor liver transplant for donor safety and successful outcome. Transplantation Proceedings. 2022;**54**(2):374-379

[34] Nakamuta M, Morizono S, Soejima Y, Yoshizumi T, Aishima S, Takasugi S, et al. Short-term intensive treatment for donors with hepatic steatosis in living-donor liver transplantation. Transplantation. 2005;**80**(5):608-612

[35] Makuuchi M, Kawasaki S, Noguchi T, Hashikura Y, Matsunami H, Hayashi K, et al. Donor hepatectomy for living related partial liver transplantation. Surgery. 1993;**113**(4):395-402

[36] Broering DC, Wilms C, Bok P, Fischer L, Mueller L, Hillert C, et al. Evolution of donor morbidity in living related liver transplantation: A single-center analysis of 165 cases. Annals of Surgery. 2004;**240**(6):1013-1024 discussions 24-6

[37] Rammohan A, Rela M. Robotic donor hepatectomy: Are we there yet? World Journal of Gastrointestinal Surgery. 2021;**13**(7):668-677

[38] Broering D, Sturdevant ML, Zidan A. Robotic donor hepatectomy: A major breakthrough in living donor liver transplantation. American Journal of Transplantation. 2022;**22**(1):14-23

[39] Au KP, Chok KSH. Minimally invasive donor hepatectomy, are we ready for prime time? World Journal of Gastroenterology. 2018;**24**(25):2698-2709

[40] Kakos CD, Papanikolaou A, Ziogas IA, Tsoulfas G. Global dissemination of minimally invasive living donor hepatectomy: What are the barriers? World Journal of Gastrointestinal Surgery. 2023;**15**(5):776-787

[41] Cho CW, Choi GS, Lee DH, Kim HJ, Yun SS, Lee DS, et al. Comparison of pure laparoscopic donor right posterior sectionectomy versus right hemihepatectomy for living donor liver transplantation. Liver Transplantation. 2023;**29**(11):1199-1207

[42] Cho CW, Choi GS, Kim KS. Surgical techniques and outcomes of pure laparoscopic donor right posterior Sectionectomy for living donor liver transplantation. Liver Transplantation. 2022;**28**(2):325-329

[43] Cherqui D, Ciria R, Kwon CHD, Kim KH, Broering D, Wakabayashi G, et al. Expert consensus guidelines on minimally invasive donor hepatectomy for living donor liver transplantation from innovation to implementation: A

joint initiative from the international laparoscopic liver society (ILLS) and the Asian-Pacific Hepato-Pancreato-biliary association (A-PHPBA). Annals of Surgery. 2021;**273**(1):96-108

[44] Hong SK, Choi Y, Yi NJ, Lee KW, Suh KS. Insights from Seoul National University Hospital's experience: A systematic review of pure laparoscopic donor hepatectomy progression. HepatoBiliary Surgery and Nutrition. 2024;**13**(2):293-300

[45] Soyama A, Eguchi S. New technical development for pure laparoscopic donor hepatectomy: Indocyanine green cholangiography and three-dimensional laparoscopy Laparoscopic Surgery 2020;**4**:17

[46] Suh KS, Hong SK, Yi NJ, Lee KW, Kim HS, Yoon KC, et al. Pure 3-dimensional laparoscopic extended right hepatectomy in a living donor. Liver Transplantation. 2016;**22**(10):1431-1436

[47] Hong SK, Suh KS, Kim HS, Yoon KC, Ahn SW, Oh D, et al. Pure 3D laparoscopic living donor right hemihepatectomy in a donor with separate right posterior and right anterior hepatic ducts and portal veins. Surgical Endoscopy. 2017;**31**(11):4834-4835

[48] Song JL, Wu H, Yang JY. Pure three-dimensional laparoscopic full left hepatectomy of a living donor for an adolescent in China. Chinese Medical Journal. 2019;**132**(2):242-244

[49] Finotti M, D'Amico F, Testa G. The current and future role of robotic surgery in liver surgery and transplantation. Minerva Surgery. 2022;**77**(4):380-390

[50] Kwon CHD, Choi GS, Joh JW. Laparoscopic right hepatectomy for living donor. Current Opinion in Organ Transplantation. 2019;**24**(2):167-174

[51] Rhu J, Kim MS, Choi GS, Kim JM, Kwon CHD, Joh JW. Laparoscopic living donor right hepatectomy regarding the anatomical variation of the portal vein: A propensity score-matched analysis. Liver Transplantation. 2021;**27**(7):984-996

[52] Shehta A, Lee JM, Lee KW, Hong SK, Cho JH, Yi NJ, et al. Pure laparoscopic living donor hepatectomy for donors with right portal vein anatomical variations. Liver Transplantation. 2019;**25**(9):1445-1454

[53] Hong SK, Hong SY, Lee JM, Choi Y, Yi NJ, Lee KW, et al. Criteria for selecting living liver donors to optimize recipient outcomes in pure laparoscopic donor right hepatectomy: A cohort study. International Journal of Surgery. 2024;**110**(6):3203-3211

[54] Adcock L, Macleod C, Dubay D, Greig PD, Cattral MS, McGilvray I, et al. Adult living liver donors have excellent long-term medical outcomes: The University of Toronto liver transplant experience. American Journal of Transplantation. 2010;**10**(2):364-371

[55] Yankol Y, Mecit N, Kanmaz T, Kalayoglu M, Acarli K. Complications and outcomes of 890 living liver donor hepatectomies at a single center: Risks of saving loved one's life. Turkish Journal of Surgery. 2020;**36**(2):192-201

[56] Takagi K, Umeda Y, Yoshida R, Watanabe N, Kuise T, Yoshida K, et al. Short-term and long-term outcomes in living donors for liver transplantation: Cohort study. International Journal of Surgery. 2020;**84**:147-153

[57] Benzing C, Schmelzle M, Oellinger R, Gruettner K, Muehlisch AK, Raschzok N, et al. Living-donor liver transplant: An analysis of postoperative outcome and health-related quality of life in liver donors. Experimental

and Clinical Transplantation. 2018;**16**(5):568-574

[58] Lee JG, Lee KW, Kwon CHD, Chu CW, Kim BW, Choi DL, et al. Donor safety in living donor liver transplantation: The Korean organ transplantation registry study. Liver Transplantation. 2017;**23**(8):999-1006

[59] Iida T, Ogura Y, Oike F, Hatano E, Kaido T, Egawa H, et al. Surgery-related morbidity in living donors for liver transplantation. Transplantation. 2010;**89**(10):1276-1282

[60] Lei J, Yan L. Donor morbidity including biliary complications in living-donor liver transplantation: A single center analysis of 283 cases. Transplantation. 2012;**94**(7):e51-e52 author reply e2-3

[61] Ozgor D, Dirican A, Ates M, Gonultas F, Ara C, Yilmaz S. Donor complications among 500 living donor liver transplantations at a single center. Transplantation Proceedings. 2012;**44**(6):1604-1607

[62] Dirican A, Ara C, Kutluturk K, Ozsoy M, Ates M, Baskiran A, et al. Donor postoperative biliary complications after living-donor liver transplant. Experimental and Clinical Transplantation. 2015;**13**(6):516-523

[63] Abecassis MM, Fisher RA, Olthoff KM, Freise CE, Rodrigo DR, Samstein B, et al. Complications of living donor hepatic lobectomy--a comprehensive report. American Journal of Transplantation. 2012;**12**(5):1208-1217

[64] Hall EC, Boyarsky BJ, Deshpande NA, Garonzik-Wang JM, Berger JC, Dagher NN, et al. Perioperative complications after live-donor hepatectomy. JAMA Surgery. 2014;**149**(3):288-291

[65] Lo CM. Complications and long-term outcome of living liver donors: A survey of 1,508 cases in five Asian centers. Transplantation. 2003;**75**(3 Suppl):S12-S15

[66] Hwang S, Lee SG, Lee YJ, Sung KB, Park KM, Kim KH, et al. Lessons learned from 1,000 living donor liver transplantations in a single center: How to make living donations safe. Liver Transplantation. 2006;**12**(6):920-927

[67] Haga J, Shimazu M, Wakabayashi G, Tanabe M, Kawachi S, Fuchimoto Y, et al. Liver regeneration in donors and adult recipients after living donor liver transplantation. Liver Transplantation. 2008;**14**(12):1718-1724

[68] Kwon KH, Kim YW, Kim SI, Kim KS, Lee WJ, Choi JS. Postoperative liver regeneration and complication in live liver donor after partial hepatectomy for living donor liver transplantation. Yonsei Medical Journal. 2003;**44**(6):1069-1077

[69] Zhang Y, Li B, He Q, Chu Z, Ji Q. Comparison of liver regeneration between donors and recipients after adult right lobe living-donor liver transplantation. Quantitative Imaging in Medicine and Surgery. 2022;**12**(6):3184-3192

[70] Kim M, Suh SW, Lee ES, Suh S, Lee SE, Choi YS. Clinical factors affecting the rate of liver regeneration in living donors after right hepatectomy. Journal of Personalized Medicine. 2024;**14**(5)

[71] Wang WC, Wu TH, Hung HC, Lee JC, Cheng CH, Wang YC, et al. Liver regeneration of living donor after liver donation for transplantation: Disparity in the left and right remnant liver. Medicine (Baltimore). 2024;**103**(14):e37632

[72] Pomfret EA, Pomposelli JJ, Gordon FD, Erbay N, Lyn Price L,

Lewis WD, et al. Liver regeneration and surgical outcome in donors of right-lobe liver grafts. Transplantation. 2003;**76**(1):5-10

[73] Marcos A, Fisher RA, Ham JM, Shiffman ML, Sanyal AJ, Luketic VA, et al. Liver regeneration and function in donor and recipient after right lobe adult to adult living donor liver transplantation. Transplantation. 2000;**69**(7):1375-1379

[74] Parikh ND, Ladner D, Abecassis M, Butt Z. Quality of life for donors after living donor liver transplantation: A review of the literature. Liver Transplantation. 2010;**16**(12):1352-1358

[75] Kroencke S, Nashan B, Fischer L, Erim Y, Schulz KH. Donor quality of life up to two years after living donor liver transplantation: A prospective study. Transplantation. 2014;**97**(5):582-589

[76] Togashi J, Sugawara Y, Tamura S, Yamashiki N, Kaneko J, Aoki T, et al. Donor quality of life after living donor liver transplantation: A prospective study. Journal of Hepato-Biliary-Pancreatic Sciences. 2011;**18**(2):263-267

[77] Ladner DP, Dew MA, Forney S, Gillespie BW, Brown RS Jr, Merion RM, et al. Long-term quality of life after liver donation in the adult to adult living donor liver transplantation cohort study (A2ALL). Journal of Hepatology. 2015;**62**(2):346-353

[78] Kousoulas L, Emmanouilidis N, Klempnauer J, Lehner F. Living-donor liver transplantation: Impact on donor's health-related quality of life. Transplantation Proceedings. 2011;**43**(10):3584-3587

[79] Makki K, Chorasiya VK, Sood G, Srivastava PK, Dargan P, Vij V. Laparoscopy-assisted hepatectomy versus conventional (open) hepatectomy for living donors: When you know better, you do better. Liver Transplantation. 2014;**20**(10):1229-1236

[80] Cho CW, Choi GS, Kim JM, Rhu J, Kwon CHD, Joh JW. Postoperative health status and quality of life after pure laparoscopic donor hepatectomy for living donor liver transplantation. Annals of Transplantation. 2022;**27**:e935611

[81] Chen PD, Wu CY, Hu RH, Ho CM, Lee PH, Lai HS, et al. Robotic liver donor right hepatectomy: A pure, minimally invasive approach. Liver Transplantation. 2016;**22**(11):1509-1518

[82] Suh SW, Lee KW, Lee JM, Choi Y, Yi NJ, Suh KS. Clinical outcomes of and patient satisfaction with different incision methods for donor hepatectomy in living donor liver transplantation. Liver Transplantation. 2015;**21**(1):72-78

[83] Soubrane O, Eguchi S, Uemoto S, Kwon CHD, Wakabayashi G, Han HS, et al. Minimally invasive donor hepatectomy for adult living donor liver transplantation: An international, multi-institutional evaluation of safety. Efficacy and Early Outcomes. Annals of Surgery. 2022;**275**(1):166-174

[84] Yamanouchi K, Takatsuki M, Hidaka M, Soyama A, Miyazaki K, Inokuma T, et al. Changes in quality of life after hepatectomy and living donor liver transplantation. Hepato-Gastroenterology. 2012;**59**(117):1569-1572

[85] LaPointe RD, DeLair S, Feeley T, Florman S, Guarrera J, Kinkhabwala M, et al. Longterm impact of living liver donation: A self-report of the donation experience. Liver Transplantation. 2019;**25**(5):724-733

[86] Hong SK, Choe S, Yi NJ, Shin A, Choe EK, Yoon KC, et al.

Long-term survival of 10,116 Korean live liver donors. Annals of Surgery. 2021;**274**(2):375-382

[87] Muzaale AD, Dagher NN, Montgomery RA, Taranto SE, McBride MA, Segev DL. Estimates of early death, acute liver failure, and long-term mortality among live liver donors. Gastroenterology. 2012;**142**(2):273-280

[88] Dew MA, Butt Z, Liu Q, Simpson MA, Zee J, Ladner DP, et al. Prevalence and predictors of patient-reported long-term mental and physical health after donation in the adult-to-adult living-donor liver transplantation cohort study. Transplantation. 2018;**102**(1):105-118

Chapter 10

Normothermic Regional Perfusion in Liver Transplantation

Tiffany Hsiung, Hetal Lad, Aditya Kasina and Arpit Amin

Abstract

There continues to be a significant mismatch between number of patients awaiting liver transplantation (LT) and number of available liver grafts that are deemed transplantable when they are preserved with static cold storage (SCS). Liver grafts from donors meeting circulatory death (DCD) preserved with SCS are discarded due to high rates of early allograft dysfunction (EAD), ischemic cholangiopathy (IC) and inferior graft survival. Normothermic regional perfusion (NRP) is an emerging in-vivo application of normothermic perfusion technology for DCD organs. NRP allows normothermic oxygenated reconditioning of multiple DCD organs (including liver grafts) and simultaneous in-vivo assessment of liver graft viability. Compared to SCS DCD LT recipients, NRP DCD LT recipients have been found to have lower rates of primary non-function (PNF), early allograft dysfunction (EAD), and ischemic cholangiopathy (IC). NRP has become an established modality for DCD liver graft preservation and evaluation in many European countries over the past decade. Significant progress has been made in increasing application of NRP to increase DCD liver graft utilization in USA over the past 5 years.

Keywords: liver transplantation (LT), donation after circulatory death (DCD), static cold storage (SCS), abdominal normothermic regional perfusion (A-NRP), thoraco-abdominal normothermic regional perfusion (TA-NRP)

1. Introduction

The number of patients waitlisted for potential liver transplantation (LT) continues to far exceed the number of available liver grafts [1]. Historically, static cold storage (SCS) has been the preferred method of liver graft preservation. However, liver grafts from donation after circulatory death criteria (DCD) preserved with SCS have been associated with high rate of early allograft dysfunction (EAD), ischemic cholangiopathy (IC) and inferior liver graft/patient survival [2]. As a result, there is high discard rate of SCS preserved DCD liver grafts [2]. To overcome limitations associated with SCS preservation for DCD liver grafts, there has been interest within the liver transplant community to evaluate application of normothermic regional perfusion (NRP) to increase utilization of DCD liver grafts and improve clinical outcomes of

DCD LT. The focus of this chapter is to describe mechanistic benefits of NRP, technical nuances associated with NRP and clinical evidence supporting application of NRP in DCD LT.

2. Normothermic regional perfusion

NRP utilizes modified extracorporeal membrane oxygenation (ECMO) circuit to perfuse DCD organs with non-pulsatile oxygenated blood at flow rates of 1.5–4 L/min to maintain physiologic temperature and acid-base homeostasis [3, 4]. With respect to DCD liver grafts, NRP allows rapid normothermic oxygenation of hepatocytes and cholangiocytes to attenuate the effects of warm ischemic injury incurred during withdrawal of life support [3, 4]. Secondly, NRP allows in-vivo functional assessment about quality of DCD liver grafts through macroscopic visual inspection, liver biopsy, serial lactate measurements, serial transaminase measurements, bile production, and bile chemistry evaluation [3, 4]. Thirdly, NRP converts the rushed super rapid recovery of DCD liver grafts to a more methodical and controlled recovery like the traditional recovery of liver grafts from donors meeting brain death criteria (DBD) [3, 4].

There are two distinct modalities of NRP, namely thoraco-abdominal NRP (TA-NRP) and abdominal NRP (A-NRP) [5, 6]. TA-NRP involves perfusion of both thoracic and abdominal organs in DCD and thereby facilitates procurement of both thoracic and abdominal organs [5, 6]. In TA-NRP, venous outflow cannula is placed within the right atrium and arterial inflow cannula is placed within the ascending aorta [5, 6]. Aortic arch vessels are ligated/vented to prevent inadvertent perfusion of brain during TA-NRP [5, 6]. TA-NRP requires dedicated cardiothoracic donor surgeon, trained ECMO perfusionist, dedicated abdominal donor surgeon, blood products, and ECMO circuit disposables [5, 6]. Given that cardiac activity is restored in TA-NRP, ethical issues and local hospital/organ procurement organization (OPO) policy may not allow TA-NRP initiation in DCD [5, 6].

A-NRP involves perfusion of abdominal organs only in DCD [6, 7]. There are different cannulation strategies available for A-NRP depending on donor hospital/OPO policy related to premortem versus postmortem cannulation and donor anatomic factors/donor abdominal surgeon expertise. If premortem A-NRP cannulation is allowed, venous sheath is placed within right femoral vein, arterial sheath is placed within right femoral artery and endovascular balloon is advanced to supraceliac aorta via left femoral artery in the intensive care unit [6, 7]. Subsequently, withdrawal of life support is commenced in the operating room and once donor meets circulatory death criteria, supraceliac endovascular balloon is inflated, venous femoral sheath exchanged over a guidewire to venous cannula and arterial femoral sheath exchanged to arterial cannula over a guidewire for A-NRP initiation [6, 7]. Due to regulatory and ethical concerns related to premortem procedural interventions in potential DCD, postmortem cannulation for A-NRP is more common [6, 7]. For postmortem A-NRP, arterial cannula may be placed within infrarenal aorta, right iliac artery, or right femoral artery for inflow [6, 7]. Venous cannula may be placed with the infrarenal inferior vena cava (IVC), right atrium, right iliac vein, or right femoral vein for outflow [6, 7]. Supraceliac aorta is clamped prior to initiation of A-NRP (**Figure 1**). Given that cardiac activity is not restored during A-NRP, it can be more easily implemented across different hospitals/OPO regions [6, 7]. A-NRP still requires a dedicated abdominal donor surgeon trained in NRP nuances, dedicated perfusionist, blood products and ECMO circuit disposables [6, 7].

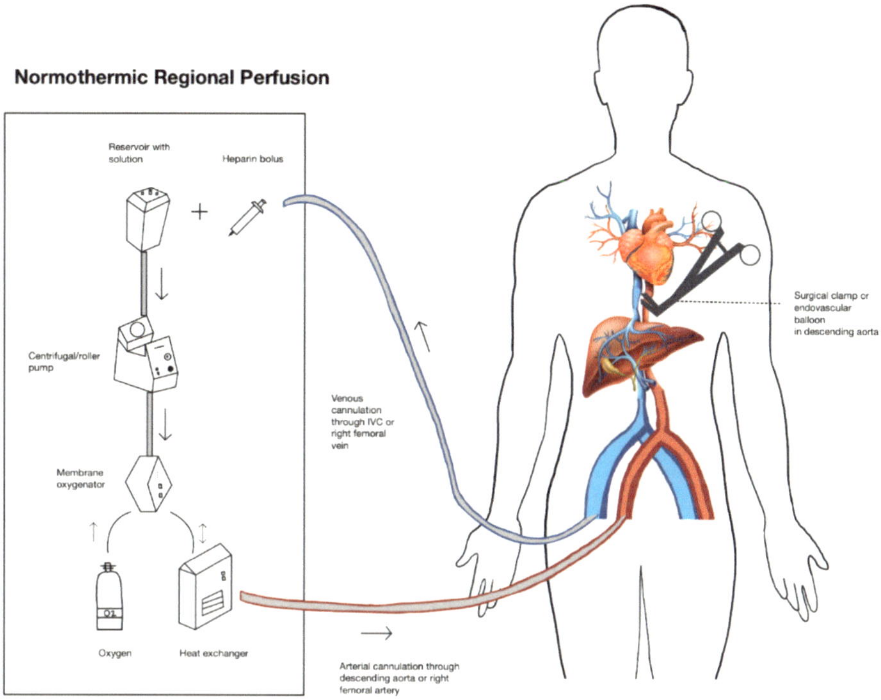

Figure 1.
Abdominal normothermic regional perfusion schematic: *To achieve abdominal normothermic regional perfusion, a venous cannula is placed through the infrarenal inferior vana cava or right femoral vein and arterial cannula is placed through the infrarenal aorta or right femoral artery. Inflow and outflow cannulas are connected to respective inflow and outflow tubing of the extracorporeal membrane oxygenation (ECMO) circuit. ECMO circuit consists of a reservoir, centrifugal pump, and membrane oxygenator that maintains the blood in a normothermic oxygenated state through the use of a heat exchanger and oxygen tank. A surgical clamp or endovascular balloon stops blood flow at the descending aorta to ensure abdominal normothermic regional perfusion.*

While evaluating clinical literature on NRP, it is, also, important to understand DCD Maastricht classification. Maastricht category 1 DCD suffer cardiac arrest outside hospital and are brought to hospital without resuscitation [8, 9]. Maastricht category 2 DCD suffer cardiac arrest outside hospital, undergo resuscitation outside/inside the hospital but resuscitation is not successful [8, 9]. Maastricht category 3 DCD undergo elective withdrawal of life support in the hospital prior to organ retrieval [8, 9]. Maastricht category 4 DCD initially meet DBD criteria but suffer from unexpected cardiac arrest [8, 9]. Masstricht category 1, 2, and 4 DCD are considered uncontrolled DCD (uDCD) while Maastricht category 3 DCD are considered controlled DCD (cDCD) [8, 9]. NRP has been utilized in both uDCD and cDCD to increase liver graft utilization.

Given definitions of "no-touch period" after asystole before declaration of death in DCD varies in different countries resulting in significantly different warm ischemia times in DCD liver procurements and unique national logistical/regulatory challenges associated with implementing NRP infrastructure. For example, "no-touch period" is 5 minutes in Spain, France, United Kingdom (UK) and United States of America (USA) compared to 20 minutes in Italy. Also, liver grafts from both uDCD and cDCD are utilized in Spain while other countries mainly utilize liver grafts from cDCD. We have summarized NRP experiences of various European countries and USA separately to appreciate finer nuances of NRP application in different countries.

3. Normothermic regional perfusion application in different countries

3.1 Normothermic regional perfusion experience (Spanish experience)

3.1.1 Uncontrolled DCD

Fondevilla et al. reported the first experience of A-NRP in uDCD in a cohort of 10 LT recipients in 2007 [8]. The Spanish donation system is founded on the principle of presumed donation consent and this allowed initiation of A-NRP via femoral cannulation in potential uDCD. Subsequently, once permission was obtained for donation from the family, donor livers from uDCD were utilized if witnessed cardiac arrest was less than 15 minutes, continuous CPR time was less than 150 minutes, A-NRP time was less than 4 hours, donor age < 65 years, donor had negative hepatitis viral serologies, transaminases were less than 4 times upper limit of normal during A-NRP, and liver biopsy excluded steatosis or fibrosis [8]. The authors reported PNF rate of 10% and biliary stricture rate of 10%. They demonstrated 1-year LT graft survival of 50% and 1-year LT patient survival of 70% with their A-NRP protocol in uDCD [8]. Fondevilla et al. reported an update on their experience of A-NRP in uDCD in a cohort of 34 LT recipients in 2012 [10]. Interestingly, there were 400 potential uDCD evaluated over the 9-year study period and only 9% were utilized for LT [10]. 8% of LT recipients developed IC. 1-year LT graft survival was 70% and 1-year LT patient survival of 82% [10].

Torres et al. reported single-center outcomes of A-NRP in uDCD in a cohort of 10 LT recipients in 2019 [11]. IC was observed in 10% of LT recipients [11]. Median LT graft survival and recipient survival was 5 years [11].

Jimenez-Ramirez et al. reported the largest series on uDCD LT in 2019 [12]. The study group included 75 uDCD LT recipients and control group included 265 DBD LT recipients [12]. Out of 265 uDCD livers, 75 livers were accepted for LT resulting in 28% liver utilization rate for uDCD [12]. PNF rate was statistically significantly higher in the uDCD LT group (8%) compared to the DBD LT group (2%) [12]. The overall rate of biliary complications was statistically significantly higher in the uDCD LT group (31%) compared to the DBD LT group (12%) [12]. Both the non-anastomotic biliary stricture (NABS) and anastomotic biliary stricture (ABS) rate was statistically significantly higher in uDCD LT group (NABS: 16%; ABS: 7%) compared to DBD LT group (NABS: 3%; ABS; 2%) [12]. 1-year LT graft survival was statistically significantly lower in the uDCD LT group (73%) compared to DBD LT group (87%) [12]. 1-year patient survival was not statistically significantly different between the uDCD LT group (83%) and DBD LT group (89%) [12]. 5-year LT graft survival was statistically significantly lower in the uDCD LT group (64%) compared to the DBD LT group (77%) [12]. 5-year patient survival was not statistically significantly different between the uDCD LT group (72%) compared to the DBD LT group (79%) [12].

In summary, unique regulatory protocols in Spain have allowed application of A-NRP in uDCD resulting in increased donor liver pool. However, A-NRP application in uDCD is still associated with high rate of biliary complications and inferior graft survival.

3.1.2 Controlled DCD

Concurrent to their uDCD A-NRP experience, Spanish centers developed cDCD A-NRP protocol to increase liver donor pool.

Rodriguez-Sanguan et al. reported single-center outcome of A-NRP in 11 cDCD LT recipients in comparison to 51 DBD LT recipients in 2019 [13]. PNF rate was not statistically significantly different between cDCD NRP LT group (9%) and DBD LT group (2%) [13]. There was no statistically significant difference in biliary stricture rate between cDCD NRP LT group (13%) compared to DBD LT group (26%) [13]. Ruiz et al. reported single-center outcome of A-NRP in 46 cDCD LT recipients in 2019 [14]. Median donor age was 59 years [14]. Median recipient MELD score was 12 [14]. EAD rate was noted in 23% of cDCD NRP LT recipients [14]. No cases of ischemic cholangiopathy were noted in cDCD NRP LT recipients [14]. 1-year LT graft survival was 100% [14].

Subsequently, Ruiz et al. reported the largest single-center outcome of A-NRP cDCD LT recipients (n = 100) to SCS DBD LT recipients (n = 200) in 2021 [15]. Of note, pre-mortem femoral cannulation was performed resulting in short median functional warm ischemia time (defined as duration from systolic blood pressure less than 60 mm Hg until NRP initiation) of 10 minutes in A-NRP group [15]. Median donor age was not statistically significantly different between 2 groups (62 years for A-NRP cDCD group and 62 years for SCS DBD group) [15]. Median recipient MELD score was not statistically significantly different between 2 groups (12 in A-NRP cDCD group and 12 in SCS DBD group) [15]. Median cold ischemia time was not statistically significantly different between 2 groups (274 minutes in A-NRP cDCD group and 264 minutes in SCS DBD group) [15]. The EAD rate was not statistically significantly different between A-NRP cDCD group (19%) and SCS DBD LT group (20%) [15]. Biliary complication rate was not statistically significantly different between A-NRP cDCD group (5%) and SCS DBD group (6%) [15]. 1-year LT graft survival was not noted to be statistically significantly different in A-NRP cDCD group (100%) compared to SCS DBD group (96%) [15]. 1-year LT patient survival was not statistically significantly different between A-NRP cDCD group (97%) and SCS DBD group (96%) [15]. Given the excellent results with A-NRP cDCD, authors reported that A-NRP cDCD livers account for 40% of LT performed at their center while having equivalent outcomes of SCS DBD livers [15].

In 2019, Munoz et al. reported single-center outcome of A-NRP cDCD LT recipients (n = 23) to SCS cDCD LT recipients (n = 22) [16]. The EAD rate was statistically significantly lower in the NRP cDCD group (30%) compared to SCS cDCD group (68%) [16]. Biliary complication rate was statistically significantly lower in NRP cDCD group (4%) compared to SCS cDCD group (23%) [16]. In 2022, these authors reported updated outcomes of A-NRP in 39 cDCD LT recipients compared to 78 SCS DBD LT recipients from their center [17]. They reported no statistically significant difference in EAD rate, PNF rate, biliary complications, and 1-yr graft/1-yr patient survival between A-NRP cDCD group and SCS DBD group [17].

In 2019, Hessheimer et al. compared multicenter outcomes of A-NRP cDCD LT recipients (n = 95) to SCS cDCD LT recipients (n = 117) performed in Spain from 2012 to 2017 [18]. 34% of cDCD NRP livers were declined while 38% of SCS cDCD were declined due to organ quality [18]. There was no statistically significant difference in median donor age (NRP: 58 years vs. SCS: 56 years) and median recipient MELD (NRP: 15 vs. SCS: 14) in both groups [18]. Median total warm ischemia time was 18 minutes for premortem NRP cannulation versus 27 minutes for postmortem NRP cannulation [18]. Median NRP duration was 120 minutes [18]. There was no statistically significant difference in EAD rate (NRP: 22% vs. SCS: 27%) and PNF rate (NRP: 2% vs. SCS: 3%) in two groups [18]. The NRP group (2%) had a statistically significantly lower rate of ischemic type biliary complications compared to the SCS group (13%) [18]. Both 1-year graft survival and 3-year graft survival were statistically significantly higher in the NRP group (88% at both 1 year and 3 years) compared to SCS group (83% at 1 year and 78% at 3 years) [18].

Subsequently, Hessheimer et al. reported an update on multicenter outcomes of A-NRP cDCD LT recipients (n = 545) to SCS cDCD LT recipients (n = 258) performed in Spain from 2012 to 2019 [18]. Median donor age was not statistically significantly different between A-NRP cDCD (59 years) and SCS cDCD group (58 years) [18]. Median recipient MELD score was not statistically significantly different between A-NRP cDCD (59 years) and SCS cDCD group (58 years) [18]. Median A-NRP duration was 111 minutes [18]. The EAD rate was statistically significantly lower in A-NRP cDCD group (15%) compared to SCS cDCD group (23%) [18]. Biliary complication rate was statistically significantly lower in A-NRP cDCD group (12%) compared to SCS cDCD group (29%) [18]. Ischemic type biliary complications were noted to be statistically significantly lower in A-NRP cDCD group (1%) compared to SCS cDCD group (29%) [18]. 1-year LT graft survival in A-NRP cDCD group (90%) was statistically significantly better compared to SCS cDCD group (79%) [18]. 3-year LT graft survival in A-NRP cDCD group (87%) was statistically significantly better compared to SCS cDCD group (68%) [18]. Cold ischemia time > 7 hours and utilization of A-NRP cDCD liver grafts in re-transplant cases was associated with increased risk of graft loss [18]. All the Spanish NRP studies have been summarized in **Table 1**.

In conclusion, cumulative Spanish experience with A-NRP cDCD LT recipients has demonstrated significantly lower rates of EAD/IC and significantly improved short and long-term LT graft survival compared to SCS cDCD LT recipients.

3.2 Normothermic regional perfusion in cDCD (Italian experience)

In Italy, there is an obligatory 20 minutes "no-touch period" after asystole following withdrawal of life support in cDCD procurements before donor organs can be procured [20–25]. As a result, cDCD liver grafts in Italy are exposed to longer warm ischemia time compared to other European and North American centers prior to initiation of procurement [20–25]. To reduce EAD and IC rates in cDCD liver grafts with long warm ischemia time (>30 minutes), Italian centers have combined utilization of NRP for in-situ liver graft assessment followed by back-to-base liver graft preservation with hypothermic oxygenated machine perfusion (HOPE), dual hypothermic oxygenated machine perfusion (dHOPE) or normothermic machine perfusion (NMP) [20–25]. Pre-mortem guidewire placement in femoral vessels is allowed in Italy to reduce time for NRP initiation after the obligatory 20 minute "no-touch period" [20–25].

De Carlis et al. published a single Italian center study highlighting outcomes of A-NRP dHOPE DCD LT recipients (uDCD:n = 14 and cDCD: n = 6) compared to matched SCS DBD LT recipients (n = 52) in 2018 [20]. The median warm ischemia time (time from extubation to NRP initiation) was 125 minutes in the DCD group [20]. The median A-NRP duration was approximately 6 hours. A-NRP DCD LT grafts were accepted if following criteria were met; recipient age < 65, witnessed cardiac arrest, WIT <160 minutes, aspartate aminotransferase (AST) < 1000 IU/L, alanine transferase (ALT) < 1000 IU/L, downward trend in serum lactate, good macroscopic liver graft appearance, graft macrosteatosis <30% and graft fibrosis Ishak score < 1 [20]. Median recipient MELD score was similar in both groups (A-NRP dHOPE DCD: 10 vs. SCS DBD: 10) [20]. There was no statistically significant difference in EAD rate (A-NRP dHOPE DCD: 24% vs. SCS DBD: 27%) and PNF rate (A-NRP dHOPE

DOI: http://dx.doi.org/10.5772/intechopen.1010806

Study	N, Donor Type	Type of NRP	Cannulation, Premortem = 0, Postmortem = 1	NRP Times (Median (IQR)), Hours	Total Warm Ischemic Time (Median (IQR)), Hours	EAD Within First Week, N (%)	Nonanastomotic Biliary Stricture Development, N (%)	Anastomotic Biliary Strictures, N (%)	1-Year Graft Survival, N (%)	1 Year Patient Survival, N (%)
Fondevila et al. Spain [8]	10 uDCD (Maastricht type 2)	A-NRP	1	3.1 (2–4)	NA	NA	0 (0)	1 (10)	5 (50)	7 (70)
Fondevila et al. Spain [10]	34 uDCD (Maastricht type 2)	A-NRP	1	6.33 (5.42–7.17)	0.5 (0.6–0.58)	NA	3 (8)	1 (2.9)	24 (70)	28 (82)
Herrero Torres et al. Spain 2019	9 uDCD (Maastricht type 2); 24 cDCD (Maastricht type 3)	A-NRP	0	uDCD: 1.83 ± 1 cDCD: 0.62 ± 0.68	0.62 ± 0.68	NA	NA	cDCD: 2 (8)	NA	NA
Rodriguez-Sanjuan et al. Spain [13]	11 cDCD (Maastricht type 3); 51 DBD	A-NRP	0	1.57 (0.33–2.5)	0.26 (0.12–0.67)	cDCD:1 (1.2) DBD: 1 (9)	cDCD: 2 (13.3) DBD: 16 (29.6)	cDCD: 10 (90)	cDCD: 10 (90)	
Ruiz et al. Spain [14]	46 cDCD (Maastricht type 3)	A-NRP	0	2.11 (1.43–2.68)	0.17 (0.1–0.37)	11 (23)	NA	4 (8.7)	46 (100)	46 (100)
Hessheimer et al. Spain [19]	95 cDCD (Maastricht type 3); 117 SRR cDCD	A-NRP	0, 1	Postmortem: 2 (1.32–2.27)	Premortem: 0.45 (0.37–0.55) Postmortem: 0.3 (0.22–0.37)	cDCD: 21 (22) SRR cDCD: 32 (27)	NA	cDCD: 5 (5.3) SRR cDCD: 16 (13.7) P = 0.0041	cDCD: 84 (88) SRR cDCD: 97 (83.6)	cDCD: 88 (92.6) SRR cDCD: 103 (88.0)

Study	N, Donor Type	Type of NRP	Cannulation, Premortem = 0, Postmortem = 1	NRP Times (Median (IQR)), Hours	Total Warm Ischemic Time (Median (IQR)), Hours	EAD Within First Week, N (%)	Nonanastomotic Biliary Stricture Development, N (%)	Anastomotic Biliary Strictures, N (%)	1-Year Graft Survival, N (%)	1 Year Patient Survival, N (%)
Jimenez Romero et al. Spain [9]	75 uDCD (Maastricht type 2)	A-NRP	0	3.41 (1.97–4.75)	2.17 (1.99–2.53)	6 (8)	12 (16)	5 (6.7)	55 (73.3)	62 (82.7)
Munoz et al. Spain [16]	23 cDCD NRP; 22 SRR DCD	A-NRP	0, 1	Postmortem: 0.9, Premortem: 0.8 hours, P = 0.418	Postmortem: 0.35, Premortem: 0.38, P = 0.418	7 (30)	cDCD NRP: 5 (22.7) SRR DCD: 1 (4.3)	NA	NA	cDCD NRP: 22 (95) SRR DCD: 18 (85)
Ruiz et al. Spain [15]	100 cDCD NRP; 200 DBD	A-NRP	0	2.02 (1.97–2.13)	0.17 (0.14–0.2)	19 (19)	cDCD NRP: 0 (0) DBD: 0 (0)	cDCD NRP: 2 (2) DBD: 6 (3)	cDCD NRP: 99 (99) DBD: 184 (92)	cDCD NRP: 99 (99) DBD: 188 (94)
Fernandez-de la Varga et al. Spain 2022	22 cDCD A-NRP; 29 cDCD SRR; 51 DBD	ANRP	0	1.77 (0.9–4.67)	0.83 ± 0.3	NA	NA	cDCD: 2 (3.9) DBD: 0 (0)	cDCD: 41 (80.4) DBD: 45 (88.2)	cDCD: 41 (80.4) DBD: 45 (88.2)
Rodriguez et al. Spain [17]	39 cDCD NRP; 78 DBD	A-NRP	0	1.5–2	0.32 (0.17–0.63)	13 (34)	NA	cDCD NRP: 0 (0) DBD: 1 (1.2)	NA	cDCD NRP: 37 (94) DBD: 66 (84)

Study	N, Donor Type	Type of NRP	Cannulation, Premortem = 0, Postmortem = 1	NRP Times (Median (IQR)), Hours	Total Warm Ischemic Time (Median (IQR)), Hours	EAD Within First Week, N (%)	Nonanastomotic Biliary Stricture Development, N (%)	Anastomotic Biliary Strictures, N (%)	1-Year Graft Survival, N (%)	1 Year Patient Survival, N (%)
Heissheimer et al. Spain 2022	545 cDCD A-NRP; 258 cDCD SRR	A-NRP	0	1.85 (1.35–2.1)	0.3 (0.22–0.38)	A-NRP: 81 (15) SRR: 6- (23)	cDCD A-NRP: 63 (12) cDCD SRR: 75 (29)		cDCD A-NRP: 468 (86) cDCD SRR: 170 (66)	cDCD A-NRP: 480 (88) cDCD SRR: 192 (74)
Feo et al. Spain 2022	82 cDCD NRP	A-NRP	0	NA	NA	NA	NA	NA	NA	76 (93)

Abbreviations: abdominal normothermic regional perfusion, A-NRP; controlled donation after circulatory death, cDCD;donation after circulatory death, DCD; interquartile range, IQR; not available, NA; super-rapid recovery, SRR; uncontrolled donation after circulatory death uDCD.

Table 1.
Spanish normothermic regional perfusion studies.

DCD: 10% vs. SCS DBD: 4%) between two groups [20]. IC rate was not statistically significantly different between A-NRP dHOPE DCD LT recipients (10%) compared to SCS DBD LT recipients (4%) [20]. 1-year LT graft survival was equivalent between A-NRP dHOPE DCD LT group (85%) and SCS DBD LT group (91%) [20]. Authors, also, noted that A-NRP dHOPE DCD LT recipients, who developed EAD had a significantly longer median cold ischemia time (9 hours) compared to NRP-dHOPE DCD LT recipients, who did not develop EAD (6.5 hours) [20]. EAD rate in A-NRP dHOPE DCD LT recipients, whose grafts demonstrated lactate drop >1.11 mmol/L, was 20% compared to 80% in ANRP dHOPE DCD LT recipients, whose grafts did not demonstrate lactate drop >1.11 mmol/L during A-NRP [20].

Oliveri et al. reported a single-center Italian case series of A-NRP dHOPE DCD LT recipients (uDCD: n = 1; cDCD = 9) in 2019 [25]. Median functional donor warm ischemia time (defined as time from systolic blood pressure < 50 mm Hg to NRP initiation) was 38 minutes [25]. Median NRP duration was 3.5 hours [25]. Median end-ischemic dHOPE duration was about 2 hours [25]. All LT recipients in the series had a MELD score between 6 and 14 [25]. DCD Liver grafts were accepted for subsequent LT if they had satisfactory uniformly perfusion macroscopic appearance on donor surgeon evaluation, demonstrated lactate clearance during NRP, had <30% macrosteatosis/no fibrosis on liver biopsy, and AST/ALT <2000 IU/L during NRP [25]. Authors reported no cases of PNF. They reported 2 cases of anastomotic biliary stricture and 2 cases of biliary leak in their cohort [25].

Ghinolfi et al. reported a dual center Italian retrospective evaluating outcomes of A-NRP dHOPE DCD LT recipients (n = 11) compared to A-NRP NMP DCD LT recipients (n = 7) in 2020 [21]. Of note, this study included 11 uDCD and 7 cDCD liver grafts [21]. Of note, DCD liver grafts were accepted for LT if they met following criteria: recipient age < 70 years, witnessed cardiac arrest, A-NRP flow rate > 2 L/min, acceptable macroscopic appearance on donor surgeon evaluation, liver biopsy showing <30% macrosteatosis/Ishak <1 fibrosis stage, total warm ischemia time (defined as time from extubation to NRP initation) less than 170 minutes, functional warm ischemia time (defined as time from systolic blood less than 50 mm Hg till NRP initiation) less than 120 minutes, ALT <1000 IU/L during A-NRP, and downward lactate trend during A-NRP [21]. Due to stringent acceptance criteria, only 56% of potential DCD liver grafts were utilized for LT [21]. There was no statistically significant difference in A-NRP duration between the two groups (A-NRP dHOPE: 6 hours vs. A-NRP NMP: 5 hours) [21]. Median total warm ischemia time was not statistically different between A-NRP dHOPE group (142 minutes) versus A-NRP NMP group (158 minutes) [21]. There was no statistically significant difference in ex-situ machine perfusion duration between two groups (A-NRP dHOPE: 5.5 hours versus A-NRP NMP: 6.2 hours) [21]. There was no PNF in either group [21]. EAD rate was not statistically significantly different between two groups (A-NRP dHOPE: 18% vs. A-NRP NMP 43%) [21]. There was no statistically significant difference in biliary complication rate in two groups (A-NRP dHOPE: 0% vs. A-NRP NMP: 14%) [21]. 6-month graft survival was not statistically significantly different between two groups (A-NRP dHOPE: 100% vs. A-NRP NMP: 86%) [21]. Authors attributed adherence to strict A-NRP criteria and liver graft protection offered by ex-situ preservation techniques (dHOPE/NMP) as critical for their excellent outcomes in DCD liver grafts with long warm ischemia times [21].

De Carlis et al. published a multicenter Italian study in 2021 comparing the outcomes of A-NRP dHOPE cDCD LT recipients (n = 37) with SCS cDCD LT recipients (n = 37) matched by donor age, donor body mass index, cold ischemia time, and recipient age [22]. Liver grafts on A-NRP were accepted if they met following criteria: recipient age ≤ 75 years, donor functional warm ischemia time (defined as time from systolic blood pressure < 50 mm Hg to NRP initiation) < 60 minutes, ALT <1000 IU/L at end of NRP, downward lactate trend during NRP, optimal macroscopic appearance (uniform perfusion; no congestion), liver biopsy with macrosteatosis <30%, and liver fibrosis Ishak score 0/1 [22]. Median functional warm ischemia time was statistically significantly longer in NRP-dHOPE cDCD LT group (40 minutes) compared to SCS cDCD LT group (18 minutes) [22]. PNF rate was not statistically significantly different between two groups (NRP-dHOPE cDCD LT group: 3% vs. SCS cDCD LT group: 3%) [22]. There was no statistically significant difference in IC rate between two groups (NRP-dHOPE LT group: 3% vs. SCS DCD LT group: 8%) [22]. Their findings suggest that A-NRP can be utilized for liver graft conditioning and functional assessment of liver grafts with prolonged warm ischemia times resulting in increased utilization and comparable outcomes to SCS DCD liver grafts with significantly shorter warm ischemia time [22].

Patrono et al. published a single center study in 2022 evaluating outcomes of A-NRP dHOPE cDCD LT recipients (n = 20) with SCS DBD LT recipients (n = 20) matched on recipient age, recipient body mass index, recipient MELD score, donor age, liver graft macrovesicular steatosis, and portal reperfusion time [23]. The median donor functional warm ischemia time was 43 minutes in A-NRP dHOPE cDCD group [23]. The median A-NRP time was 246 minutes and median end-ischemia dHOPE time was 205 minutes in the A-NRP dHOPE cDCD group [23]. EAD rate was not statistically significantly different between A-NRP dHOPE cDCD group (5%) and SCS DBD group (15%) [23]. There was no statistically significant difference in the IC rate between A-NRP dHOPE cDCD group (5%) and SCS DBD group (2%) [23]. There was no statistically significant difference in 1-year graft survival between A-NRP dHOPE cDCD group (90%) and SCS DBD group (95%) [23]. Their findings are remarkable in that combination of A-NRP and dHOPE appears to confer protective effects on cDCD liver grafts with long functional warm ischemia time resulting in equivalent outcomes of SCS DBD liver grafts [23].

Camagmi et al. published a single center Italian study in 2023 reporting their outcomes of A-NRP cDCD LT recipients (n = 24) [24]. Femoral cannulation was performed along with placement of endovascular aortic balloon to establish A-NRP [24]. Their A-NRP involved additional placement of ipsilateral limb perfusion cannula or ligation of ipsilateral common iliac vein to prevent leakage of anoxic blood from non-perfused extremity [24]. Median donor age was 59 years and median functional warm ischemia time was 43 minutes [24]. Median A-NRP time was 4 hours [24]. Liver graft was accepted for LT as long as there was steady decrease in lactate on A-NRP (accepted liver grafts demonstrated median lactate clearance of 60% from start of A-NRP to end of A-NRP) [24]. Median cold ischemia time was 5 hours [24]. Median recipient MELD was 16 [24]. No PNF was observed [24]. EAD rate was reported to be 8% [24]. Authors reported no cases of IC in their cohort [24]. 1-year graft survival was noted to be 87% and 1-year patient survival was 92% [24]. Based on their experience, the authors advocated that A-NRP allowed reconditioning of liver graft from hypoxic injury during life support withdrawal and subsequent liver graft viability assessment during DCD procurement. Authors reported that A-NRP alone may be sufficient for DCD liver graft preservation even in cases with prolonged functional warm ischemia time as long as liver graft demonstrates adequate viability during A-NRP and logistics allow short duration of cold ischemia time [24].

All of the Italian NRP studies have been summarized in **Table 2**. Italian experience with A-NRP in cDCD liver grafts with prolonged warm ischemia times (>30 minutes)

Study	N, Donor Type	Type of NRP	Cannulation, Premortem = 0, Postmortem = 1	NRP Times (Median (IQR)), Hours	Total Warm Ischemic Time (Median (IQR)), Hours	EAD Within First Week, N (%)	Nonanastomotic Biliary Stricture Development, N (%)	Anastomotic Biliary Strictures, N (%)	1-Year Graft Survival, N (%)	1 Year Patient Survival, N (%)
De Carlis et al. Italy [20]	14 uDCD (Maastricht type 2); 6 cDCD (Maastricht type 3)	A-NRP + HMP	1	5.87	2.08	DCD: 4 (24) DBD: 13 (27) P > 0.99	DCD: 4 (20)* DBD: 7 (13) P = 0.65		85	95
Oliveri et al. Italy [25]	10 cDCD	A-NRP + HMP	1	4.21 (0.83–10.4)	0.6	0 (0)	1 (10)	1 (10)	100	100
Ghinolfi et al. Italy [21]	18 cDCD NRP	A-NRP + HMP or NMP	1	5.88 (5–6.27) p = 0.096	2.51 (2.33–2.73), p = 0.920	5 (28)	1 (5.6)*		17 (94)	17 (94)
De Carlis et al. Italy [22]	44 cDCD ANRP; 19 uDCD	A-NRP	1	4.17 (0.88–7.72)	0.67 (0.33–1.33)	cDCD ANRP: 1 (3)	cDCD ANRP: 1(2)	cDCD ANRP: 5(12)	cDCD ANRP: 40 (91)	cDCD ANRP: 43 (97.7)
Patrono et al. Italy [23]	20 cDCD A-NRP + HOPE; 555 DBD	A-NRP + HOPE	1	4.1 (3.68–4.48)	0.72 (0.67, 0.8)	cDCD A-NRP: 1 (5) DBD: 6 (15)	cDCD A-NRP + HOPE: 2 (10) DBD: 75 (14)	cDCD A-NRP + HOPE: 3 (15) DBD: 85 (15)	cDCD A-NRP + HOPE: 13 (65) DBD: 476 (85.8)	cDCD A-NRP + HOPE: 15 (75) DBD: 490 (88.3)
Camagni et al. Italy [24]	24 cDCD	A-NRP	0	242 (223–265)	0.85 (0.77–0.92)	4 (16.7)	0 (0)	6 (25)	85.7	90.5

**Overall Biliary Complications.*
Abbreviations: abdominal normothermic regional perfusion, A-NRP; controlled donation after circulatory death, cDCD;donation after circulatory death, DCD; hypothermic oxygenated machine perfusion, HOPE; interquartile range, IQR; not available, NA; super-rapid recovery, SRR; uncontrolled donation after circulatory death uDCD.

Table 2.
Italian normothermic regional perfusion studies.

has been mainly performed in context of complementary ex vivo machine perfusion (HOPE/dHOPE/NMP). Excellent results have been demonstrated in terms of low EAD rates/IC rates and acceptable 1-year LT graft survival in Italian cDCD LT recipients with prolonged warm ischemia times when A-NRP has been utilized with complementary ex vivo machine perfusion. Additional studies are required to determine if A-NRP alone or A-NRP in combination with ex-vivo machine perfusion (HOPE/dHOPE/NMP) is required for cDCD liver grafts with prolonged warm ischemia time (>30 minutes), especially if cold ischemia times are subsequently kept short (<6 hours).

3.3 Normothermic regional perfusion (French experience)

LT using A-NRP in uDCD was initiated in France in 2005 [26]. Savier et al. published a multicenter French retrospective study in 2015 reporting outcomes of a series of 13 LT recipients, who received uDCD liver grafts [26]. Of note, a total of 299 uDCD donors were evaluated and subsequently 13 liver grafts were utilized from uDCD donors resulting in a 4% utilization rate [26]. Authors reported PNF in 3 out of 13 cases (23%) and EAD in 4 out of 13 cases (31%) [26]. IC rate was 20% [26]. 1-year LT graft survival was 69% [26]. French experience with low uDCD liver graft utilization despite A-NRP application mirrors the Spanish experience and reflects the logistical challenges of coordinating donor family consent and availability of A-NRP infrastructure for uDCD donors.

A- NRP in cDCD liver donors was introduced in France in 2015. Premortem femoral venous and arterial lines are allowed in France to facilitate expeditious A-NRP initiation once donor has been pronounced dead [27]. Savier et al. published a multicenter French experience in 2020 evaluating outcomes of A-NRP cDCD LT recipients (n = 50) compared to DBD LT recipients (n = 100) matched based on donor age, recipient age, and LT indication [27]. French A-NRP cDCD liver graft acceptance protocol mandated functional warm ischemic time less than 30 minutes, donor age < 66 years, transaminases <200 IU/L during A-NRP, liver biopsy with less than 20% macrosteatosis, and A-NRP duration of 1 to 4 hours [27]. Median functional warm ischemia time was 22 minutes [27]. Median cold ischemia time was 6 hours [27]. EAD rate was not statistically significantly different between NRP cDCD LT recipients (18%) and DBD LT recipients (32%) [27]. Biliary complication rate was not statistically significantly different between two groups (NRP cDCD: 16% vs. DBD: 17%) [27]. There was no statistically significant difference in 2-year LT graft survival between two groups (NRP cDCD: 91% vs. DBD: 88%) [27]. 2-year patient survival was not statistically significant between NRP cDCD LT group (98%) and DBD group (91%) [27]. Their findings demonstrate that A-NRP cDCD LT recipients with short cold ischemia times (<6 hours) can have equivalent outcomes to SCS DBD LT recipients due to cDCD liver graft repair during A-NRP and functional cDCD liver graft viability assessment during A-NRP [27].

Babier et al. published a multicenter French experience in 2022 evaluating outcomes of A-NRP cDCD LT recipients (n = 156) with a focus on A-NRP duration and outcomes [3]. Donor liver acceptance criteria included donor age < 65 years, donor agonal phase <180 minutes, functional warm ischemia time < 30 minutes, transaminases <200 iU/L at two different points on NRP, and liver biopsy with <20% steatosis/fibrosis grade < 1 [3]. All liver grafts were preserved with SCS after NRP. Recipient characteristics included recipient age < 65 years, first LT, no portal vein thrombosis, no prior supramesocolic surgery, and cold ischemia time < 8 hours [3]. PNF rate was

2%, EAD rate was 19%, and IC rate was 4% [3]. Mean A-NRP duration was 180 minutes [3]. Authors reported that there was no correlation between A-NRP duration and liver graft outcomes (EAD rate, IC rate, graft survival) [3]. Their findings highlight that optimal duration of A-NRP for cDCD liver graft preservation is likely between 1 to 4 hours [3]. A-NRP duration can be flexible depending on factors like possibility of thoracic organ procurement and recipient operating room logistics [3]. All of the French NRP studies have been summarized in **Table 3**.

3.4 Normothermic regional perfusion [UK experience]

Oniscu et al. first reported a multicenter UK experience in 2014 evaluating outcomes of A-NRP cDCD LT recipient (n = 11) [28]. A-NRP was established postmortem via infrarenal aortic and infrarenal vena caval cannulation [28]. A-NRP was maintained for 2 hours [28]. Donor liver acceptance criteria were based on maintaining functional warm ischemia time (defined as time from systolic blood pressure < 50 mm Hg to A-NRP initiation) < 30 minutes, transaminases <4 times upper limit of normal at end of A-NRP, macroscopic appearance of liver/small bowel/gallbladder/bile duct during A-NRP, pump flow of 1.7-4 L/min, and no steatosis/fibrosis in donor liver graft [28]. Median functional warm ischemia time was 26 minutes [28]. PNF rate was 9% [28]. EAD rate was 27% [28]. None of the patients developed IC [28].

Watson et al. reported updated UK multicenter outcomes of NRP cDCD LT recipients (n = 43) compared to SCS cDCD LT recipients (n = 187) in 2019 [29]. Of note, UK DCD risk index score was similar between the two groups (1.9 in both groups) [29]. Amongst NRP cohort, A-NRP was used in 33 cases and TA-NRP was used in 10 cases [29]. Median NRP duration was 2 hours [29]. Median cold ischemia time was statistically significantly shorter in NRP cDCD LT group (6 hours 22 minutes) compared to SCS cDCD LT group (7 hours 24 minutes) [29]. No cases of PNF were reported in NRP group [29]. EAD rate was statistically significantly lower in NRP cDCD LT group (12%) compared to SCS cDCD LT group (32%) [29]. Biliary anastomotic stricture rate was statistically significantly lower in NRP cDCD LT group (7%) compared to SCS cDCD LT group (27%) [29]. IC rate was statistically significantly lower in NRP cDCD LT group (0%) compared to SCS cDCD LT group (27%) [29]. 3-month death censored graft survival was not statistically different between NRP cDCD LT group (98%) compared to SCS DCD LT group (90%) [29]. Authors reported that non-NRP cDCD liver grafts, lower recipient sodium at time of LT, older donor age, and donor location outside the local recipient hospital were independent factors associated with development of IC [29]. Their study demonstrated that both A-NRP and TA-NRP can be utilized depending on local expertise to condition cDCD liver grafts after warm ischemic injury resulting in minimal IC and low EAD rates in NRP cDCD LT recipients compared to SCS cDCD LT recipients [29].

Watson and colleagues subsequently reported their single-center experience comparing outcomes of SCS DCD LT recipients (n = 97), NRP DCD LT recipients (n = 69), and NMP DCD LT recipients (n = 67) in 2022 [32]. UK donor risk index was score was similar between the three groups (SCS: 1.9, NRP 2, NMP 1.9) [32]. Median functional warm ischemia time was statistically significantly longer in NRP group (19 minutes) compared to SCS group (15 minutes) and NMP group (15 minutes) [32]. The median cold ischemia time was statistically significantly longer in SCS group (7 hours 10 minutes) compared to NRP group (6 hours 39 minutes) and NMP group (6 hours 36 minutes) [32]. There was no statistically significant difference in EAD

Study	N, Donor Type	Type of NRP	Cannulation, Premortem = 0, Postmortem = 1	NRP Times (Median (IQR)), Hours	Total Warm Ischemic Time (Median (IQR)), Hours	EAD Within First Week, N (%)	Nonanastomotic Biliary Stricture Development, N (%)	Anastomotic Biliary Strictures, N (%)	1-Year Graft Survival, N (%)	1 Year Patient Survival, N (%)
Oniscu et al. UK [28]	11 cDCD (Maastricht type 3)	A-NRP	0	2 (0.57–2.6)	0.53 (0.38–1.18)	4 (36)	NA	1 (9)	NA	9 (81.8)
Savier et al. France [26]	13 uDCD (Maastricht type 2)	A-NRP	1	4	0.82 (0.75–0.88)	4 (30.8)	1 (7.7)	1 (7.7)	9 (69)	11 (85)
Hagness et al. Norway 2019	8 cDCD	A-NRP	1	1.57 (1.22–3.68)	0.48 (0.27–1.6)	0	0 (0)	1 (12.5)	8 (100)	8 (100)
Watson et al. UK [29]	43 cDCD NRP (Maastricht type 3); 187 SRR cDCD	A-NRP or TA-NRP	1	2.05 (1.72–2.17)	0.5 (0.43–0.6)	cDCD NRP: 5 (12) SRR cDCD: 55 (32)	NA	cDCD NRP: 3 (7) SRR cDCD: 46 (27)	cDCD NRP: 39 (90.1) SRR cDCD: 153 (81.8)	cDCD NRP: 39 (90.1) SRR cDCD: 153 (81.8)
Antoine et al. 2020 France	123 cDCD (Maastricht type 3)	A-NRP	1	3.1 (2.68–3.45)	0.37 (0.3–0.43)****	5 (4)	NA	NA	100 (81.3)	109 (88.6)
Muller et al. Europe [30]	132 cDCD NRP; 93 cDCD HOPE	A-NRP vs. HOPE	1	3.07 (2.65–3.45)	0.52 (0.44–0.6), p < 0.001	cDCD NRP: 26 (20) cDCD HOPE: 63 (68)	cDCD NRP: 6 (4.5) cDCD HOPE: 8 (8.6)	cDCD NRP: 14 (10.6) cDCD HOPE: 24 (25.8)	cDCD NRP: 114 (86.4) cDCD HOPE: 69 (74.2)	cDCD NRP: 114 (86.4) cDCD HOPE: 87 (93)
Savier et al. France [27]	50 cDCD; 100 DBD	A-NRP	1	3.17 (2.52–3.72)		cDCD: 9 (18) DBD: 32 (32)	cDCD: 8 (16)** DBD: 17 (17)		cDCD: 44 (88)****** DBD: 85 (85)	cDCD: 48 (96)****** DBD: 96 (96)
Maroni et al. Europe [31]	19 cDCD A-NRP + D-HOPE; 16 cDCD A-NRP only	A-NRP + HOPE vs. A-NRP	1	3.79 ± 1.14 vs. 3.32 ± 0.79 (p = 0.185)	0.94 ± 0.34 vs. 0.65 ± 0.36 (p = 0.021)	cDCD A-NRP + D-HOPE: 4 (21) cDCD A-NRP only: 4 (25)	cDCD A-NRP + D-HOPE: 0 (0) cDCD A-NRP: 2 (12.5)	cDCD A-NRP + D-HOPE: 0 (0) cDCD A-NRP: NA	NA	NA
Babier et al. France [3]	156 cDCD A-NRP	A-NRP	1	2.98 (±0.72)	0.37 (±0.08)	30 (19)	6 (3.9)	20 (12.8)	150 (96)	150 (96)

Study	N, Donor Type	Type of NRP	Cannulation, Premortem = 0, Postmortem = 1	NRP Times (Median (IQR)), Hours	Total Warm Ischemic Time (Median (IQR)), Hours	EAD Within First Week, N (%)	Nonanastomotic Biliary Stricture Development, N (%)	Anastomotic Biliary Strictures, N (%)	1-Year Graft Survival, N (%)	1 Year Patient Survival, N (%)
Gaurav et al. UK [32]	69 cDCD NRP; 67 cDCD NMP; 97 cDCD SCS	A-NRP	1	2.22 (2.02–2.38)	0.48 (0.38–0.55)	cDCD NRP: 10 (14) cDCD NMP:7 (11) cDCD SCS: 19 (21)	cDCD NRP: 4 (6) cDCD NMP:12 (19) cDCD SCS: 22 (25)	cDCD NRP: 5 (8) cDCD NMP:13 (21) cDCD SCS: 15 (17)	cDCD NRP: 57 (82.6) cDCD NMP:50 (74.6) cDCD SCS: 81 (83.5)	cDCD NRP: 58 (84.1) cDCD NMP:54 (80.6) cDCD SCS: 91 (93.8)
Schurink et al. Netherlands [33]	20 cDCD	A-RNP	1	2 (1.83–2.13)	0.48 (0.43–0.55)	5 (25)	11 (55)	NA	18 (90)	19 (95)
Mohkam et al. Europe [34]	68 cDCD NRP; 34 cDCD NMP	A-NRP vs. NMP	1	NA	0.37 (0.32–0.43)	cDCD NRP: 14 (21) cDCD NMP: 30 (8.8)	cDCD NRP: 1 (1.5) cDCD NMP: 1 (2.9)	cDCD NRP: 6 (8.8) cDCD NMP: 6 (17.6)	cDCD NRP: 64 (93.9) cDCD NMP: 30 (88.2) P = 0.516	cDCD NRP: 65 (94.1) cDCD NMP: 30 (88.2) P = 0.523

*Total Ischemia Time.
**Overall Biliary Complications.
***Overall Biliary Strictures.
****Functional Warm Ischemia Time.
*****Overall Survival.
******2-Year Survival.
Abbreviations: abdominal normothermic regional perfusion, A-NRP; controlled donation after circulatory death, cDCD;donation after circulatory death, DCD; hypothermic oxygenated machine perfusion, HOPE; interquartile range, IQR; not available, NA; normothermic regional perfusion, NRP; super-rapid recovery, SRR; thoracoabdominal normothermic regional perfusion, TA-NRP; uncontrolled donation after circulatory death uDCD.

Table 3.
Rest of European normothermic regional perfusion studies (France, UK, Netherlands, pan European).

rate and PNF rate in three groups [32]. NRP DCD LT recipients (6%) had a statistically significantly lower IC rate compared to SCS DCD LT recipients (25%) and NMP DCD LT recipients (19%) [32]. 6-month death censored graft survival was similar between SCS DCD LT group (91%), NRP DCD LT group (97%) and NMP DCD LT group (92%) [32]. Their findings are highly impactful and suggest that outcomes of NRP DCD LT recipients in terms of IC development are significantly better compared to NMP DCD LT recipients or SCS DCD LT recipients as long as cold ischemia time is kept short (<7 hours) [32]. Given significant cost associated with NMP circuits and equivalent outcomes in cDCD liver grafts with short functional warm ischemia times (<30 minutes), NRP may be a more cost-effective strategy when anticipated subsequent cold ischemia times are short (<7 hours). All of the UK NRP cohort studies have been summarized in **Table 3**.

3.5 Normothermic regional perfusion (Dutch experience)

Schurink et al. described the Dutch experience with salvaging DCD liver grafts, which were declined by all centers in Euro transplant region, using A-NRP in 2022 [33]. Livers with functional warm ischemia time (mean arterial pressure < 50 mm Hg) up to 60 minutes were considered for A-NRP [33]. Liver was considered suitable for LT after at least 1 hr. of A-NRP if transaminases were < 200 U/L, peak glucose >10 mmol/L, decreasing lactate trend (with last lactate <5 mmol/L), quality bile production (bile pH > 7.45 and bile glucose <3 mmol/L), and absence of fibrosis/cirrhosis on liver biopsy [33]. Out of 45 offered donor livers, eventually 25 livers were successfully evaluated with A-NRP while 20 livers could not be evaluated with A-NRP due to failure of donor to expire within 120 minutes of life support withdrawal (n = 15), finding of malignancy in donor (n = 1), pre-mature donor cardiac arrest before A-NRP team was available (n = 1), and technical failure to establish A-NRP (n = 3) [33]. Amongst the 25 livers evaluated on A-NRP, 20 liver grafts (80%) were eventually transplanted [33]. Authors reported that the declined liver grafts had statistically significantly higher transaminase levels during A-NRP [Median ALT 367 (range, 318–488) and median AST 363 (range, 349–486)] compared to accepted liver grafts [Median ALT 53 (range, 34–68) and median AST 71 (41–137)] [33]. Median functional warm ischemia time was 29 minutes [33]. Median cold ischemia time was about 6 hours in A-NRP LT recipients [33]. The median MELD of A-NRP LT recipients was 11 [33]. When compared to contemporary DCD LT recipients (n = 49, of which 19 received end-ischemic dHOPE while remaining 30 were SCS preserved), A-NRP DCD LT recipients (n = 20, of which 5 received end-ischemic dHOPE while remaining 15 were SCS preserved), there was no statistically significant difference in EAD rate between two groups (45% vs. 25%) [33]. When dHOPE LT recipients were excluded from both groups, authors found that IC rate was statistically significantly lower in A-NRP group (7%) compared to SCS group (26%) [33]. There was no statistically significant difference in 1-year graft survival between A-NRP DCD LT recipients (90%) and SCS DCD LT recipients (82%) [33]. Authors recommended that liver grafts meeting hepatocellular functional viability criteria (decreasing lactate trend without any discrete absolute cutoff, glucose production>10 mmol/L or > 180 mg/dL, bile production), low level liver ischemic injury (terminal transaminase cutoff <200 IU/L during A-NRP) and cholangiocyte functional viability criteria [bile pH > 7.45, bile glucose <3 mmol/L, delta bile to serum bicarbonate [bile bicarbonate – serum bicarbonate] > 5 mmol/L or > 90 mg/dL, and delta bile pH (bile pH – serum pH > 0.1)) should be considered for eventual LT [33]. While additional prospective studies are required to confirm their assessment criteria, this study was the first to include cholangiocyte functional viability criteria during A-NRP in addition to traditional hepatocellular viability/ischemic injury assessment markers [33].

3.6 Normothermic regional perfusion (pan-European experience)

Muller et al. compared outcomes of A-NRP DCD LT recipients (n = 132) in France to HOPE DCD LT recipients (n = 93) in Switzerland in 2020 [30]. LT graft utilization was statistically significantly lower in A-NRP group (63%) compared to HOPE DCD group (81%) [30]. The functional warm ischemia time was statistically significantly lower in A-NRP group (22 minutes) compared to HOPE group (31 minutes) [30]. Median donor risk index was statistically significantly lower in A-NRP group (2) compared to HOPE group (2.5) [30]. Recipient median MELD score was not statistically significantly different between two groups (A-NRP: 12 vs. HOPE: 12) [30]. Median cold ischemia time was not statistically significantly different between A-NRP group (5.7 hours) and HOPE group (6.4 hours) [30]/EAD rate was statistically significantly lower in A-NRP group (20%) compared to HOPE group (62%) [30]. IC rate was not statistically significantly lower in A-NRP group (5%) compared to HOPE group (9%) [30]. 1-year graft survival was not statistically significantly different in A-NRP group (93%) compared to HOPE group (86%) [30]. Findings of this study suggest that both A-NRP and HOPE appear to provide DCD LT graft protection resulting in excellent outcomes and may be utilized depending on logistical factors at individual transplant center.

Maroni et al. compared outcomes of A-NRP HOPE DCD LT recipients in Italy (n = 19) to A-NRP SCS DCD LT recipient in France (n = 17) in 2022 [31]. Both groups were well-matched based on donor age, recipient age, and MELD score (median MELD score < 15). Functional warm ischemia time (defined as systolic blood pressure < 50 mm Hg till A-NRP initiation) was statistically significantly higher in in NRP-HOPE DCD LT recipients (42 minutes) compared to NRP SCS DCD LT recipients (26 minutes) [31]. Median cold ischemia time was not statistically significantly different between NRP-HOPE DCT LT recipients (8 hours) compared to NPR SCS DCD LT recipients (6.5 hours) [31]. PNF rate (NRP-HOPE: 5% vs. NRP-SCS: 6%, EAD rate (NRP-HOPE: 21% vs. NRP-SCS: 25%) and IC rate (NRP-HOPE: 0% vs. NRP-SCS: 12%) was not statistically significantly different between two groups [31]. Findings of this international study mirror findings of Italian studies that combination of NRP-HOPE may provide complimentary protection to DCD LT graft exposed to extended functional warm ischemia times (>30 minutes) [31].

Mokham et al. compared outcomes of propensity matched A-NRP DCD LT recipients (n = 68) to NMP DCD LT recipients (n = 34) using A-NRP data from six French centers and NMP data from six European centers (UK, Spain, Germany, Belgium) in 2022 [34]. The groups were well-matched in terms of donor functional warm ischemia time (A-NRP: 21 minutes versus NMP: 20 minutes), UK DCD risk score [A-NRP: 5 points (high-risk) vs. NMP: 5 points (high-risk)], and recipient MELD score [NRP: 12 vs. NMP: 12, 34]. Median cold ischemia time was 346 minutes in A-NRP group. There was no statistically significant difference in EAD rate between NRP group (21%) and NMP group (9%) [34]. There was no statistically significant difference in clinically relevant IC rate between NRP group (2%) and NMP group (3%) [34]. 1-year LT graft survival was not statistically significantly different between the two groups (NRP: 94% vs. NMP: 88%) [34]. Findings of this study suggest that both NRP and NMP provide equivalent results in DCD LT recipients and utilization of NRP or

NMP can be dictated based on logistical and financial factors at local center. All of the pan-European studies have been summarized in **Table 3**.

3.7 Normothermic regional perfusion (north American experience)

3.7.1 Abdominal normothermic regional perfusion (A-NRP)

Magliocca et al. first described the application of A-NRP at University of Michigan in United States of America (USA) via premortem cannulation in potential DCD donors in 2005 [35]. They initially reported outcomes with NRP DCD kidneys in 24 kidney transplant recipients with low delayed graft function rates of 8% [35]. Subsequently, Rojas Pena et al. from the same center reported an update in 2015 about outcomes of A-NRP DCD LT recipients (n = 13) [36]. PNF was noted in 1 LT recipient and IC cholangiopathy was observed in 1 LT recipient [36]. 1-year LT graft survival was noted to be 86% [36].

Subsequently, Croome et al. first reported the application of a portable A-NRP circuit for cDCD liver procurement in USA in 2023 [7]. Their protocol involved postmortem arterial cannulation of infrarenal aorta, venous cannulation of infrarenal vena cava and placement of occluding balloon in supraceliac aorta to ensure abdominal only perfusion [7]. When institutional policies allowed, premortem arterial/venous femoral cannulation and placement of endovascular supraceliac deflated balloon catheter was performed [7]. They reported their outcomes of 11 A-NRP cDCD LT recipients [7]. Dedicated trained perfusionist accompanied the procurement team for all A-NRP procurements [7]. Mean donor age was 47 years. Mean donor BMI was 30. A-NRP duration was restricted to 60–90 minutes. Liver grafts were accepted for LT if lactate clearance was demonstrated [7]. Median recipient MELD score was 26 [7]. EAD was observed in 1 LT recipient [7]. No cases of IC were noted at 3-month follow-up [7]. 3-month LT graft survival was 100% [7]. They reported disposable cost of $6344 associated with A-NRP [7]. There has been increasing momentum at individual transplant center level and OPO level to establish A-NRP infrastructure to facilitate increased cDCD liver graft utilization in USA.

3.7.2 Thoraco-abdominal normothermic regional perfusion (TA-NRP)

Merani et al. first reported single center North American experience of cDCD liver procurement using TA-NRP resulting in three liver transplants in 2022 [37]. Their center's primary intention was to utilize TA-NRP to expand cDCD heart utilization and this resulted in secondary utilization of additional abdominal organs [37]. Two livers were declined due to concern related to prolonged total warm ischemia time and liver quality on assessment [37]. These DCD livers fell in high-risk category (>5) based on UK DCD liver risk score and were transplanted in recipients with median MELD score 16 [37]. The authors reported no PNF or IC in any of the TA-NRP DCD LT recipients [37]. The authors reported 100% patient and graft survival in all three TA-NRP DCD LT recipients [37].

Sellers et al. then described the application of TA-NRP during cDCD procurement in USA in 2022 across 8 separate OPO [38]. The authors reported the outcomes of 13 TA-NRP DCD LT recipients in their case series [38]. Venous cannulation was performed in right atrium, arterial cannulation was performed in ascending aorta and innominate/left carotid/left subclavian artery were stapled/vented [38]. Median donor age was 25 years [38]. Median donor functional warm ischemia time was

13 minutes [38]. Median NRP duration was 56 minutes [38]. Median recipient MELD score was 21 [38]. EAD occurred in 3 LT recipients [38]. No IC was noted in any LT recipient [38]. 6-month LT graft survival was 100% [38]. Authors concluded that post-mortem TA-NRP application maybe scalable more easily across various OPOs in USA compared to initiative to establish pre-mortem femoral cannulation given varied hospital/OPO policies [38].

Wall et al. then described early USA experience with TA-NRP DCD LT recipients (n = 56) compared to SCS DCD LT recipients (n = 64) procurement using the United Network for Organ Sharing (UNOS) database in 2023 [39]. Median donor age was not statistically significantly different between two groups (TA-NRP: 26 vs. SCS: 29) [39]. Median cold ischemia time was not statistically significantly different between two groups (TA-NRP: 4.8 hours vs. SCS: 5 hours) [39]. Median recipient MELD score was not statistically significantly different between two groups (TA-NRP: 19 vs. SCS: 18) [39]. They reported no IC complications in either group [39]. 6-month LT graft survival was not statistically significantly different between two groups (TA-NRP: 92% vs. SRR: 95%) [39].

Brubaker et al. then described outcomes of 16 TA-NRP DCD LT recipients at multiple centers in USA in 2023 [5]. Median donor age was 32 years and median donor BMI was 27 [5]. Peak/terminal donor transaminases were less than 200 IU/L at the time of procurement [5]. Median total warm ischemia time was 25 minutes [5]. Median recipient MELD score was 22 [5]. Median cold ischemia time was 4.9 hours [5]. PNF rate was 0% and EAD rate was 19% [5]. Anastomotic biliary strictures occurred in 19% of cases and were successfully managed with endoscopic stenting [5]. No cases of IC were noted [5]. 3-month LT graft and patient survival was 100% [5]. However, TA-NRP results in reinitiation of cardiac activity, which has restricted its broader adoption due to ethical concerns.

Lastly, Brubaker et al. published outcomes of NRP DCD LT recipients (n = 106) compared to SCS DCD LT recipients (n = 136) from 17 different LT centers in USA in 2024 [40]. Amongst the NRP group, 79 livers were procured using TA-NRP and 27 livers were procured using A-NRP [40]. Median donor age was statistically significantly younger in NRP group (30 years) compared to SCS group (36 years) [40]. Median functional warm ischemia time was statistically significantly longer in NRP group (22 minutes) compared to SCS group (19 minutes) [40]. Median recipient MELD-Na score was not statistically significantly different between two groups (NRP: 289 minutes vs. SCS: 299 minutes) [40]. Median cold ischemia time was not statistically significantly different between groups (NRP: 289 minutes vs. SCS: 299 minutes) [40]. PNF rate was not statistically significantly different between two groups (NRP: 0% vs. SCS: 1.5%) [40]. EAD rate was statistically significantly lower in NRP group (36%) compared to SCS group (56%) [40]. IC rate was statistically significantly lower in NRP group (0%) compared to SCS group (9%) [40]. Biliary anastomotic strictures were statistically significantly lower in NRP group (7%) compared to SCS group (22%) [40]. 1-year LT graft survival was not statistically significantly different between two groups (NRP group: 100% vs. SCS group: 90%) [40]. This study demonstrated that TA-NRP and A-NRP can be feasibly and safely applied at different liver transplant centers in different OPO regions across USA with excellent outcomes in NRP DCD LT recipients (lower EAD/lower IC rates) compared to SCS DCD LT recipients. All the relevant USA NRP studies have been summarized in **Table 4**.

DOI: http://dx.doi.org/10.5772/intechopen.1010806

Study	N and Donor Type	Type of NRP	Cannulation, Premortem = 0, Postmortem = 1	NRP Times, Median (IQR), Hours	Total Warm Ischemic Time Median (IQR), Hours	EAD Within First Week, N (%)	Nonanastomotic Biliary Stricture Development, N (%)	Anastomotic Biliary Strictures, N (%)	1-Year Graft Survival, N (%)	1 Year Patient Survival, N (%)
Rojas Pena et al. USA [36]	13 cDCD (Maastricht type 3)	A-NRP	0	10.2	0.5–0.75	4 (31)	1 (14.3)	1 (14.3)	11 (85.7)	NA
Sellers et al. USA[38]	13 cDCD	TA-NRP	1	0.93 (0.7–1.18)	0.35 (0.23–0.47)	3 (23)	0 (0)	1 (7.7)	12 (92)	12 (92)
Wisel et al. USA 2023	133 TA-DCD	TA-NRP	0	1.83 (1.27–2.5)	1.7 (1.28–2.37), $p < 0.001$	NA	NA	NA	120 (90.1)	123 (92.3)
Croome et al. USA [7]	11 cDCD	A-NRP	0	1.13	NA	1 (9.1)	0 (0)	0 (0)	11 (100)*	11 (100)*

**At median follow up of 142 days.*
Abbreviations: abdominal normothermic regional perfusion, A-NRP; controlled donation after circulatory death, cDCD;donation after circulatory death, DCD; interquartile range, IQR; not available, NA; normothermic regional perfusion, NRP; thoracoabdominal normothermic regional perfusion, TA-NRP.

Table 4.
North American normothermic regional perfusion studies.

4. Conclusion

Both TA-NRP and A-NRP cDCD LT recipients have been demonstrated to have low rates of EAD, IC and graft loss compared to SCS cDCD LT recipients across multiple European and North American studies. NRP allows in-situ cDCD liver graft repair after warm ischemic injury and simultaneous cDCD liver graft functional assessment, which aids LT teams in selecting cDCD liver grafts for eventual LT. NRP has the potential to be utilized in complimentary fashion with ex-vivo machine perfusion technologies (HOPE/dHOPE and NMP) to further increase cDCD liver graft utilization, especially in cases with prolonged warm ischemia times and/or prolonged cold ischemia times. Future areas of research need to be focused on refining functional assessment criteria of cDCD liver grafts on NRP. Additionally, both individual transplant centers and OPO need to invest in NRP infrastructure so that cDCD liver graft utilization can be maximized to reduce the LT waitlist mortality. Rapid adoption of NRP occurred in cDCD liver donors in European countries and similar trend can be anticipated in USA over the next few years given excellent outcomes in NRP cDCD LT recipients.

Conflict of interest

The authors declare no conflict of interest.

Notes/thanks/other declarations

Not applicable.

Author details

Tiffany Hsiung†, Hetal Lad†, Aditya Kasina and Arpit Amin*
Department of Surgery, Rutgers New Jersey Medical School, Newark, NJ, USA

*Address all correspondence to: arpit.amin@rutgers.edu

† These authors contributed equally.

References

[1] Kwong AJ, Kim WR, Lake JR, Schladt DP, Schnellinger EM, Gauntt K, et al. OPTN/SRTR 2022 annual data report: Liver. American Journal of Transplantation. 2024;**24**(2s1):S176-s265

[2] Croome KP, Mathur AK, Aqel B, Yang L, Taner T, Heimbach JK, et al. Classification of distinct patterns of ischemic cholangiopathy following DCD liver transplantation: Distinct clinical courses and long-term outcomes from a multicenter cohort. Transplantation. 2022;**106**(6):1206-1214

[3] Barbier L, Guillem T, Savier E, Scatton O, Donder F, Si Larbi AG, et al. Impact of the duration of normothermic regional perfusion on the results of liver transplant from controlled circulatory death donors: A retrospective, multicentric study. Clinical Transplantation. 2022;**36**(2):e14536

[4] Oniscu GC, Mehew J, Butler AJ, Sutherland A, Gaurav R, Hogg R, et al. Improved organ utilization and better transplant outcomes with in-situ normothermic regional perfusion in controlled donation after circulatory death. Transplantation. 2023;**107**(2):438-448

[5] Brubaker AL, Taj R, Jackson B, Lee A, Tsai C, Berumen J, et al. Early patient and liver allograft outcomes from donation after circulatory death donors using thoracoabdominal normothermic regional perfusion: A multi-center observational experience. Frontiers in Transplantation. 2023;**2**:1184620

[6] Silpe S, Martinez E, Wall A. Normothermic regional perfusion procurement for abdominal organ donors: Techniques and troubleshooting. Current Opinion in Organ Transplantation. 2024;**29**(3):200-204

[7] Croome KP, Brown TE, Mabrey RL, Sonnewald SL, Burns JM, Mao SA, et al. Liver Transplantation. 2023;**29**(12):1282-1291

[8] Fondevila C, Hessheimer AJ, Ruiz A, Calatayud D, Ferrer J, Charco R, et al. Liver transplant using donors after unexpected cardiac death: Novel preservation protocol and acceptance criteria. American Journal of Transplantation. 2007;7(7):1849-1855

[9] Jimenez-Romero C, Manrique A, Calvo J, Caso O, Marcacuzco A, Gacia-Sesma A, et al. Liver transplantation using uncontrolled donors after circulator death: A 10-year single-center experience. Transplantation. 2019;**103**(12):2497-2505

[10] Fondevila C, Hessheimer AJ, Flores E, Ruiz A, Mestres N, Calatayud D, et al. Applicability and results of Maastricht type 2 donation after cardiac death liver transplantation. American Journal of Transplantation. 2012;**12**(1):162-170

[11] Torres MA, Bastante MD, Raya AM, Herrera MT, Massare AB, Jimenez AP, et al. Eight years of extracorporeal membrane oxygenation in liver transplantation: Our experience. Transplantation Proceedings. 2020;**52**(2):572-574

[12] Jimenez-Romero C, Manrique A, Calvo J, Caso O, Marcacuzco A, Garcia-Sesma A, et al. Liver transplantation using uncontrolled donors after circulatory death: A 10-year single-center experience. Transplantation. 2019;**103**(12):2497-2505

[13] Rodriguez-Sanjuan JC, Ruiz N, Minambres E, Toledo E, Gonzalez-Noreiga M, Fernandez-Santiago R, et al. Liver transplant from controlled cardiac death donors using normothermic regional perfusion: Comparison with liver transplants from brain dead donors. Transplantation Proceedings. 2019;**51**(1):12-19

[14] Ruiz P, Gastaca M, Bustamante FJ, Ventoso A, Palomares I, Prieto M, et al. Favorable outcomes after liver transplantation with normothermic regional perfusion from donors after circulatory death: A single-center experience. Transplantation. 2019;**103**(5):938-943

[15] Ruiz P, Valdivieso A, Palomares I, Prieto M, Ventoso A, Salvador P, et al. Similar results in liver transplantation from controlled donation after circulatory death donors with normothermic regional perfusion and donation after brain death donors: A case-matched single-center study. Liver Transplantation. 2021;**27**(12):1747-1757

[16] Munoz DC, Perez BS, Martinez MP, Diaz FJ, Aguilar JL, Daga JA, et al. Does normothermic regional perfusion improve the results of donation after circulatory death liver transplantation. Transplantation Proceedings. 2020;**52**(5):1477-1480

[17] Rodriguez RP, Perez BS, Daga JA, Diaz FJ, Aguilar JL, Munoz MA, et al. Outcome of liver transplants usings donors after cardiac death with normothermic regional perfusion. Transplantation Proceedings. 2022;**54**(1):37-40

[18] Hessheimer AJ, Rosa G, Gastaca M, Ruiz P, Otero A, Gomez M, et al. Abdominal normothermic regional perfusion in donation after circulatory determination of death liver transplantation: Outcomes and risk factors for graft loss. American Journal of Transplantation. 2022;**22**(4):1169-1181

[19] Hessheimer AJ, Coll E, Torres F, Ruiz P, Gastaca M, Rivas JI, et al. Normothermic regional perfusions vs super-rapid recovery in controlled donation after circulatory death liver transplantation. Journal of Hepatology. 2019;**70**(4):658-665

[20] De Carlis R, Sandro S, Lauterio A, Botta F, Ferla F, Andorno E, et al. Liver grafts from donors after circulatory death on regional perfusion with extended warm ischemia compared with donors after brain death. Liver Transplantation. 2018;**24**(11):1523-1535

[21] Ghinolfi D, Dandossola D, Rreka E, Lonati C, Pezzati D, Cacciatoinsilla A, et al. Sequential use of normothermic regional and ex situ machine perfusion in donation after circulatory death liver transplant. Liver Transplantation. 2021;**27**(3):385-402

[22] De Carlis R, Schlegel A, Frassoni S, Oliveri T, Ravaioli M, Camagni S, et al. How to preserve liver grafts from circulatory death with long warm ischemia? A retrospective Italian cohort study with normothermic regional perfusion and hypothermic oxygenated perfusion. Transplantation. 2021;**105**(11):2385-2396

[23] Patrono D, Zanierato M, Vergano M, Magaton C, Diale E, Rizza G, et al. Normothermic regional perfusion and hypothermic oxygenated machine perfusion for livers donated after controlled circulatory death with prolonged warm ischemia time: A matched comparison with livers from brain-dead donors. Transplant International. 2022;**35**:10390

[24] Camagni S, Amaduzzi A, Grazioli L, Ghitti D, Pasulo L, Pinelli D, et al.

Extended criteria liver donation after circulatory death with prolonged warm ischemia: A pilot experience of normothermic regional perfusion and no subsequent ex-situ machine perfusion. HPB: The Official Journal of the International Hepato Pancreato Biliary Association. 2023;**25**(12):1494-1501

[25] Olivieri Y, Magistri P, Guidetti C, Baroni S, Rinaldi S, Assirati G, et al. University of Modena experience with liver grafts from donation after circulatory death: What really matters in organ selection? Transplantation Proceedings. 2019;**51**(9):2967-2970

[26] Savier E, Dondero F, Vibert E, Eyraud D, Brisson H, Riou B, et al. First experience of liver transplantation with type 2 donation after cardiac death in France. Liver Transplantation. 2015;**21**(5):631-643

[27] Savier E, Lim C, Rayar M, Orlando F, Boudjema K, Mohkam K, et al. Favorable outcomes of liver transplantation from controlled circulatory death donors using normothermic regional perfusion compared to brain death donors. Transplantation. 2020;**104**(9):1943-1951

[28] Oniscu GC, Randle LV, Muiesan P, Butler AJ, Currie IS, Perera MT, et al. In situ normothermic regional perfusion for controlled donation after circulatory death – The United Kingdom experience. American Journal of Transplantation. 2014;**14**(12):2846-2854

[29] Watson CJ, Hunt F, Messer S, Currie I, Large S, Sutherland A, et al. In situ normothermic perfusion of livers in controlled circulatory death donation may prevent ischemic cholangiopathy and improve graft survival. American Journal of Transplantation. 2019;**19**(6):1745-1758

[30] Muller X, Mohkam K, Mueller M, Schlegel A, Dondero F, Sepulveda A, et al. Hypothermic oxygenated perfusion versus normothermic regional perfusion in liver transplantation from controlled donation after circulatory death: First international comparative study. Annals of Surgery. 2020;**272**(5):751-758

[31] Maroni L, Musa N, Ravaioli M, Dondossola DE, Germinario G, Sulpice L, et al. Normothermic with or without hypothermic oxygenated perfusion for DCD before liver transplantation: European multicentric experience. Clinical Transplantation. 2021;**35**(11):e14448

[32] Gaurav R, Butler AJ, Kosmoliaptsis V, Mumford L, Fear C, Swift L, et al. Liver transplantation outcomes from controlled circulatory death donors: SCS vs in situ NRP vs ex situ NMP. Annals of Surgery. 2022;**275**(6):1156-1164

[33] Schurink IJ, de Goeij FHC, Habets LJM, van de Leemkolk FEM, van Dun CAA, Oniscu GC, et al. Salvage of declined extended criteria DCD livers using in situ normothermic regional perfusion. Annals of Surgery. 2022;**276**(4):e223-e230

[34] Mohkam K, Nasralla D, Mergental H, Muller X, Butler A, Jassem W, et al. In situ normothermic regional perfusion versus ex situ normothermic machine perfusion in liver transplantation from donation after circulatory death. Liver Transplantation. 2022;**28**(11):1716-1725

[35] Magliocca JF, Magee JC, Rowe SA, Gravel MT, Chenault RH, Merion RM, et al. Extracorporeal support for organ donation after cardiac death effectively expands the donor pool. The Journal of Trauma. 2005;**58**(6):1095-1101

[36] Rojas-Pena A, Sall LE, Gravel MT, Cooley EG, Pelletier SJ, Bartlett RH, et al. Donation after circulatory determination

of death: The University of Michigan experience with extracorporeal support. Transplantation. 2014;**98**(3):328-334

[37] Merani S, Urban M, Um JY, Maskin A, Vargas LM, Castleberry AW, et al. A north American single-center experience with liver transplantation using thoraco-abdominal normothermic regional perfusion for donation after circulatory death. American Journal of Transplantation. 2022;**22**(2):666-668

[38] Sellers MT, Nassar A, Alebrahim M, Sasaki K, Lee DD, Bohorquez H, et al. Early United States experience with liver donation after circulatory determination of death using thoraco-abdominal normothermic regional perfusion: A multi-institutional observational study. Clinical Transplantation. 2022;**36**(6):e14659

[39] Wall A, Rosenzweig M, McKenna GJ, Ma TW, Asrani S, Testa G. Six-month abdominal transplant recipient outcomes from donation after circulatory death heart donors: A retrospective analysis by procurement technique. American Journal of Transplantation. 2023;**23**(7):987-995

[40] Brubaker AL, Sellers MT, Abt PL, Croome KP, Merani S, Wall A, et al. US liver transplant outcomes after normothermic regional perfusion vs standard super rapid recovery. JAMA Surgery. 2024;**159**(6):677-685

Chapter 11

Hypothermic Oxygenated Machine Perfusion in Donor Hearts

Nafiye Busra Celik, Mohammad Alomari, Vivienne Pham, Pankaj Garg and Si Pham

Abstract

Heart transplantation remains the definitive treatment for end-stage heart diseases. The rising demand for heart transplants underscores the need to expand the donor pool by using marginal and long-distant donors with the potential of increasing the rate of primary graft dysfunction. On-going ischemia under static cold storage (SCS) contributes to myocardial injury, severe primary graft dysfunction, and increased mortality, highlighting the necessity for improved graft preservation strategies. Hypothermic oxygenated machine perfusion (HOPE) offers a promising solution by continuously delivering oxygenated, nutrient-rich cardioplegic fluid under hypothermic conditions. This chapter will review the pre-clinical and clinic studies using HOPE to preserve donor hearts for transplantation. Mechanistic studies demonstrates that HOPE increases ischemia tolerance by enhancing succinate clearance, preserving ATP levels, and minimizing free radical formation. Pre-clinical and clinical studies have reinforced HOPE's potential to attenuate tissue injury and reduce primary graft dysfunction. Initial clinical studies suggest that HOPE is safe and has favorable impact on heart transplant outcomes. Despite the promising outcomes, most existing clinical studies on HOPE are limited by small sample sizes and a lack of randomization, which could affect the generalizability of the results. Future research should focus on conducting larger, randomized controlled trials to provide more robust evidence on the efficacy and safety of HOPE. Furthermore, future integration of HOPE with innovative technologies such as real-time monitoring of tissue metabolism, pharmacologic or biological modifications of the donor heart during HOPE may lead to better outcomes.

Keywords: heart donors, hypothermic oxygenated machine perfusion, heart transplants, primary graft dysfunction, cold static storage, ischemia

1. Introduction

Heart transplantation remains the preferred treatment option for end-stage heart failure. In recent years, the increasing demand for heart transplantation underscores the necessity to expand the donor pool by using marginal and long-distant donors that are more susceptible to primary graft dysfunction. Additionally, the traditional method of heart donor preservation involves static cold storage (SCS) with limited duration of donor ischemic time. These challenges highlights the need for more effective strategies to preserve donor hearts [1]. Among all transplanted solid organs the heart is most sensitive to ischemia. During SCS, the donor's heart undergoes a period of ischemia due to ongoing low-grade metabolism in the absence of oxygen and nutrients. This ongoing metabolic activity forces the myocardial cells to adapt to anaerobic metabolism resulting in intracellular acidosis and energy stress due to ATP depletion and lactate accumulation. Subsequent reperfusion of ischemic myocardium leads to the activation of the immune system resulting in cell death by apoptosis and necrosis, known as ischemia-reperfusion injury [2]. Hypothermic oxygenated machine perfusion (HOPE) has recently been investigated as an alternative to SCS. HOPE mitigates the fundamental problem of SCS by continuous perfusion of the heart with oxygenated and nutrient-hormone-rich cardioplegic fluid, while hypothermia ensures myocardial protection by maintaining the metabolism to the lowest. In a donor-after-circulatory death (DCD) rat model, Wyss et al., recently demonstrated the importance of both hypothermic perfusion and oxygenation of DCD hearts prior to normothermic perfusion [3]. The authors proposed that succinate accumulates in the mitochondria during SCS and rapid succinate oxidation during normothermic reperfusion plays an important role in ischemia-reperfusion injuries by reverse electron transfer from complex II (succinate dehydrogenase) to complex I and subsequently inducing oxidative stress and cellular injury. On the other hand, during HOPE, hypothermia and low-flow delivery of oxygen are believed to reduce oxygen-induced return of mitochondrial proton motive force, thereby decreasing the susceptibility for reverse electron transfer upon succinate oxidation, while promoting ATP production via oxidative phosphorylation. Further, perfusion may itself promote succinate washout [3]. There is an ongoing debate about the optimum oxygen requirement for the donor hearts during hypothermia. Because the cellular metabolism at 4°C is only 12% of normothermia, higher oxygen delivery during HOPE may generate free radicals and tissue damage [4]. On the other hand, ATP levels in the tissue can only be preserved when an adequate amount of oxygen is supplied, even during hypothermia.

The rationale for ex-vivo HOPE of the heart include the following: (a) homogeneous cooling of the heart below 10 degree Celsius (°C) and reduction in myocardial metabolic requirements, (b) prevention of ATP depletion by continuous infusion of the nutrient-enriched solution, (c) continuous elimination of the toxic metabolites including lactate, and (d) extension of safe ischemia time. The International Society for Heart and Lung Transplantation (ISHLT) registry data has shown that ischemia of more than 200 minutes is associated with higher mortality after heart transplant [5]. By extending the safe ischemic period HOPE may permit the transportation of the hearts procured from more distant sites as well as enable physical human leukocyte antigen (HLA) matching between donors and recipients. Currently, physical HLA-matching is not routine in heart transplantation because of time constraints, however, it has been shown to improve survival in heart transplantation [6]. Hearts receiving HOPE also showed preserved tissue ATP stores and architecture of the mitochondria. Published studies reported that HOPE reduced endothelial dysfunction (lower endothelin-1 levels) and apoptosis in the hearts preserved for 12 hours at 4°C compared to hearts stored by SCS [7, 8]. Collectively, available data suggest that the benefits of HOPE could potentially translate into better short-term (less primary graft failure) and long-term (less cardiac allograft vasculopathy) outcomes after heart transplantation [9].

2. Evolution of hypothermic machine perfusion for donor organ preservation

The field of hypothermic machine perfusion has evolved significantly over the last 4 decades as a method for organ preservation, moving from initial applications in renal transplants to the more complex preservation of livers and hearts. This method has transformed the landscape of organ transplantation by improving graft viability and extending preservation times, ultimately enhancing transplant outcomes.

2.1 Kidney preservation

Hypothermic machine perfusion was first applied in the preservation of kidneys, addressing limitations associated with static cold storage (SCS). Pioneering studies in the mid-twentieth century demonstrated that continuous perfusion at hypothermic temperatures could reduce ischemic injury and improve post-transplant outcomes. The introduction of pulsatile perfusion systems in the 1960s allowed better maintenance of microcirculatory flow and cellular metabolism [10, 11].

2.2 Liver preservation

Success in kidneys paved the way for its application of HOPE in liver transplants, where the risks associated with ischemia-reperfusion injury were significant higher. Early research faced challenges due to the liver's complex vascular structure and metabolic demands. However, by the early 2000s, significant strides were made with the development of specialized perfusion devices that supported continuous oxygenation and metabolic conditioning. Studies have demonstrated that HOPE could enhance bile production, reduce hepatic enzyme release, and improve graft survival compared to traditional SCS [12–15].

Recently, dual hypothermic oxygenated perfusion (D-HOPE), which provides oxygenation to both the portal vein and hepatic arteries and shows less biliary complications, has emerged as an advanced technique that may improve outcomes in marginal liver donors [16, 17].

2.3 Heart preservation

The use of HOPE for heart preservation has been the most challenging due to the organ's reliance on continuous mechanical activity and its sensitivity to ischemic damage. Initial studies in heart preservation focused on cold static storage, but research in HOPE gained traction in the late twentieth century, driven by the need for extending ischemic times and reducing graft dysfunction. The development of systems capable of providing continuous perfusion with oxygen and metabolic substrates has shown promising results [18–21].

Recent studies have indicated that HOPE can significantly reduce primary graft dysfunction [22] and safely extended donor ischemic time [23–25].

3. Available systems for hypothermic perfusion of donor hearts

Currently none of the systems for hypothermic perfusion system of donor hearts has received approval from the Food and Drug Administration (FDA) in the United States or Conformité Européene (CE) mark in Europe.

3.1 XVIVO heart assist transport™ system

The XVIVO Heart Assist Transport™ system, as illustrated in **Figure 1**, is equipped with various essential components including a reservoir, pressure-controlled roller pump, oxygenator, arterial-leukocyte filter, heat-exchange unit, gas mixer, oxygen and carbon dioxide containers, and sensors; all are integrated into a programmable control system. The reservoir is filled with 2.5 liters of perfusion solution and approximately 500 milliliters (mL) of compatible, irradiated, leukocyte-reduced packed red blood cells, to achieve a hematocrit level of around 15%. The specific composition of the perfusion solution is detailed in **Table 1**. The system perfuses the coronary arteries antegradely through an aortic cannula. After retrieval, the donor heart is carefully inspected. If the foramen ovale is patent, it should be closed. The distal ascending aorta is cannulated with a double-lumen, self-deairing XVIVO aortic cannula to facilitate de-airing. Additionally, a tube is placed in the coronary sinus to allow for blood gas sampling. The aortic cannula, supplying preservation solution to the aorta, is mounted vertically, with the heart fully submerged in the preservation solution.

During perfusion, pressure in the aorta is maintained at 20 millimeters of mercury (mmHg) with pressure-regulated flow (typically between 150 and 200 mL/min), and the temperature is maintained at 8°C. To prevent left ventricular distension during perfusion, a silastic split tube is inserted through the mitral valve into the left ventricle and secured to the left atrial wall. Both the superior and inferior vena cava, along with the pulmonary artery, remain open to provide a free outlet for the perfusate exiting from the coronary sinus. The XVIVO Heart Assist Transport™ system's display shows real-time pressure, flow patterns, and temperature, and these parameters are recorded in the computer system [20, 23].

3.2 LifeCradle heart perfusion system

The LifeCradle Heart Perfusion System, which was developed by Bridge to Life, Ltd., (Illinois, USA) and recently acquired by TransMedics, Inc. (Andover, MA), is a device that delivers temperature-regulated, oxygenated perfusate to the donor heart in an anterograde or retrograde fashion. Perfusate flows, pressures, and temperatures are monitored continuously. Technically, cardioplegic perfusate is delivered in an

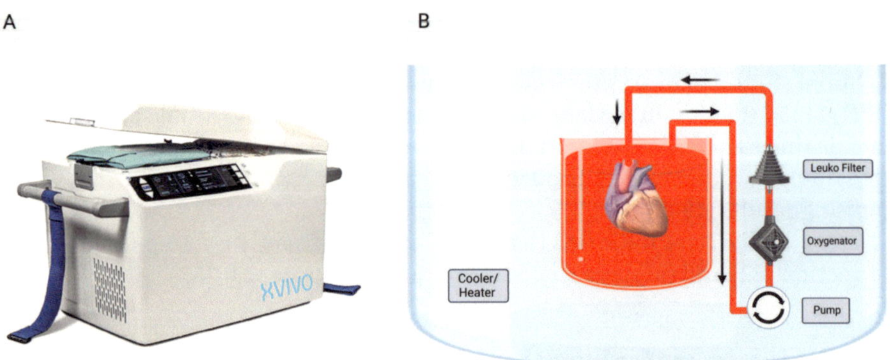

Figure 1.
XVIVO heart assist transport™ system. (A) Portable XVIVO device, (B) Schematic rendition of the temperature-regulated hypothermic oxygenated perfusion system in the device. (Published with permission from XVIVO Perfusion AP, 2024).

Constituents	Concentration
Sodium (Na+)	136 mmol/L
Potassium (K+)	2.3 mmol/L
Calcium (Ca^{2+})	1.3 mmol/L
Magnesium (Mg^{2+})	8.0 mmol/L
Chloride (Cl^-)	142 mmol/L
Bicarbonate (HCO_3^-)	25 mmol/L
Phosphate (PO_4^{2-})	1.3 mmol/L
Dextrose	6.3 mmol/L
Albumin	75 g /L
Dextran-40	1 g/L
Cocaine	6 nmol/L
Noradrenaline	6 nmol/L
Adrenaline	6 nmol/L
Triiodothyronine (T3)	3 nmol/L
Cortisol	420 nmol/L
Insulin	8U/L
Imipenem	20 mg/L
Erythrocytes (Hct)	15%
Gas 95% O_2 + 5% CO_2	0.2 U/min

O_2, oxygen; CO_2, carbon dioxide.

Table 1.
Composition of heart perfusate for hypothermic oxygenated machine perfusion [20].

anterograde fashion through the ascending aorta at a flow rate of 10 ml/100 g heart weight/min at 5 ± 2°C. Retrograde cardioplegia perfusion is carried out using a retrograde cardioplegia cannula sewn into the coronary sinus at a flow rate of 13–20 ml/100 g/min, also at 5 ± 2°C. This device has been tested in the porcine donation-after-brain-death (DBD) and canine donation-after-circulatory-death (DCD) heart models and has shown superior myocardial preservation compared to SCS [26, 27]. A study using human donor hearts that were not suitable for transplantation showed that this system preserved the aerobic metabolism of the heart equally well irrespective of whether the heart was perfused anterogradely through the aorta or retrogradely through the coronary sinus [28]. In 2022, the device received "Breakthrough Device Designation" from the FDA, but it is still not approved by the FDA and Conformite Europeenne (CE) to date.

3.3 The HEARTPORT© system

The HeartPort© System is a modified version of the LifePort© System (Organ Recovery Systems©, Itasca, IL, USA) that was originally designed for kidney graft perfusion and preservation. This system is intended for hypothermic perfusion of donor hearts [28, 29]. In this setup, the explanted heart is submerged in a reservoir and suspended vertically via a cannula inserted into the distal ascending aorta. The distal stump of the ascending aorta is clamped, and the cannula is connected to a temperature-controlled perfusion circuit, enabling antegrade perfusion of the coronary arteries. The perfusate exiting from the coronary sinus is collected back into the reservoir and recycled through the system. An external oxygenator connected to the circuit ensures oxygenation of the perfusate.

The perfusate consists of 1 liter of asanguineous preservation solution (KPS-1©, Organ Recovery Systems©, Itasca, IL, USA). It is oxygenated using an oxygenator (Minimax Oxygenation System©, Medtronic, Inc., Minneapolis, MN, USA), chilled to 4°C with a heat exchanger, and circulated using a pulsatile roller pump. The system's data reporting unit allows for continuous monitoring of temperature, perfusion pressure, and flow.

A published animal study using the HeartPort System © showed that after hearts that were perfused with the HeartPort© system for 4 hours had lower lactate and high energy phosphates, and more successful functional recovery than those with static ice storage [28, 29].

4. Cardiac function after hypothermic oxygenated perfusion

Since the hearts preserved by HOPE are kept in a non-beating state, functional assessment of the heart is possible only by either reanimating them in-vitro on a normothermic machine perfusion (NMP) system or after transplantation. However, HOPE has been shown beneficial in terms of preserved myocardial function [26, 29] as well as prolonged duration of heart preservation in preclinical studies and has been utilized successfully in human DBD heart transplantation [19, 20, 22, 23]. In a recent DCD porcine model, post-transplantation, biventricular contractility was better preserved with HOMP compared to in-situ or ex-situ normothermic machine perfusion [30]. In addition, need for inotropic support and signs of myocardial damage were lower with HOPE. Achievement of this excellent outcome has been attributed to the following mechanisms:

a. Hearts preserved by HOPE do not suffer from energy stress, tissue acidosis, or hyper contracture as they generate sufficient ATP through aerobic metabolism.

b. Due to reduced ischemic injury, these hearts produce less free oxygen radicals after reperfusion.

c. Continuous perfusion of the heart results in better-preserved endothelium and myocardium cellular structures and less cellular death due to apoptosis or necrosis.

These findings underscore HOPE's potential for improving heart transplant outcomes by providing enhanced myocardial protection during preservation.

5. Hypothermic oxygenated machine perfusion in heart transplantation: Pre-clinical studies

Numerous experimental studies conducted on large animal models suggest that Hypothermic Oxygenated Perfusion (HOPE) can mitigate tissue injuries and enhance cardiac function post-transplant when compared to Static Cold Storage (SCS). Despite these findings, the clinical adoption of HOPE is constrained by challenges in reliable functional assessment, as the graft is maintained in a non-beating state.

For instance, in a canine model, hearts preserved for 24 hours with HOPE displayed equivalent outcomes in terms of duration of cardiopulmonary bypass (CPB) support, inotropic support, cardiac output, and survival when compared to those preserved with SCS for four hours [31]. Additionally, another study indicated superior systolic function recovery in a canine model using a Lutgendorf system after 24 hours of HOPE, as opposed to 8hours with SCS [32]. This aligns with another preclinical study showing better cardiac functional recovery, increased ATP levels, decreased levels of caspase-3 (marker of apoptosis), malondialdehyde, and endothelin-1, in HOPE-preserved hearts versus those preserved with SCS [33].

In a more elaborate study, Steen et al., investigated the effectiveness of HOPE in extended preservation time (24 hours) of porcine DBD hearts using pulsed perfusion at 8°C, with intervals of 15 minutes of perfusion followed by 60 minutes without. The perfusate was a hyper-oncotic cardioplegic nutrition solution enriched with hormones and erythrocytes [19]. Their results showed that all HOPE-preserved hearts were successfully transplanted and maintained stability over 24 hours post-transplant without adverse effects on myocardial function. Moreover, hearts in the HOPE group were more easily weaned off CPB compared to the SCS controls, which had difficulties in weaning from cardiopulmonary bypass and subsequent failure shortly thereafter [19].

Further experimental research by Qin et al., on the impact of HOPE on donor hearts in a porcine model demonstrated that the coronary artery endothelium maintained normal function in terms of vascular contractility and relaxation after 8hours of HOPE [34]. Prolonged HOPE (24 hours) on six pig hearts utilized a hyper-oncotic solution comprising albumin, a cardioplegic nutrition-hormone solution, and blood, maintaining a hematocrit of 10%. Control hearts used were fresh cardioplegic hearts from 11 pigs. This study showed no significant changes in endothelium-dependent relaxation, contraction force, potentiation, and calcium recirculation fraction, or myocardial edema (as indicated by water content) in HOPE-preserved hearts [35]. Additional studies highlight HOPE's efficacy in preserving myocardial energetics. Michel and Madsen reported that HOPE led to less depletion of ATP stores and improved preservation of mitochondrial structure in a porcine heart model [2].

In another recent study by Moeslund et al., using a Swedish porcine DCD heart model, three heart donation techniques were compared: thoraco-abdominal normothermic regional perfusion (TA-NRP) followed by SCS, TA-NRP followed by HOPE with the XVIVO Heart Preservation System, and direct procurement and HOPE. The findings indicated that HOPE significantly improved biventricular contractility 2 hours post-cardiopulmonary bypass (CPB) and required a lower dose of inotropes compared to SCS. Diastolic function was preserved in all groups. Moreover, myocardial injury, as indicated by increased plasma troponin T, was significantly less in the HOPE groups compared to those preserved with SCS [30].

One of the most notable findings is the immunodepleting phenomenon after HOPE. Using a porcine DBD heart model, Critchley et al., compared hearts preserved with SCS for 2 hours to those preserved with HOPE for 8hours. In addition to showing that the HOPE hearts exhibited reduced ischemia-reperfusion injury and cell death, along with better maintenance of myocardial viability, there was a significant loss of leukocytes in the myocardium after 8hours with HOPE. These cells consist of a across a range of phenotypes, including lymphocytes, monocytes/macrophages, and granulocytes. These findings suggesting a unique immunodepleting phenomenon that could result in reduced organ rejection [36]. Langin et al., expanded on this by demonstrating how this immunodepleting phenomenon could benefit xenotransplantation [37]. Their study categorized genetically modified α1,3-galactosyltransferase-knockout pig hearts into three groups for xenotransplantation to baboons. Group I, with hearts preserved in SCS, had only one animal survived past 3 days. In contrast, all animals in Group II, with hearts preserved in HOPE, survived for 30 or more days. Remarkably, with the addition of post-transplant care adjustments, all animals in Group III survived up to 6 months [37].

In summary, these studies highlight the potential advantages of HOPE in cardiac preservation by reducing tissue injury, maintaining cellular structure and energy storage, and potentially decreasing post-transplant immunogenicity, thus supporting its clinical application for enhanced transplant outcomes.

6. Hypothermic oxygenated machine perfusion in heart transplantation: Clinical results

Since 1984, four small to moderate-sized clinical studies (excluding case reports) have explored the impact of HOPE on heart preservation using various perfusion solutions (see **Table 2**). Wicomb et al., conducted the first series of clinical heterotopic heart transplantations using hearts stored in a portable HOPE device, perfused with a cold crystalloid cardioplegic solution for 6 to 15 hours, achieving a survival rate of three out of four patients for over three months [38]. Hill et al., between May 1989 and April 1990, perfused 22 DBD hearts with Cardiosol I heart preservation solution; nine of these were perfused with HOPE during transport, while 13 were transported using SCS. The ischemic time for hearts managed with HOPE was notably longer than those in the SCS group. Initially, all transplanted hearts functioned well and were successfully weaned off CPB, although one heart in the HOPE group required defibrillation. The pH of Cardiosol I in the coronary effluent in the HOPE group decreased from 7.4 to 6.96 by the end of the microperfusion period, remaining higher than that in the SCS group. Likewise, LDH release into the coronary effluent was lower in the HOPE group by the end of 221 minutes of microperfusion. One mortality was reported in the first year post-transplant in the HOPE group, with the remaining eight patients surviving for seven years [39].

In 2020, Nilsson and colleagues conducted a non-randomized, open-label clinical trial comparing HOPE with SCS in heart transplantation [20]. In this study, six patients received standard-criteria DBD hearts preserved by HOPE and perfused with a hyper-oncotic cardioplegic solution supplemented with hormones and erythrocytes, while twenty-five patients received hearts preserved by SCS. The median preservation time for HOPE was 223 minutes, compared to 194 minutes for SCS. All patients in the HOPE group survived six months post-transplant, and all exhibited event-free survival (freedom from severe PDG, ECMO, acute cellular rejection ≥2R), contrasting with 72% in the SCS group. This study demonstrated the safety and potential benefits of HOPE in clinical cardiac transplantation.

Recently, McGriffin et al. conducted a multicenter, nonrandomized, single-arm study in Australia and New Zealand, examining the effects of prolonged donor heart storage using HOPE with the XVIVO Heart Preservation System [23]. The study, which involved 36 patients, evaluated the impact of 6–8 hours of donor heart preservation on 30-day recipient survival and allograft function post-transplant.

Each center had to complete 1 or 2 patients with short preservation time before enrolling patients with long preservation time, resulting in a total of 7 patients in the former group and 29 in the latter. Patient survival was compared with a control group from the International Society of Heart Lung Transplantation (ISHLT) Registry. The

DOI: http://dx.doi.org/10.5772/intechopen.1008546

Study	Subjects	Size (n)	Perfusion temp.	Preservation duration	Perfusate	Follow-up	Key findings
Wicomb et al. 1984 [38]	DBD	4	4–10°C	6–15 hr	Clear hyper osmolar solution	Weeks after heterotopic Tx	The hearts with shorter preservation time had a better function for longer periods after Tx.
Hill et al. 1997 [39]	DBD	1) 9	4–10 °C	221mins	Cardiosol I	7 Years	pH of the coronary effluent decreased from 7.4 to 6.96 by the end micro perfusion. Less LDH release into the coronary effluent compared to group 2.
		2) 13	SCS	185 mins	Cardiosol I	7 Years	pH decreased more than group1. LDH release was much higher than group1.
		3) 50	SCS	187 mins	mSTS	7 Years	Survival lower (70%) compared to other groups (100%) in 7 years.
Nilsson et al. 2020 [20]	DBD	1) 6	8 °C	223 min	XHS	6 months after Tx	Survival was 100% at180 days. No difference in early graft dysfunction, inotropic requirement.
		2) 25	SCS	194 min	Crystalloid cardioplegic solution		Survival was 72% in 180 days. Two recipients developed PGD within 24 hours of Tx. One recipient required ECMO within 7 days. One recipient died, and 4 developed ACR of ≥2R within 180 days.
McGiffin et al. 2023 [23]	DBD	29 Long Preserv-ation	8°C	414 min	XHS	30-day after Tx	30-days survival was 100%. Survival superior to the ISHLT comparator group. Two patients had graft dysfunction and needed mechanical circulatory support.
		7 Short Preserv-ation	8 °C	252 min	XHS	30-day after Tx	30-days survival was 100%. One patient developed PGD and required ECMO.

ACR, acute cellular rejection; DBD, donation after brain death; DCD, donation after circulatory death; ECMO, extracorporeal membrane oxygenation; hr., hour; ICU, intensive care unit; LV, left ventricle; min, minute; mSTS, modified St Thomas' cardioplegic solution; PGD, primary graft dysfunction; SCS, static cold storage; Tx, Transplantation; XHS, XVIVO Heart Solution; ISHLT, International Society of Heart and Lung Transplantation.

Table 2.
Summary of hypothermic oxygenated machine perfusion in clinical heart transplantation.

mean preservation time for long preservation cases was 414 ± 53 minutes, with the longest being 527 minutes. The recipient and graft survival at 30 days was 100% and exceeded that of the ISHLT comparator group. Two recipients in the long- and one in the short-preservation group needed temporary mechanical circulatory support post-transplant. This study demonstrated that HOPE provides effective preservation for donor hearts for up to nearly 9 hours, facilitating the retrieval of donor hearts from remote locations and potentially enhancing the donor pool and transplant outcomes.

As of November 2024, the only randomized study on HOPE in DBD heart preservation was recently published [22]. Conducted by Rega and colleagues, this multicenter, controlled, open-label trial involved 229 adult heart transplant candidates across 15 centers in eight European countries. Participants were randomly assigned to receive donor hearts preserved by either HOPE or SCS. The primary outcome was the occurrence of a composite endpoint within 30 days post-transplant, including cardiac-related death, moderate or severe primary graft dysfunction (PGD), acute cellular rejection grade 2R or higher, or graft failure necessitating mechanical support or re-transplantation. The incidence of primary endpoint events was 19% in the HOPE group versus 30% in the SCS group, indicating a 44% risk reduction, but not statistically significant. The incidence of PGD was also significantly lower in the HOPE group. While the study did not achieve statistical significance for the primary composite endpoint, the significant reductions in PGD and other complications support HOPE as an effective and safe option for donor heart preservation in clinical transplantation.

In summary, these clinical studies, while small to moderate in scale and predominantly non-randomized, show that HOPE can extend ischemic times, allowing for the utilization of donor hearts across longer distances and potentially improving transplant outcomes. Notably, these studies highlighted improved physiological parameters such as better pH stability and lower lactate dehydrogenase (LDH) release during perfusion, alongside enhanced post-transplant survival and event-free outcomes compared to SCS. Despite these encouraging findings, there remains a clear need for further research. Larger, randomized clinical trials are necessary to provide more definitive evidence of the benefits and potential risks associated with HOPE. Such studies would help clarify the impact of extended preservation times enabled by HOPE on long-term recipient outcomes and further assess the procedure's effectiveness in reducing primary graft dysfunction and other complications. By expanding the evidence base, the clinical adoption of HOPE could be accelerated, potentially transforming standard practices in heart transplantation to achieve better patient outcomes globally.

7. Ongoing and future trials

To better assess the relative benefits of heart HOPE compared to static cold storage (SCS) in donor hearts, further clinical data are required. **Table 3** lists ongoing trials registered at ClinicalTrials.gov (https://clinicaltrials.gov).

As of November 2024, four trials are ongoing. A randomized European trial (NCT03991923) is enrolling 230 heart transplant recipients receiving hearts preserved by either HOPE or SCS. The primary outcome is mortality at 1 month and 12 months, with graft dysfunction at those same time points as a secondary outcome. Another randomized trial from Sweden (NCT04066127), with 66 patients, has a primary outcome of survival free of acute cellular rejection and re-transplantation

DOI: http://dx.doi.org/10.5772/intechopen.1008546

NCT number	Institution	Study phase/ Design	Starting date–Estimated completion date	Estimated number of enrolled patients	Study arms	Outcome measures (Time period)
NCT03991923	Total eight centers in Europe	Multicenter, randomized	November 2020–August 2024	230	HOMP, SCS	Primary outcome: mortality and graft dysfunction (30 days); secondary outcomes: mortality and graft dysfunction (12 months)
NCT04066127	Skane University Hospital, Sweden	Randomized	June 2020–December 2026	66	HOMP, SCS	Primary outcome: survival free of acute cellular rejection and re-transplantation (12 months); secondary outcomes: I/R-tissue injury, early allograft dysfunction, and health status.
NCT05881278	Total fifteen centers in USA	Multicenter, non-randomized	October 2023-March 2026 (primary completion) March 2030	141	HOMP	Primary outcomes: percentage of patient survival (post-operative day 365), and percentage of patient treatment success rate (30 days post-Tx).
NCT06485596	Belgium, Netherland-total four centers	Multicenter, proof-of-concept	July 2024–June 2026	20	HOMP	Primary outcome: patient survival in 30 days; secondary outcomes: cardiac related mortality at 6 months, incidence of MCS, incidence of severe PGD at 24 hours, cardiac function as assessed by LVEF at 24 hours and 30 days, incidence of perfused hearts which are not used for transplantation, total duration of ICU stay (days), incidence of biopsy proven rejection >1 ACR, number of days until hospital discharge from index procedure.

HOMP, *Hypothermic oxygenated machine perfusion;* **PGD**, *primary graft dysfunction;* **post-Tx**, *post-transplantation;* **SCS**, *static cold storage;* **MCS**, *mechanical circulatory support;* **LVEF**, *left ventricular ejection fraction.*

Table 3.
Ongoing clinical trials using hypothermic oxygenated machine perfusion. (https://clinicaltrials.gov/).

at 12 months. A non-randomized, multicenter US trial with 141 HOPE patients has a primary outcome of patient survival at 365 days and a treatment success rate at 30 days. Finally, a non-randomized, proof-of-concept trial from Belgium involving 20 patients receiving HOMP hearts has a primary outcome of patient survival at 30 days post-transplant. Further details of these ongoing projects are listed in **Table 3**.

8. Conclusion

In summary, hypothermic oxygenated machine perfusion represents a promising strategy to address the challenges of prolonged ischemic times and ischemia-reperfusion injuries in heart transplantation. Preclinical and clinical studies collectively demonstrate that hypothermic oxygenated machine perfusion of donor hearts, as compared with static cold storage, can extend the ischemic time, facilitate the use of donor hearts over longer distances, reduce ischemia-reperfusion injury, enhance graft function, expand donor pools, and potentially improve transplant success rates and survival outcomes.

Despite the promising outcomes, most existing clinical studies on HOPE are limited by small sample sizes and a lack of randomization, which could affect the generalizability of the results. Future research should focus on conducting larger, randomized controlled trials to provide more robust evidence on the efficacy and safety of HOPE. This will help to definitively determine its benefits over traditional preservation methods like SCS.

Furthermore, exploring the integration of HOPE with innovative technologies such as real-time monitoring of tissue metabolism, pharmacologic or biological modifications of the donor heart during perfusion may further refine the evaluation and conditioning of cardiac allografts. This comprehensive and innovative approach will enable more effective and individualized care, leading to improved short- and long-term outcomes for patients with end-stage heart diseases.

Conflict of interest

None.

Author details

Nafiye Busra Celik[1], Mohammad Alomari[1], Vivienne Pham[2], Pankaj Garg[1] and Si Pham[3]*

1 Department of Cardiothoracic Surgery, Mayo Clinic Florida, Jacksonville, FL, USA

2 College of Medicine, Ohio State University, Columbus, OH, USA

3 Donald and Barbara Zucker School of Medicine at Hofstra University/Northwell, Hempstead, NY, USA

*Address all correspondence to: spham2@northwell.edu

References

[1] Ughetto A, Roubille F, Molina A, Battistella P, Gaudard P, Demaria R, et al. Heart graft preservation technics and limits: An update and perspectives. Frontiers in Cardiovascular Medicine. 2023;**10**:1248606

[2] Michel SG, Madsen JC. Current perspectives in transplant medicine: Hypothermic oxygenated perfusion. Transplant Research and Risk Management. 2016;**8**:25-30

[3] Wyss RK, Méndez Carmona N, Arnold M, Segiser A, Mueller M, Dutkowski P, et al. Hypothermic, oxygenated perfusion (HOPE) provides cardioprotection via succinate oxidation prior to normothermic perfusion in a rat model of donation after circulatory death (DCD). American Journal of Transplantation. 2021;**21**(3):1003-1011

[4] Fuller BJ, Gower JD, Green CJ. Free radical damage and organ preservation: Fact or fiction? A review of the interrelationship between oxidative stress and physiological ion disbalance. Cryobiology. 1988;**25**(5):377-393

[5] Taylor DO, Stehlik J, Edwards LB, Aurora P, Christie JD, Dobbels F, et al. Registry of the international society for heart and lung transplantation: Twenty-sixth official adult heart transplant report-2009. The Journal of Heart and Lung Transplantation. 2009;**28**(10):1007-1022

[6] Kaczmarek I, Deutsch MA, Rohrer ME, Beiras-Fernandez A, Groetzner J, Daebritz S, et al. HLA-DR matching improves survival after heart transplantation: Is it time to change allocation policies? The Journal of Heart and Lung Transplantation. 2006;**25**(9):1057-1062

[7] Michel SG, La Muraglia GM, Madariaga MLL, Titus JS, Selig MK, Farkash EA, et al. Twelve-hour hypothermic machine perfusion for donor heart preservation leads to improved ultrastructural characteristics compared to conventional cold storage. Annals of Transplantation. 2015;**20**:461-468

[8] Fitton TP, Barreiro CJ, Bonde PN, Wei C, Gage F, Rodriguez R, et al. Attenuation of DNA damage in canine hearts preserved by continuous hypothermic perfusion. The Annals of Thoracic Surgery. 2005;**80**(5):1812-1820

[9] Taylor MJ, Baicu SC. Current state of hypothermic machine perfusion preservation of organs: The clinical perspective. Cryobiology. 2010;**60**(3 Suppl):S20-S35

[10] Belzer FO, Southard JH. Principles of solid-organ preservation by cold storage. Transplantation. 1988;**45**(4):673-676

[11] Kang M, Kim S, Choi JY, Kim KS, Jung YK, Park B, et al. Ex vivo kidney machine perfusion: Meta-analysis of randomized clinical trials. The British Journal of Surgery. 2024;**111**(4):1-6

[12] Dutkowski P, Schlegel A, de Oliveira ML, Müllhaupt B, Clavien PA. HOPE for human liver grafts obtained from donors after cardiac death. Journal of Hepatology. 2015;**63**(2):388-396

[13] Parente A, Tirotta F, Pini A, Eden J, et al. Machine perfusion techniques for liver transplantation—A meta-analysis of the first seven randomized-controlled trials. Journal of Hepatology. 2023;**79**(5):1201-1213

[14] Guarrera JV. Donation: Where are our opportunities for expansion? Liver Transplantation. 2014;**20**(Suppl. 2):S2-S4

[15] Lee-Riddle GS, Panayotova GG, Guarrera JV. Using organ perfusion to optimize donor livers. Current Opinion in Organ Transplantation. 2023;**28**(2):95-103

[16] Pereyra D, Dingfelder J, Riha M, et al. Dual hypothermic oxygenated machine perfusion of the liver reduces post-transplant biliary complications—A retrospective cohort study. International Journal of Surgery. 2024;**110**(12):7909-7918. DOI: 10.1097/JS9.0000000000002115 [Epub ahead of print]

[17] Panayotova GG, Rosado J, Paterno F, et al. Novel oxygenation technique for hypothermic machine perfusion of liver grafts: Validation in porcine donation after cardiac death (DCD) liver model. American Journal of Surgery. 2020;**220**(5):1270-1277

[18] Michel SG, La Muraglia GM, Madariaga MLL, et al. Preservation of donor hearts using hypothermic oxygenated perfusion. Annals of Transplantation. 2014;**19**:409-416

[19] Steen S, Paskevicius A, Liao Q, Sjöberg T. Safe orthotopic transplantation of hearts harvested 24 hours after brain death and preserved for 24 hours. Scandinavian Cardiovascular Journal. 2016;**50**(3):193

[20] Nilsson J, Jernryd V, Qin G, et al. A nonrandomized open-label phase 2 trial of nonischemic heart preservation for human heart transplantation. Nature Communications. 2020;**11**(1):2976

[21] Qin G, Jernryd V, Sjöberg T, Steen S, Nilsson J. Machine perfusion for human heart preservation: A systematic review. Transplant International. 2022;**35**:10258

[22] Rega F, Lebreton G, Para M, et al. Hypothermic oxygenated perfusion of the donor heart in heart transplantation: The short-term outcome from a randomised, controlled, open-label, multicentre clinical trial. The Lancet. 2024;**404**(10453):670-682

[23] McGiffin DC, Kure CE, Macdonald PS, et al. Hypothermic oxygenated perfusion (HOPE) safely and effectively extends acceptable donor heart preservation times: Results of the Australian and New Zealand trial. The Journal of Heart and Lung Transplantation. 2024;**43**(3):485-495

[24] Lebreton G, Leprince P. Successful heart transplant after 12 h preservation aboard a commercial flight. Lancet. 2024;**403**(10431):1019

[25] Lechiancole A, Sponga S, Benedetti G, et al. Graft preservation in heart transplantation: Current approaches. Frontiers in Cardiovascular Medicine. 2023;**10**:1253579

[26] Rosenbaum DH, Peltz M, DiMaio JM, et al. Perfusion preservation versus static preservation for cardiac transplantation: Effects on myocardial function and metabolism. The Journal of Heart and Lung Transplantation. 2008;**27**(1):93-99

[27] Schipper DA, Marsh KM, Ferng AS, et al. The critical role of bioenergetics in donor cardiac allograft preservation. Journal of Cardiovascular Translational Research. 2016;**9**(3):176-183

[28] Van Caenegem O, Beauloye C, Bertrand L, et al. Hypothermic continuous machine perfusion enables preservation of energy charge and functional recovery of heart grafts in an ex vivo model of donation following circulatory death. European Association for Cardio-Thoracic Surgery. 2016;**49**(5):1348-1353

[29] Van Caenegem O, Beauloye C, Vercruysse J, et al. Hypothermic

continuous machine perfusion improves metabolic preservation and functional recovery in heart grafts. Transplant International. 2015;**28**(2):224-231

[30] Moeslund N, Ertugrul IA, Hu MA, et al. Ex-situ oxygenated hypothermic machine perfusion in donation after circulatory death heart transplantation following either direct procurement or in-situ normothermic regional perfusion. The Journal of Heart and Lung Transplantation. 2023;**42**(6):730-740

[31] Fitton TP, Wei C, Lin R, et al. Impact of 24 h continuous hypothermic perfusion on heart preservation by assessment of oxidative stress. Clinical Transplantation. 2004;**18**(Suppl. 12): 22-27

[32] Poston RS, Gu J, Prastein D, et al. Optimizing donor heart outcome after prolonged storage with endothelial function analysis and continuous perfusion. The Annals of Thoracic Surgery. 2004;**78**(4):1362-1370

[33] Ozeki T, Kwon MH, Gu J, et al. Heart preservation using continuous ex vivo perfusion improves viability and functional recovery. Circulation Journal. 2007;**71**(1):153-159

[34] Qin G, Sjöberg T, Liao Q, Sun X, Steen S. Intact endothelial and contractile function of coronary artery after 8 hours of heart preservation. Scandinavian Cardiovascular Journal. 2016;**50**(5-6):362-366

[35] Qin G, Wohlfart B, Zuo L, Hu J, Sjöberg T, Steen S. Intact coronary and myocardial functions after 24 hours of non-ischemic heart preservation. Scandinavian Cardiovascular Journal. 2020;**54**(1):59-65

[36] Critchley WR, Stone JP, Liao Q, et al. Non-ischemic heart preservation via hypothermic cardioplegic perfusion induces immunodepletion of donor hearts resulting in diminished graft infiltration following transplantation. Frontiers in Immunology. 2020;**11**:1621

[37] Längin M, Mayr T, Reichart B, et al. Consistent success in life-supporting porcine cardiac xenotransplantation. Nature. 2018;**564**(7736):430-433

[38] Wicomb WN, Cooper DK, Novitzky D, Barnard CN. Cardiac transplantation following storage of the donor heart by a portable hypothermic perfusion system. The Annals of Thoracic Surgery. 1984;**37**(3):243-248

[39] Hill DJ, Wicomb WN, Avery GJ, Portnoy VF, Collins GM. Evaluation of a portable hypothermic microperfusion system for storage of the donor heart: Clinical experience. Transplantation Proceedings. 1997;**29**(8):3530-3531

Chapter 12

Xenotransplantation: Current Situation and Future Perspective

Manuel Quiroz-Flores, Marc Leon, Ali Own, Akash Shah, Samuel Jacob and Chawannuch Ruaengsri

Abstract

This chapter aims to explore the history of xenotransplant, contemporary practices, ethical considerations, and the challenges associated with xenotransplantation. Due to the persistent scarcity of donor organs available for transplantation, various alternative sources are under investigation, one of which is xenotransplantation—transplanting organs from one species to another. Among nonhuman primates, porcine is considered the most suitable species for organ usage, as they grow to human size in just a few months. Significant progress has been made in the genetic engineering of pigs, whose hearts closely resemble human hearts in both structure and function. Genetic engineering plays a crucial role in overcoming immune barriers in xenotransplantation, helping to prevent T-cell-mediated and hyperacute rejection. Although using large animal models for orthotopic heart transplants presents technical challenges, the approach holds promise. Despite some religious prohibitions on pork, leaders in Muslim and Jewish traditions generally consider porcine organ donation ethical, as it saves lives. While technological advances have reduced the risk of xenografts transmitting novel viruses, this danger remains and has serious implications for the informed consent process in clinical xenotransplantation research.

Keywords: xenotransplant, xenograft, genetic engineering, genetic modification, organ preservation, rejection

1. Introduction

Approximately 6.7 million Americans aged over 20 years have heart failure (HF), with estimates suggesting a rise to 8.5 million Americans by 2030. The lifetime risk has escalated to 24%, implying that approximately one in four individuals will encounter HF at some stage in their lives [1].

For patients with end-stage heart failure, the most effective treatment is receiving a heart transplant from either a brain death or circulatory death donor. To tackle the shortage of donated hearts, alternative sources are being explored. Many countries have implemented large-scale organ recovery programs, either voluntary or mandatory, with sophisticated allocation systems to ensure fair distribution and optimal outcomes [2].

The limited availability of donors is a significant barrier to heart transplantation. To expand the donor pool, hearts from extended criteria donors, such as those of advanced age, left ventricular hypertrophy, hepatitis B or C infection, donor-recipient size mismatch, and prolonged ischemic times, are frequently utilized with the satisfactory outcomes [3].

The scarcity of donor organs and tissues continues to be the most significant obstacle to expanding transplantation, despite numerous advancements in the field over recent decades. In the United States, the national transplant waiting list currently include over 100,000 individuals, with 3% of them being heart failure patients; in contrast, only 3.659 heart transplants are performed annually, indicating that nearly half of the patients will not receive a heart transplant [4].

One potential solution to bridge the gap between the supply and demand for donor hearts is xenotransplantation. Xenotransplantation involves the transplantation of organs from one to another species. Pigs are considered the most suitable species for xenotransplantation due to their anatomical and physiological similarities to humans, their low risk of transmitting xenozoonoses, and their compatibility with genetic engineering techniques that help reduce the risk of organ rejection. Despite these advantages, the genetic differences between pigs and humans have posed challenges, such as immune rejection and the potential transmission of diseases [5]. While primates are genetically closer to humans, their use is ethically and ecologically unsustainable, as many are endangered. Pigs, on the other hand, are widely bred and consumed, making them a more viable ethical option for harvesting organs to treat human diseases [6, 7].

2. Xenotransplantation in the mythology

Before the idea of xenotransplantations emerged, folklore already contained tale of being that were part of human, part animal. Prehistoric cave art seldom depicts humans, but in France's Lascaux cave, dating back to around 15,000 BC, a unique depiction shows a human with a bird's head. Ancient Egyptian deities are often illustrated with human bodies and animal heads. Anubis has a jackal's head and the Great Sphinx of Giza from about 2500 BC is portrayed as a lion with a woman's head. A first account of xenotransplantation appears in Indian mythology, found in Sanskrit text from the twelfth century BC [7]. According to the legend, Indian gods Shiva and Parvati had a child named Ganesha while Shiva was away hunting. Like many mythical figures, Ganesha was born a giant, and upon his return, Shiva mistakenly beheaded him, thinking he was a stranger. Parvati threatened to destroy the universe unless Shiva revived their son. Since Shiva could not replace Ganesha's head, he instructed his servants to retrieve the head of the first creature they encounter, resulting in Ganesha being revived with an elephant's head [8].

In Ancient Greek mythology, the Minotaur is depicted as having a man's body with a bull's head, while the Sphinx is a winged lion with a woman's head, and Centaurs have the body of a horse and the torso and head of a man. In Homer's "Odyssey" written around 750 BC, Ulysses's crew is magically turned into half-human, half-swine creatures by the sorceress Circe. More recent legends of werewolves and vampires, which involve transformations from human to animal, also reflect these hybrid beings [8]. The late Keith Reemtsma suggested an early example of xenotransplantation might be Daedalus and his son Icarus' attempt to fly from Crete to Greece using wings attached to their arms. Though Icarus failed, potentially due to what Reemtsma humorously referred to as hyperacute rejection or adhesive failure, Daedalus succeed, marking a 50% success rate for the venture [9, 10].

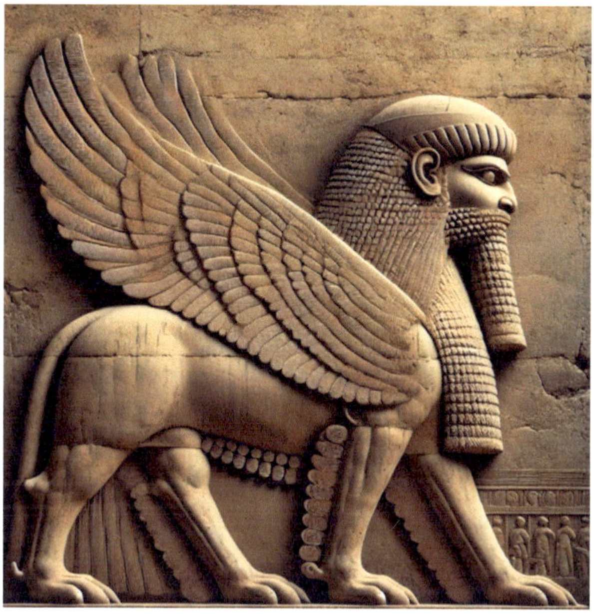

Figure 1.
Lamassu, the mythological creature with a human head, the body of a bull or lion, and the wings of an eagle. It stands majestically in an ancient Assyrian setting.

The Lamassu (**Figure 1**), a mythological creature from ancient Mesopotamian art, features a human head, the body of a lion or bull, and the wings of an eagle. Regarded as a protective deity, it was often positioned at city or palace entrances to guard against evil. These statues are primarily associated with the Assyrian Empire, especially in cities like Nineveh and Nimrud. The Lamassu has been chosen as the emblem for the International Xenotransplantation Association and its scientific journal, "Xenotransplantation" [11].

2.1 History of cardiac xenotransplantation

Early xenotransplantation involved cells and tissues, such as blood, bone, skin, and testicular tissue. However, the transplantation of whole organs was delayed due to the lack of techniques to manage bleeding after the removal of a diseased organ and to effectively restore blood circulation following transplantation [10–12].

In the seventeenth century, the earliest documented instance of xenotransplantation (as well as blood transfusion) to humans was performed by Jean-Baptiste Denis, who transfused lamb's blood into a 15-year-old boy [11].

In 1838, Sharp-Kissam conducted the first corneal transplant by placing a pig's cornea into the eye of a 35-year-old man. During the nineteenth century, scientists began experimenting with skin xenografts from a variety of animals, including pigs, sheep, frogs, pigeons, and chickens, for biological dressings, as well as using bovine embryonic skin grafts for skin dressings [10].

In the twentieth century, Voronoff attempted to "rejuvenate" elderly men by conducting several chimpanzee and baboon testicular transplants purportedly thereby elevating energy levels in patients. In the 1960s, Reemtsma carried out 13 chimpanzee-to-human kidney xenotransplants, most of which failed within 4–8 weeks due to rejection or infections, except for one that lasted for 9 months [11].

Alexis Carrel transformed organ transplantation by creating the triangulation technique for vascular anastomosis [13, 14]. Throughout the twentieth century, multiple efforts at xenotransplantation were undertaken, utilizing organs from nonhuman primates as well as mammals such as rabbits, sheep, and pigs.

In 1906, Mathieu Jaboulay conducted the initial documented effort to transplant pig and goat kidneys into individuals suffering from chronic kidney disease, but both operations were unsuccessful due to graft thrombosis [15]. Similarly, in 1909, Ernst Unger's attempt to use a macaque kidney ended in failure [16]. These early efforts were largely unsuccessful due to the lack of effective immunosuppression and were discontinued until the 1960s [5]. At that time, Keith Reemtsma used immunosuppressive drugs and full-body radiation to successfully graft a monkey kidney into a human patient, who survived for 2 months before dying of pneumonia. Reemtsma continued his research, with one patient surviving up to 9 months [17–19].

In 1964, James Hardy, a cardiac surgeon in Jackson, Mississippi, performed the first non-human to primate (NHP) heart transplant at the University of Mississippi using a chimpanzee heart on a 68-year-old patient suffering from heart failure with left leg gangrene and shock. However, the chimp's heart was too small to meet the demands of the patient body, requiring manual cardiac massage and pumping for only an hour before the patient lost consciousness and expired. An autopsy and histopathological exam later revealed that antibody-mediated graft rejection was the primary cause of death [20, 21].

In 1967, Christian Barnard conducted the initial human heart transplant on Louis Washansky, who lived for 18 days afterward. The second individual survived for 19 months, while the fifth and sixth patients lived for 13 and 24 years, respectively [22, 23]. Following Barnard's groundbreaking transplant, there was a surge in heart transplants worldwide, with over 100 performed across 24 countries, temporarily shifting attention away from xenotransplantation [24]. Dr. Barnard also performed two xenotransplantations in 1977. The first patient was a 25 years old female with history of prior severe aortic stenosis underwent Bjork-Shiley aortic valve replacement and had severe hemolysis from the mechanical valve. She subsequently underwent a redo aortic valve replacement with aortoventriculoplasty. The patient was not able to wean off cardiopulmonary bypass. Dr. Barnard decided to perform a heterotrophic heart transplant using a baboon heart. However, both hearts developed ventricular fibrillation and not recovered [21]. Dr. Barnard later performed a second heterotrophic xenotransplant in the same year, using a chimpanzee heart transplanted to a 60 years old male underwent aortic valve replacement who had cardiogenic shock and was unable to wean from cardiopulmonary bypass. This patient survived 4 days postoperatively, but the heart function gradually declined. The patient expired from severe graft rejection [21].

After Barnard's achievement, many mammalian hearts were used in transplants, with one notable case of Stephanie Fae Beauclair, also known as "Baby Fae," a pediatric patient diagnosed with hypoplastic left heart syndrome. Leonard Lee Bailey and the team from Loma Linda University Medical Center transplanted a baboon heart into Baby Fae on October 26, 1984 and she survived for 20 days, marking the first recorded pediatric heart xenotransplant [21, 25, 26].

2.2 Current status of xenotransplantation

In January 2022, a groundbreaking medical procedure was performed when David Bennett Sr., a 57-year-old man suffering from heart failure, became the first patient to receive a heart transplant from a genetically modified pig. This operation was carried out by Dr. Bartley P. Griffith, Dr. Muhammad M. Mohiuddin, and their team at the University of Maryland Medical Center. Bennett's health had declined so severely that he was dependent on mechanical circulatory support and extracorporeal membrane oxygenation (ECMO). Due to non-compliance with medications and medical recommendations, he was ineligible for a human heart transplant or LVAD therapy because of an irregular heart rhythm. As this procedure was not included in a clinical trial, the medical team requested special authorization from the FDA under "compassionate use." Initially, Bennett showed signs of recovery—he could communicate with family, watch TV, and work with a physical therapist during his stay in the hospital. After about 40 days, his condition worsened, and he passed away on March 8, 2022 [27], two months after the transplant [28, 29].

The team discovered the presence of a virus known as porcine cytomegalovirus (CMV) in the transplanted heart. The donor pig had been genetically modified to reduce the risk of Bennett's body rejecting the organ, and it had undergone multiple screenings for infections. Despite these precautions, concerns remain about the possibility of viruses being transmitted from animals to humans during xenotransplantation. Experts, however, believe the virus found in Bennett's donor pig is not capable of infecting human cells. Although Bennett did not survive, the procedure was considered a milestone in xenotransplantation, and researchers aim to continue exploring the use of animal organs to save human lives [27].

This procedure marked a breakthrough, as it was the first pig heart transplant to sustain life for 2 months, significantly longer than previous attempts. The pig's heart had been heavily genetically modified, with 10 gene alterations [28]. These modifications included knocking out the galactose α-1,3-galactose (Gal) gene, creating genetically engineered α1,3-galactosyltransferase gene-knockout (GTKO) pigs. Human complement regulatory proteins (CRPs), including human membrane cofactor (CD46) expression, human decay-accelerating factor (CD55) expression, and membrane attack complex inhibitor protein (CD59), were added to prevent the human immune system from attacking the pig tissue [30, 31]. Additionally, human antithrombotic genes were introduced to prevent thrombotic microangiopathy. Immunosuppressive therapies were used to reduce T and B cell activities and prevent heart muscle hypertrophy [6, 32, 33]. A new experimental drug, KPL-404, was also administered to inhibit communication between T and B cells, reducing anti-porcine antibodies [28]. Improved preservation techniques, such as *ex vivo* heart storage, helped reduce perioperative cardiac xenograft dysfunction (PCXD), a common cause of graft failure within the first couple days after transplantation [6, 34].

Lawrence Faucette, a 58-year-old man, was the second person to receive a pig heart transplant on September 20, 2023. He was suffering from end-stage heart failure and was not eligible for a human heart transplant due to severe peripheral vascular disease and other comorbidities. Based on the first pig to human heart transplant, the team considered better screening to identify the presence of porcine viruses and administer intravenous immunoglobulin G (IVIG) to remove anti-pig antibodies [35]. Faucette was continuing to recover and was able to sit up in the chair after 2 days postoperatively and lived for nearly 6 weeks after transplant. Faucette passed away on October 30, 2023 from graft rejection (**Table 1**) [35].

Genetic engineering plays a crucial role in overcoming immune barriers for successful xenotransplantation by addressing issues such as T cell-mediated rejection and hyperacute rejection. However, conducting orthotopic, life-sustaining heart transplants using large animal models remains a technical challenge. Most cardiac

Year	Author	Place	Animal source	Patient description	Survival	References
1964	Hardy	Jackson, MS, USA	Chimpanzee	68-year-old man	90 min	[20]
1968	Ross	London, UK	Pig	48-year-old man	4 min	[9]
1968	Cooley	Austin, TX, USA	Sheep	48-year-old man	10 min	[36]
1969	Marion	Lyon, France	Chimpanzee	Young woman	"Quickly"	[37]
1977	Barnard	Cape Town, South Africa	Baboon	25-year-old woman	5 h 30 min	[38]
1977	Barnard	Cape Town, South Africa	Chimpanzee	60-year-old man	4 days	[38]
1984	Bailey	Loma Linda, CA, USA	Baboon	14-day-old baby	20 days	[26]
1992	Religa & Czaplicki	Sosnowiec, Poland	Pig	31-year-old man	23 h	[39]
1996	Baruah	Sonapur, India	Pig	32-year-old man	7 days	[9]
2022	Bartley Griffith	Maryland, USA	Pig	57-year-old man	60 days	[29]
2022	Nader Moazami	NYU, USA	Pig	72- year-old man*	72 h**	[21]
2022	Nader Moazami	NYU, USA	Pig	64-year-old women*	72 h**	[21]
2023	Bartley Griffith	Maryland, USA	Pig	58-year-old man	30 days	[35]

There have been 13 heart xenograft experiments. Donors were chimpanzees in three cases, baboons in two cases, pigs in seven cases, and sheep in one case.
**These recipients were brain death patients, and they were part of experimentation.*
***As part of the research protocol, the observation period was set to 72 h.*

Table 1.
History of heart xenotransplantation.

xenografts are heterotopic, meaning they are connected to the recipient's major blood vessels in the abdominal cavity and function more like an appendage rather than a fully functional heart. These heterotopic grafts are not responsible for sustaining the recipient's life. Yet, with long-term immunosuppression, xenografts engineered with porcine GalT KO, human complement regulatory proteins (CRPs), and thrombomodulin genes have survived in baboons for several years after transplant [6, 32].

More recent advancements have taken orthotopic heart xenotransplantation further. In baboon models, life-sustaining grafts have survived for over 6 months when using GalT KO, human membrane cofactor protein (CD46), and human thrombomodulin pig hearts, combined with a regimen of immunosuppressive therapies such as rituximab, antithymocyte globulin (ATG), inhibition of CD40-CD154 (CD40 Ligand) costimulatory pathway, mycophenolate mofetil, and steroids. These developments signal an exciting leap forward in the potential for heart xenotransplantation [6, 33].

The production of transgenic hA20, a zinc finger protein enzyme activated by tumor necrosis factor (TNF), suppresses nuclear factor-kB activation and prevents TNF-induced apoptosis. Although there was no significant enhancement in organ survival, the expression of this transgene was confined to the pig heart and seemed to slightly decrease ischemia-reperfusion injury [6, 40]. Additionally, human thrombomodulin (CD141), an anticoagulant protein located on the surface of endothelial cells, was produced transgenically. This modification was one of the crucial transgenic alterations in pig hearts that helped prolong the survival of heterotopic heart xenotransplants in baboons [6, 41].

Mohiuddin and colleagues reported that GTKO.hCD46.hTBM pig heart xenografts, transplanted heterotopically into baboons, survived for over a year. Their immunomodulatory strategy included the use of anti-CD40 antibodies, which successfully reduced the production of antipig antibodies, minimized thrombotic microangiopathy in the organ, and lowered the incidence of systemic consumptive coagulopathy [6, 42].

Additionally, Mohiuddin and colleagues tested a modified immunomodulation method, focusing on the anti-CD154-CD40 costimulation pathway in baboon recipients of GTKO.hCD46.hTBM pig hearts. The findings revealed that ongoing treatment with the anti-CD40 (2C10R4) antibody successfully prevented xenograft rejection, leading to graft survival of over 2 years. This approach may hold potential for pig-to-human xenotransplantation (**Figure 2** and **Table 2**) [6, 35, 43].

2.3 Religious condition and community perspectives

Several factors we should consider for the ideal animal heart donor include anatomically like human heart, proper size to support human circulation, immunological compatibility, easy to breed, less cost of animal care, and low zoonotic disease spreading [21]. Baboons were used in the first attempt of heart xenotransplantation

Gene	Modification	Function
Gal	Inactivation	Preventing synthesis of the αGal antigen.
ß4GalNT2	Inactivation	Preventing synthesis of the SDa antigen.
CMAH	Inactivation	Preventing synthesis of the Neu5Gc antigen.
GHr	Inactivation	Regulating animal growth by inactivating the growth hormone receptor.
hCD46	Insertion	Encoding a complement pathway inhibitor (membrane cofactor protein).
hCD55	Insertion	Encoding a complement pathway inhibitor (decay accelerating factor).
THBD	Insertion	Encoding thrombomodulin, an inhibitor of coagulation and thrombosis in vascular endothelium.
EPCR	Insertion	Encoding a receptor with anticoagulant properties.
CD47	Insertion	Encoding a protein that inhibits macrophage-mediated immune responses.
HO1	Insertion	Encoding heme oxygenase 1, with anti-inflammatory properties.

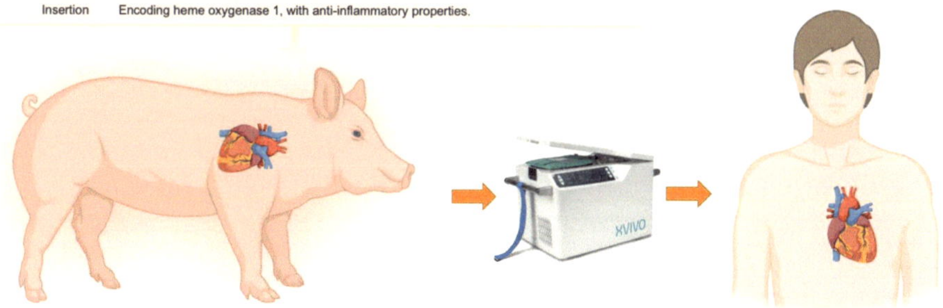

Figure 2.
Gene-edited pigs for human heart transplantation.

Gene	Gene product	GE	Native function	Xeno-strategy
Controlling rejection				
1. *GGTA1* (α1,3-galactosyltransferase)	Gal (Galactose-alpha-1,3-galactose)	Knockout	Carbohydrate antigen on cell surface	Decrease preformed antibody binding and HAR
2. *B4GalNT2* (β1,4-nacetylgalactosyltransferase)	SDa (SD antigen)	Knockout	Cell membrane antigen	Decrease preformed antibody binding and HAR
3. *CMAH* (N-acetylneuraminic acid hydroxylase)	Neu5Gc (N-glycolylneuraminic acid)	Knockout	Glycocalyx component	Decrease preformed antibody binding and HAR
Preventing complement activation				
4. *CD46*	CD 46 (membrane cofactor protein)	Human transgene	Cleaves C3b and C4b	Decrease complement activation
5. *CD55*	CD55 (decay accelerating factor)	Human transgene	Dissociates C3 and C5 convertases	Decrease complement activation
Controlling coagulopathy				
6. *TBM*	TBM (thrombomodulin)	Human transgene	Sequesters thrombin from fibrinogen, activates protein C	Decrease coagulability
7. *EPCR*	EPCR (endothelial protein C receptor)	Human transgene	Positions protein C for activation	Decrease coagulability
Controlling inflammation				
8. *CD47*	CD47	Human transgene	Binds SIRP-α on macrophages, preventing phagocytosis	Decrease macrophage activity
9. *HO-1*	HO-1 (heme oxygenase-1)	Human transgene	Degrades free heme	Proactive ischemia reperfusion response
Controlling excessive growth				
10. *Growth hormone receptor*	Growth hormone receptor	Knockout	Diverse effects on growth and metabolism	Match porcine graft growth with primate recipient

Table 2.
Components of the 10-GE pig.

due to similarity of immunology and anatomy. Nevertheless, there are some concerns about high cost and ethical considerations. Baboons are now widely adopted for animal-to-human heart xenotransplantation [21]. Pigs are considered an ideal species for organ utilization compared to primates, as they grow and enlarge to human size within just a few months. Moreover, significant progress has been made in the genetic engineering of pigs, whose hearts are structurally and functionally like human hearts [44]. However, xenotransplantation raises various concerns, including zoonotic risks, ethical dilemmas, and religious issues [45]. Social approval of xenotransplantation remains uncertain. Religious objections have also emerged, particularly within Jewish and Muslim traditions, which historically prohibit the use of pigs. Nonetheless, some reconciliation has been observed when xenotransplantation is performed to save human lives or prevent worsening of diseases [6, 46].

Although certain religious traditions, such as Judaism and Islam, prohibit the consumption of pork, some religions find the donation of porcine organs acceptable when it serves to save human lives. Dietary restrictions for Jews and Muslims do not extend to tissue implantation perspective. Approximately half of Seventh-day Adventists and more than a third of Buddhists practice vegetarianism, which may lead to refusal of xenogeneic tissue. While many Hindus prohibit the use of both human and animal tissue, there are some who accept human tissue and organ donations. Vegans typically favor human (allogeneic) tissue over animal (xenogeneic) tissue. Scientologists, Lutherans, Baptists, Evangelicals, and Catholics usually accept both allogeneic and xenogeneic acellular grafts. In contrast, Jehovah's Witnesses, Methodists, and members of The Church of Jesus Christ of Latter-day Saints allow individuals to make their own choices regarding these matters [6, 46, 47].

One potential solution to these concerns is to clarify that only a small portion of transplant patients would benefit from xenotransplantation. In the meantime, some patients might explore alternative treatments that do not require animal involvement. As a result, the justification for utilizing animals in this manner is that only a small number of animals would be necessary as organ donors, since they are the only feasible solution for a particular group of patients requiring transplants [6, 47].

Communities of animal rights have opposed the use of animals as organ sources due to concerns about their intelligence, sentience, and capacity for suffering. The debate over whether donor animals have rights remains unclear. Animal rights advocates view pigs as complex, intelligent beings and argue that they should not be sacrificed for human organs, despite their long history of being used for meat consumption [48]. Similar to nonhuman primates, especially baboons, which exhibit advanced social behaviors, the use of these animals in research and organ donation raises ethical issues. However, the use of porcine tends to be less controversial. Organizations like People for the Ethical Treatment of Animals (PETA) have expressed their opposition to the use of animals and animal-derived tissues for medical training, experimentation, and clinical treatments. This includes their opposition to using biologic meshes derived from animals for the repair of soft tissues [6, 37].

2.4 Infectious disease

The risk of transmitting infections from swine to human is a major concern in xenotransplantation. Instances, such as HIV/AIDS, Ebola, swine flu (influenza A/H1N1), and avian flu (influenza A/H5N1), demonstrate how infections can be transferred from animals to humans. Pigs can carry several viral pathogens, including the hepatitis E virus, swine lymphotropic herpesviruses, and cytomegalovirus (CMV) [40]. While many of these issues can be mitigated by breeding pathogen-free pigs, porcine endogenous retroviruses (PERV) remain a problem as they are embedded in the genomes of all pigs and cannot be eliminated through breeding alone. There are worries that PERVs might infect human cells, mutate, cause cancer, or merge with other viruses to form new infections. Recent developments, like the gene-editing elimination of all proviruses in pig genomes, have considerably lessened, but not completely eradicated, these risks. Endogenous retroviruses in pigs, which can potentially spread to human cells and cause illness, have been partially addressed by gene-knockout techniques that significantly lower the risk [37].

Porcine endogenous retroviruses (PERVs) are categorized into three subtypes, PERV-A, PERV-B, and PERV-C [49]. While all pig breeds carry PERV-A and PERV-B, PERV-C is only present in a few breeds [50]. The recombinant virus PERV-A/C has shown increased infectivity in human cells [51]. Therefore, the International Xenotransplantation Association suggests donor pigs used for xenotransplantation be free from PERV-C [52]. Several *in vitro*, but not *in vivo* studies have demonstrated the transmission of PERVs from pigs to human cells and between human cells, though only specific cell types were affected, as many lack the necessary receptors for PERVs infection [53]. In 2017, Niu and colleagues used somatic cell nuclear transfer to deactivate all PERVs in a swine primary cell line, leading to the development of healthy, PERV-free pigs [54]. While these pigs offer a promising new approach to xenotransplantation with reduced PERVs risk, their susceptibility to reinfection remains unknown. Although CRISPR/Cas9-modified PERV-inactivated cell lines produced non-infectious virus particles, they were no longer capable of spreading the virus, protecting the mutant cells from reinfection [55].

Despite advances in reducing the risk of xenografts causing a novel virus outbreak, the danger persists and has important implications for the informed consent process in heart xenotransplantation clinical trials. Recipients of swine hearts may pose a health risk to themselves, their families, and the broader public. Therefore, as mandated by U.S. Public Health Service regulations for xenotransplantation, the informed consent process must clearly outline these risks. Since many zoonotic diseases such as HIV and Creutzfeldt-Jakob disease can have long-latency periods before symptoms appear, patients must be informed about the need for periodically and lifelong laboratory and clinical monitoring. Additionally, privacy concerns, such as the mandatory reporting of sexual contacts and the requirement for an autopsy upon death, should be communicated thoroughly to patients and their relatives [56].

3. Organ preservation

The current gold standard for heart preservation involves antegrade flushing of the coronary arteries with a cardioplegic solution, followed by cold ischemic storage at 4 degree Celsius [57]. Ischemic times <4 h are linked to a higher chance of survival, while ischemia extending >6 h significantly increases the risk of 1-year mortality. To improve outcomes, better organ preservation techniques are needed to reduce cell metabolism and minimize ischemia reperfusion injury [58].

Steen and his collaborators effectively conducted orthotopic allotransplantation of pig hearts following 24 h of preservation. They accomplished this by perfusing the donor hearts with an oxygenated, cold (8°C) hyperoncotic cardioplegic solution that included hormones and erythrocytes, utilizing a heart preservation system (XVIVO heart assist transport, Sweden). The hearts were kept in this preservation system for an additional 24 h before transplantation into recipient pigs [59]. A similar preservation method was utilized during the first pig-to-human heart transplant earlier this year. In this case, a technique developed by Lund University was adapted, using an *ex vivo* device to preserve the pig heart, which was submersed in a fluid containing hormones such as epinephrine and cortisol, as well as dissolved cocaine. This approach demonstrated good preservation of the heart, which maintained proper function after being transplanted [28].

Although traditional cold antegrade flushing of cardioplegia solution has been effective in human allotransplantation for decades, Längin and colleagues noted that these methods were ineffective and insufficient for pig hearts transplanted into baboons. Ischemic storage resulted in significant deterioration of heart function and decreased oxygen delivery to tissues, leading to multi-organ dysfunction in many trials. In contrast, cold, nonischemic preservation with continuous perfusion consistently prevented primary graft failure, highlighting the need for stable perioperative survival in long-term experimental xenotransplantation studies [60].

4. The future of xenotransplantation

The field of xenotransplantation has made significant strides over the past decade, thanks to advancements in immunosuppression, genetic engineering, and a deeper understanding of cross-species incompatibilities. Consequently, cardiac xenografts have achieved survival rates of over 3 years [61]. With the right immunosuppressive protocols, the longevity of xenografts can be further extended. Acute humoral xenograft rejection, a slower form of rejection driven by antibodies, is now uncommon, and acute cellular rejection is no longer the main reason for graft failure. Instead, the primary challenge seems to be coagulation issues between the donor and recipient, appearing as thrombotic microangiopathy in pig-to-human heart transplants. This leads to ischemic damage to the myocardial cell and subsequently causes consumptive coagulopathy [62]. Despite these challenges, the future of xenotransplantation looks promising.

5. Conclusions

Xenotransplantation holds promise for the future, offering the potential to reduce or even eliminate organ transplant waiting lists by expanding the donor pool. However, the technique still faces significant challenges that must be addressed before it can transition from an experimentation to a standard practice. While it has the capacity to increase the availability of donor hearts, several critical issues remain unresolved. Ongoing research continues to bring this innovation closer to becoming a viable option for transplantation.

Author details

Manuel Quiroz-Flores, Marc Leon, Ali Own, Akash Shah, Samuel Jacob and Chawannuch Ruaengsri*
Stanford University, Stanford, California, United States

*Address all correspondence to: noot@stanford.edu

References

[1] Heidenreich PA, Bozkurt B, Aguilar D, Allen LA, Byun JJ, Colvin MM, et al. 2022 AHA/ACC/HFSA guideline for the management of heart failure: Executive summary: A report of the American College of Cardiology/American Heart Association Joint Committee on Clinical Practice Guidelines. Journal of the American College of Cardiology. 2022;**79**(17):1757-1780

[2] Cooper DKC, Gaston R, Eckhoff D, Ladowski J, Yamamoto T, Wang L, et al. Xenotransplantation-the current status and prospects. British Medical Bulletin. 2018;**125**(1):5-14

[3] Chambers DC, Perch M, Zuckermann A, Cherikh WS, Harhay MO, Hayes D Jr, et al. The International Thoracic Organ Transplant Registry of the International Society for Heart and Lung Transplantation: Thirty-eighth adult lung transplantation report - 2021; focus on recipient characteristics. The Journal of Heart and Lung Transplantation. 2021;**40**(10):1060-1072

[4] Carrier AN, Verma A, Mohiuddin M, Pascual M, Muller YD, Longchamp A, et al. Xenotransplantation: A new era. Frontiers in Immunology. 2022;**13**:900594

[5] Cooper DK, Gollackner B, Sachs DH. Will the pig solve the transplantation backlog? Annual Review of Medicine. 2002;**53**:133-147

[6] Wadiwala IJ, Garg P, Yazji JH, Alamouti-Fard E, Alomari M, Hussain MWA, et al. Evolution of xenotransplantation as an alternative to shortage of donors in heart transplantation. Cureus. 2022;**14**(6):e26284

[7] Groth CG. The potential advantages of transplanting organs from pig to man: A transplant Surgeon's view. Indian Journal of Urology. 2007;**23**(3):305-309

[8] Kahan BD. Ganesha: The primeval Hindu xenograft. Transplantation Proceedings. 1989;**21**(3 Suppl. 1):1-8

[9] Deschamps JY, Roux FA, Sai P, Gouin E. History of xenotransplantation. Xenotransplantation. 2005;**12**(2):91-109

[10] Jaulin P, Lefrere JJ. First French transfusions (1667-1668). Transfusion Clinique et Biologique. 2010;**17**(4):205-217

[11] Cooper DK. A brief history of cross-species organ transplantation. Proceedings (Baylor University. Medical Center). 2012;**25**(1):49-57

[12] Hernigou P. Bone transplantation and tissue engineering, part I. Mythology, miracles and fantasy: From chimera to the miracle of the black leg of saints Cosmas and Damian and the cock of John hunter. International Orthopaedics. 2014;**38**(12):2631-2638

[13] Merchant J, Tan SY. Alexis carrel (1873-1944): Pioneer of vascular surgery and organ transplantation. Singapore Medical Journal. 2013;**54**(11):602-603

[14] Vernon G. Alexis carrel: 'father of transplant surgery' and supporter of eugenics. The British Journal of General Practice. 2019;**69**(684):352

[15] Laios K, Bontinis V, Bontinis A, Mavrommatis E, Lytsikas-Sarlis P, Tsoucalas G, et al. Mathieu Jaboulay (1860-1913) and his innovations in vascular and general surgery. Surgical Innovation. 2020;**27**(1):120-123

[16] Brosig W. Nierentransplantation Langenbecks Archiv für klinische. Chirurgie. 1966;**316**(1):233

[17] Tandukar S, Hariharan S. Xenotransplantation. Organogenesis. 2018;**14**(4):159-162

[18] Reemtsma K, McCracken BH, Schlegel JU, Pearl MA, Pearce CW, Dewitt CW, et al. Renal Heterotransplantation in man. Annals of Surgery. 1964;**160**(3): 384-410

[19] Reemtsma K. Renal heterotransplantation from nonhuman primates to man. Annals of the New York Academy of Sciences. 1969;**162**(1):412-418

[20] Hardy JD, Kurrus FD, Chavez CM, Neely WA, Eraslan S, Turner MD, et al. Heart transplantation in man. Developmental studies and report of a case. Journal of the American Medical Association. 1964;**188**:1132-1140

[21] Hess NR, Kaczorowski DJ. The history of cardiac xenotransplantation: Early attempts, major advances, and current progress. Frontiers in Transplantation. 2023;**2**:1125047

[22] Cooper DKC. Christiaan Barnard-the surgeon who dared: The story of the first human-to-human heart transplant. Global Cardiology Science & Practice. 2018;**2018**(2):11

[23] Barnard CN, Cooper DK. Clinical transplantation of the heart: A review of 13 years' personal experience. Journal of the Royal Society of Medicine. 1981;**74**(9):670-674

[24] Hoffenberg R. Christiaan Barnard: His first transplants and their impact on concepts of death. BMJ. 2001;**323**(7327):1478-1480

[25] Cooper DKC, Hara H, Banks CA, Cleveland D, Iwase H. The "baby Fae" baboon heart transplant-potential cause of rejection. Xenotransplantation. 2019;**26**(4):e12511

[26] Bailey LL, Nehlsen-Cannarella SL, Concepcion W, Jolley WB. Baboon-to-human cardiac xenotransplantation in a neonate. Journal of the American Medical Association. 1985;**254**(23):3321-3329

[27] Mohiuddin MM, Singh AK, Scobie L, Goerlich CE, Grazioli A, Saharia K, et al. Graft dysfunction in compassionate use of genetically engineered pig-to-human cardiac xenotransplantation: A case report. Lancet. 2023;**402**(10399):397-410

[28] Kobashigawa J. Pig-to-human heart transplantation: Culmination of technology and ingenuity. The Annals of Thoracic Surgery. 2022;**113**(3):711

[29] Reardon S. First pig-to-human heart transplant: What can scientists learn? Nature. 2022;**601**(7893):305-306

[30] Sandrin MS, Loveland BE, McKenzie IF. Genetic engineering for xenotransplantation. Journal of Cardiac Surgery. 2001;**16**(6):448-457

[31] Murthy R, Bajona P, Bhama JK, Cooper DK. Heart xenotransplantation: Historical background, experimental Progress, and clinical prospects. The Annals of Thoracic Surgery. 2016;**101**(4):1605-1613

[32] Langin M, Mayr T, Reichart B, Michel S, Buchholz S, Guethoff S, et al. Consistent success in life-supporting porcine cardiac xenotransplantation. Nature. 2018;**564**(7736):430-433

[33] Mohiuddin MM, Corcoran PC, Singh AK, Azimzadeh A, Hoyt RF Jr, Thomas ML, et al. B-cell depletion extends the survival of GTKO.hCD46Tg pig heart xenografts in baboons for up to 8 months. American Journal of Transplantation. 2012;**12**(3):763-771

[34] Goerlich CE, Griffith B, Singh AK, Abdullah M, Singireddy S, Kolesnik I, et al. Blood Cardioplegia induction, perfusion storage and graft dysfunction in cardiac xenotransplantation. Frontiers in Immunology. 2021;**12**:667093

[35] Cooper DKC, Cozzi E. Clinical pig heart xenotransplantation-where do we go from here? Transplant International. 2024;**37**:12592

[36] Cooley DA, Hallman GL, Bloodwell RD, Nora JJ, Leachman RD. Human heart transplantation. Experience with twelve cases. The American Journal of Cardiology. 1968;**22**(6):804-810

[37] Siems C, Huddleston S, John R. A brief history of xenotransplantation. The Annals of Thoracic Surgery. 2022;**113**(3):706-710

[38] Barnard CN, Wolpowitz A, Losman JG. Heterotopic cardiac transplantation with a xenograft for assistance of the left heart in cardiogenic shock after cardiopulmonary bypass. South African Medical Journal. 1977;**52**(26):1035-1038

[39] Czaplicki J, Blońska B, Religa Z. The lack of hyperacute xenogeneic heart transplant rejection in a human. The Journal of Heart and Lung Transplantation. 1992;**11**(2 Pt 1):393-397

[40] Niemann H, Petersen B. The production of multi-transgenic pigs: Update and perspectives for xenotransplantation. Transgenic Research. 2016;**25**(3):361-374

[41] Singh AK, Chan JL, DiChiacchio L, Hardy NL, Corcoran PC, Lewis BGT, et al. Cardiac xenografts show reduced survival in the absence of transgenic human thrombomodulin expression in donor pigs. Xenotransplantation. 2019;**26**(2):e12465

[42] Mohiuddin MM, Singh AK, Corcoran PC, Hoyt RF, Thomas ML, 3rd, Ayares D, et al. Genetically engineered pigs and target-specific immunomodulation provide significant graft survival and hope for clinical cardiac xenotransplantation. The Journal of Thoracic and Cardiovascular Surgery 2014;148(3):1106-13; discussion 13-4

[43] Mohiuddin MM, Singh AK, Corcoran PC, Thomas Iii ML, Clark T, Lewis BG, et al. Chimeric 2C10R4 anti-CD40 antibody therapy is critical for long-term survival of GTKO.hCD46. hTBM pig-to-primate cardiac xenograft. Nature Communications. 2016;7:11138

[44] Sade RM, Mukherjee R. Ethical issues in xenotransplantation: The first pig-to-human heart transplant. The Annals of Thoracic Surgery. 2022;**113**(3):712-714

[45] Cooper DK, Keogh AM, Brink J, Corris PA, Klepetko W, Pierson RN, et al. Report of the Xenotransplantation Advisory Committee of the International Society for heart and lung transplantation: The present status of xenotransplantation and its potential role in the treatment of end-stage cardiac and pulmonary diseases. The Journal of Heart and Lung Transplantation. 2000;**19**(12):1125-1165

[46] Jenkins ED, Yip M, Melman L, Frisella MM, Matthews BD. Informed consent: Cultural and religious issues associated with the use of allogeneic and xenogeneic mesh products. Journal of the American College of Surgeons. 2010;**210**(4):402-410

[47] Paris W, Seidler RJH, FitzGerald K, Padela AI, Cozzi E, Cooper DKC. Jewish, Christian and Muslim theological perspectives about xenotransplantation. Xenotransplantation. 2018;**25**(3): e12400

[48] Denner J. Recent progress in xenotransplantation, with emphasis on virological safety. Annals of Transplantation. 2016;**21**:717-727

[49] Ericsson T, Oldmixon B, Blomberg J, Rosa M, Patience C, Andersson G. Identification of novel porcine endogenous betaretrovirus sequences in miniature swine. Journal of Virology. 2001;**75**(6):2765-2770

[50] Blusch JH, Patience C, Martin U. Pig endogenous retroviruses and xenotransplantation. Xenotransplantation. 2002;**9**(4):242-251

[51] Denner J. Recombinant porcine endogenous retroviruses (PERV-A/C): A new risk for xenotransplantation? Archives of Virology. 2008;**153**(8): 1421-1426

[52] Hawthorne WJ, Cowan PJ, Buhler LH, Yi S, Bottino R, Pierson RN 3rd, et al. Third WHO global consultation on regulatory requirements for xenotransplantation clinical trials, Changsha, Hunan, China December 12-14, 2018: "the 2018 Changsha communique" the 10-year anniversary of the international consultation on xenotransplantation. Xenotransplantation. 2019;**26**(2):e12513

[53] Denner J, Specke V, Thiesen U, Karlas A, Kurth R. Genetic alterations of the long terminal repeat of an ecotropic porcine endogenous retrovirus during passage in human cells. Virology. 2003;**314**(1):125-133

[54] Niu D, Wei HJ, Lin L, George H, Wang T, Lee IH, et al. Inactivation of porcine endogenous retrovirus in pigs using CRISPR-Cas9. Science. 2017;**357**(6357):1303-1307

[55] Godehardt AW, Fischer N, Rauch P, Gulich B, Boller K, Church GM, et al. Characterization of porcine endogenous retrovirus particles released by the CRISPR/Cas9 inactivated cell line PK15 clone 15. Xenotransplantation. 2020;**27**(2):e12563

[56] Bloom ET. Xenotransplantation: Regulatory challenges. Current Opinion in Biotechnology. 2001;**12**(3):312-316

[57] Minasian SM, Galagudza MM, Dmitriev YV, Karpov AA, Vlasov TD. Preservation of the donor heart: From basic science to clinical studies. Interactive Cardiovascular and Thoracic Surgery. 2015;**20**(4):510-519

[58] Mohiuddin MM, Reichart B, Byrne GW, McGregor CGA. Current status of pig heart xenotransplantation. International Journal of Surgery. 2015;**23**(Pt B):234-239

[59] Steen S, Paskevicius A, Liao Q, Sjoberg T. Safe orthotopic transplantation of hearts harvested 24 hours after brain death and preserved for 24 hours. Scandinavian Cardiovascular Journal. 2016;**50**(3):193-200

[60] Langin M, Reichart B, Steen S, Sjoberg T, Paskevicius A, Liao Q, et al. Cold non-ischemic heart preservation with continuous perfusion prevents early graft failure in orthotopic pig-to-baboon xenotransplantation. Xenotransplantation. 2021;**28**(1):e12636

[61] Chan JL, Mohiuddin MM. Heart xenotransplantation. Current Opinion in Organ Transplantation. 2017;**22**(6):549-554

[62] Houser SL, Kuwaki K, Knosalla C, Dor FJ, Gollackner B, Cheng J, et al. Thrombotic microangiopathy and graft arteriopathy in pig hearts following transplantation into baboons. Xenotransplantation. 2004;**11**(5): 416-425